Ethics in HIV-Related
PSYCHOTHERAPY

Ethics in HIV-Related PSYCHOTHERAPY

CLINICAL DECISION MAKING IN COMPLEX CASES

Edited by
John R. Anderson
and Bob Barret

AMERICAN PSYCHOLOGICAL ASSOCIATION
WASHINGTON, DC

Published by
American Psychological Association
750 First Street, NE
Washington, DC 20002

Copies may be ordered from
APA Order Department
P.O. Box 92984
Washington, DC 20090-2984

In the UK and Europe, copies may be
ordered from
American Psychological Association
3 Henrietta Street
Covent Garden, London
WC2E 8LU England

Typeset in Goudy by World Composition Services, Inc., Sterling, VA

Printer: Edwards Brothers, Inc., Ann Arbor, MI
Cover designer: Kathleen Simms Graphic Design, Washington, DC
Project Manager: Debbie K. Hardin, Charlottesville, VA

The opinions and statements published are the responsibility of the authors, and such opinions and statements do not necessarily represent the policies of the APA.

Library of Congress Cataloging-in-Publication Data

Ethics in HIV-related psychotherapy : clinical decision making in complex cases / edited by John R. Anderson and Robert L. Barrett.
    p. ; cm.
Includes bibliographical references and index.
ISBN 1-55798-722-X (hardcover : alk. paper)
  1. AIDS (Disease)—Patients—Counseling of—Moral and ethical aspects. 2. HIV-positive persons—Counseling of—Moral and ethical aspects. 3. Psychotherapists—Professional ethics. 4. Psychotherapists—Legal status, laws, etc.—United States.
I. Anderson, John R., 1953-   II. Barrett, Robert L.
  [DNLM: 1. HIV Infections—psychology. 2. Psychotherapy—methods.
3. Confidentiality. 4. Decision Support Techniques. 5. Ethics, Medical.
6. Psychotherapy—legislation & jurisprudence. WC 503.7 E84 2000]
RC607.A26 E85 2000
174'.2—dc21
                                       00-059350

Printed in the United States of America
First Edition

CONTENTS

CONTRIBUTORS

John R. Anderson, PhD, American Psychological Association, Washington, DC

Bob Barret, PhD, University of North Carolina at Charlotte

Lynn Bonde, JD, MSW, Calvert Hospice, Prince Frederick, MD

Vivian B. Brown, PhD, PROTOTYPES, Culver City, CA

Scott Burris, JD, Temple Law School, Philadelphia, PA

Tom Eversole, MS, Oregon Health Division, Portland

Sally Jue, MSW, Los Angeles, CA

Karen Strohm Kitchener, PhD, University of Denver, CO

Sandra Y. Lewis, PsyD, Montclair State University, Montclair, NJ

Sara R. Stevenson, PhD, University of Denver, CO

Robert A. Washington, PhD, William Wendt Center for Loss and Healing, Washington, DC

PREFACE

In the spring of 1996, the American Psychological Association (APA) Office on AIDS received funding from the Center for Mental Health Services (CMHS) of the Substance Abuse and Mental Health Services Administration (SAMHSA)[1] to develop a training curriculum that would teach mental health practitioners how to use a systematic decision-making process for dealing with ethical challenges posed by clients with HIV/AIDS. Following the successful development and pilot testing of the curriculum (Anderson, Eversole, & Jue, 1996), the APA Office on AIDS asked the group of experts who assisted in the development of the curriculum to begin working on the book that you are about to read. The multiethnic, multicultural group of experts who contributed to the book includes several mental health practitioners, a psychologist–ethicist and former chair of the APA Ethics Committee, and a professor of law who specializes in legal issues of the HIV/AIDS mental health practitioner. The practitioners contributing to this volume include psychologists, social workers, and a master's-level counselor. These seasoned HIV/AIDS mental health clinicians have extensive experience with various populations: adults, children, men who have sex with men, heterosexual partners of injection drug users, active drug users, individuals in recovery, the worried well, and the persistently mentally ill.

Contributors to the book were convened for a two-day meeting and asked to articulate and integrate their wisdom in ways that were both maximally accessible and practically useful to the "garden-variety" mental health practitioner just beginning to work with people with HIV/AIDS. The ensuing dialogue served to sharpen the focus of the overview chapters

---

[1] Contract # 280-95-0001; "HIV/AIDS Education and Training of Psychologists."

in the first part of the book, and it led to refinement of the decision-making model applied in case discussions in the second part of the book.

The contributors were forced to reckon with the inherent tension among personal, clinical, ethical, and legal perspectives. They examined how personal reactions and cultural biases shape clinical judgments. They wrestled with the fact that ethical analysis seems cumbersome and time consuming to clinicians who feel pressured to act quickly when worried about the possibility of risk transmission or lawsuits. The contributors confronted the reality that legal analysis based on conflicting laws and statutes, both within and across states, may result in equivocal advice that leaves clinicians feeling bewildered, helpless, or scared. They found ways to cope with the fact that clinicians, ethicists, and lawyers have different vocabularies, different analytical strategies, and distinctly different goals.

The contributors to this volume are to be commended for their long-term commitment to this project as well as their assiduous attention to quality, practicality, and verisimilitude. They managed "to keep it real" while thoughtfully attending to the complexities of ethics, law, and rapid changes in the treatment of people with HIV/AIDS. Like so many HIV/AIDS providers, they are a wise and dedicated bunch.

The editors and other contributors to this volume are especially indebted to Margaret Schlegel of APA Books for her thoughtful guidance and her generous encouragement. Margaret is not only smart and highly competent, she is personable and fun. Others deserve to be acknowledged as well. Mel Hass and Barbara Silver of CMHS were instrumental in supporting the development of the training curriculum on which this book is based. Ann Rutherford and Leah Stockett were integral to the early stages of the developing book. Ida Audeh performed yeoman service in working through early drafts of the manuscript and offering assistance in terms of both copyediting and substantive editorial advice. Stan Jones, formerly the director of the APA Ethics Office, worked very hard to vet the manuscript from the standpoint of APA's 1992 Ethical Principles of Psychologists and Code of Conduct. Stan's amazing attention to detail kept the contributors on our toes and ensured that the book displays the type of thorough professionalism required of books dealing with ethics and the law. David Martin, director of the HIV Mental Health Service at Harbor/UCLA Medical Center, did an outstanding job of providing expert review of the manuscript. David's breadth of experience as an HIV/AIDS mental health practitioner, researcher, administrator, educator, and case consultant made him the perfect reviewer for this volume. His comments were consistently insightful, practical, and to the point.

Last, we wish to thank the APA for publishing the book. The editors and contributors sincerely appreciate the APA's willingness to publish a volume that realistically describes HIV/AIDS-related psychotherapy, which so commonly requires mental health practitioners to "bend the frame" of traditional psychotherapeutic practice.

REFERENCE

Anderson, J. R., Eversole, T., & Jue, S. (1996). *Ethical issues and HIV/AIDS mental health services*. Washington, DC: American Psychological Association.

DISCLAIMER

This book does not represent the views of the American Psychological Association (APA), the APA Office of Ethics, the APA Office on AIDS, the APA Ethics Committee, the APA Revision Comments Subcommittee, or any other APA administrative, legal, or governance group. The cases are wholly the creations of the chapter authors. They are not intended to serve as standards for application of the APA's 1992 "Ethical Principles of Psychologists and Code of Conduct" (see appendix), nor do they add to or reduce any requirements of the APA Ethics Code. All cases are fictional, and any similarity to actual persons or situations is coincidental and unintended by the authors. Where any conflict is perceived in interpreting the Ethical Standards or judging professional conduct, the official APA Ethics Code always controls.

INTRODUCTION

In the past two decades since the outbreak of the human immunodeficiency virus/acquired immune deficiency syndrome (HIV/AIDS) epidemic, therapists and other health care providers have been routinely challenged by a diverse and complex array of ethical dilemmas associated with psychotherapy for people living with HIV disease. Although many articles, books, and workshop presentations have been developed to help both new and seasoned practitioners understand the clinical issues of HIV/AIDS mental health care, there has been little work devoted to practical strategies for dealing with ethical situations presented by HIV-positive clients. *Ethics in HIV-Related Psychotherapy* was written for that purpose.

As discussed in the preface, the idea for the book arose from interactions with workshop participants of continuing education programs sponsored by the American Psychological Association (APA) Office on AIDS during the period of 1988 through 1999.[1] During those 12 years, more than 12,000 mental health providers were trained through APA Office on AIDS programs. The single most urgent and consistent concern expressed by those 12,000 workshop participants was, "What do I do if someone in my psychotherapy practice is having unsafe sex with someone else and they won't stop?"

Anticipatory anxiety about the possibility of being confronted with this type of situation is extraordinarily high. The root of the anxiety most often seems to be fear about getting sued for failing to warn a potential victim. Unfortunately, fears about being sued, worries about anticipated

---

[1] Support for these continuing education programs was provided by a grant from the National Institute of Mental Health (NIMH-ES-87-0008, 1989–1991) and by three contracts with the Center for Mental Health Services of the Substance Abuse and Mental Health Services Administration (Contract #280-91-0009, 1991–1994); Contract #280-95-0001, 1995–1998; and Contract #280-98-8011, 1998–2001).

ethical dilemmas, homophobia, negative attitudes toward those who abuse drugs, and unexamined anxiety about dealing with chronic illness and death cause some practitioners to exercise poor judgement in clinical situations involving persons with HIV/AIDS.

In part, this book was written to illuminate how underlying beliefs, distortions, and fears can lead to professional behavior that is clinically ethically, or legally unsound. Another reason for writing the book is that models of psychological treatment learned in graduate school often do not apply to HIV/AIDS work. Hospital and home visits blur the safe boundary between the practitioner and patient. Responding to suicidal ideation is different when working with clients with chronic or terminal illnesses. Stigma associated with the disease and with populations most commonly affected by it changes the dynamics of building rapport and trust. Multiple losses and grief change the nature of the work. Graduate courses seldom deal with many of the thorny questions that routinely confront HIV/AIDS mental health practitioners: Do I inform my client's sex partner that she is HIV-positive when I know that such disclosure might cause her partner to beat her, abandon her, and leave her to the streets? Should my seriously mentally ill HIV-positive client who has a history of discontinuing medications and engaging in unsafe sex be allowed to leave the hospital? What do I say to my 13-year-old client with AIDS who asks me what is wrong with him and his guardians have refused to let anyone disclose the nature of his illness? What do I do when my client with AIDS dismisses my concerns about the effects of his cognitive impairment on his capacity to drive a car? What should I say to the chaotic client who wants to begin a complex combination therapy regimen that may produce multidrug resistance if medications are not taken exactly as prescribed?

For many aspiring HIV/AIDS practitioners, the development of professional confidence and competence in dealing with the foregoing questions can seem daunting. This is particularly true when there is a dearth of published information with practical strategies for dealing with HIV-related ethical dilemmas. Although there are many resources for those interested in the psychosocial issues facing people with HIV disease, there is not a single book devoted to ethical issues in HIV-related psychotherapy. A few book chapters and journal articles have addressed ethics and HIV, but none provides the type of practical suggestions that clinicians seek. Most publications on the topic of ethics and HIV tend to be legalistic, overly abstract, disjointed, or just plain simplistic.

A recent article from the professional literature (Melchert & Patterson, 1999) on the topic of duty to warn with HIV-positive clients serves to illustrate. The authors allocated the first four pages of a six-page article to separate, and seemingly unrelated, sections about general laws on the limits of confidentiality, professional association policies, and data pertaining to HIV risk transmission. The authors do offer ideas for dealing with an HIV-positive client who is engaging in high-risk behavior with a partner who is unaware of the client's HIV status, but their suggestions are of little practical help to clinicians struggling with the complex array of clinical, ethical, and legal issues. For example, the authors suggested the following course of action:

> Therapists should first attempt to obtain the client's agreement to cease the high-risk behavior or to notify his or her partner(s) of their risk for HIV infection. If the client will not agree to either of these alternatives, the therapist should consider various steps such as directly warning the partners, requesting that a health department warn the partners, or notifying the police. (p. 183)

It is not that the foregoing suggestions are wrong, it is just that the real world is messy and ethical practice requires an individually tailored decision-making process that involves a more comprehensive and integrated examination of clinical issues, ethical obligations, and legal realities. A more sophisticated and practical analysis is needed.

We believe that *Ethics in HIV-Related Psychotherapy: Clinical Decision-Making in Complex Cases* offers the type of thorough, practical analysis that therapists seek. The book is intended to provide guideposts for practitioners less familiar with the field and yet also serve as a critical resource for those well-versed in mental health service delivery for people with HIV/AIDS. The book can also serve as a key textbook for ethics courses taught in graduate programs in psychology, counseling, social work, and other mental health professions and in schools of medicine, nursing, and allied health professions. It is our belief that the issues and situations outlined in this book are woven into the fabric of our multicultural, sexually active, substance-using society and thus are very likely to arise in the context of mental health practice in the new millennium.

The book is divided into two parts. Part I is intended to provide readers with a solid working knowledge of personal, professional, ethical, cultural, and legal issues that affect the decision making of mental health practitioners who work with people with HIV/AIDS.

The first chapter of the book, "HIV-Related Psychotherapy: Personal and Career Influences," discusses the many challenges inherent in clinical work with HIV-positive clients and how those challenges have transformed the personal and professional life of one clinician. The transformation Bob Barret describes is not an uncommon one. In fact, his story is offered as the opening chapter to the book precisely because it illustrates a common experience of seasoned clinicians who frequently report how their attitudes and decision-making processes about HIV-related cases have changed with experience and across time.

In the next chapter, "Ethical Issues in the Practice of Psychology With Clients With HIV and AIDS," Sara R. Stevenson and Karen Strohm Kitchener review the clinical and empirical literature on ethical issues associated with mental health services for people with HIV disease. Here the reader learns about confidentiality and HIV-disease and the implications of the *Tarasoff* case in California for HIV-related psychotherapy (*Tarasoff v. Board of Regents of University of California*, 1976). Other topics covered include the duty to warn, assisted suicide, working with minors and hospitalized psychiatric patients, and issues surrounding perinatal transmission.

In chapter 3, "Thinking Well About Doing Good in HIV-Related Practice: A Model of Ethical Analysis," Karen Strohm Kitchener and Bob Barret review the American Psychological Association's (1992) Ethics Code and discuss its application to HIV-related clinical work. They then discuss several foundational ethical principles and how they can be used to analyze ethical dilemmas and formulate a plan of action.

"Cultural Considerations in HIV Ethical Decision-Making: A Guide for Mental Health Practitioners" (chapter 4) by Sally Jue and Sandra Y. Lewis provides readers with an overview of how cultural differences in understandings about life, death, medical treatment, healing, and disease can affect clinical judgment and decision-making. This chapter will sensitize the reader to the complex interplay of cultural values and treatment decisions in work with people with HIV/AIDS.

The intense emotional impact of establishing an intimate professional relationship with a client who may be terminally ill can be overwhelming to someone who has not been close to death. HIV-related psychotherapy routinely exposes the practitioner to clients who may sicken and die. "The Effects of Grief and Loss on Decision Making in HIV-Related Psychotherapy" (chapter 5) by Lynn Bonde helps the reader develop an understanding of these dynamics and the many subtle ways they can affect clinical decision making.

In chapter 6, "Clinical Decision Making in the Shadow of Law," Scott Burris reviews the major laws pertaining to HIV-related psychotherapy and provides a legal context that will assist the student and practitioner in understanding the kinds of legal issues that help define the boundaries of ethical practice. Burris also provides information that will assist the practitioner in assessing the degree of risk of malpractice in HIV-related clinical practice.

Background information covered in the first six chapters of Part I provides both the context and rationale for the clinical decision-making model used in the cases presented in Part II. Part II offers 10 HIV-related case examples in which the clinical decision-making model is systematically applied. All cases are written by a mental health clinician, an ethicist, and an attorney. The specific circumstances of each case were developed by a mental health clinician to reflect commonly occurring ethical challenges faced by mental health providers. All cases follow the same format. The mental health clinician summarizes the ethical issues posed by the case, presents the case, and discusses initial personal reactions to the case. The clinician then outlines a tentative plan of action and obtains a consultation about ethical and legal issues. The ethical consultation is written by the ethicist, and the legal consultation is written by the attorney. The case discussion is then completed by the clinical author who first considers and weighs the information gathered from the consultations and then develops, implements, and evaluates a plan of action.

This format enables readers to consider cases in practical terms that mirrors what the clinical decision-making model calls for in the "real world." According to the model, when faced with an ethical challenge, clinicians should consult with knowledgeable colleagues and carefully consider both ethical and legal issues. In the cases presented in this book, the clinicians have the benefit of consulting with two "knowledgeable colleagues" who happen to be a former chair of the APA Ethics Committee and an expert in HIV/AIDS mental health law. Because the "real world" does not always afford the opportunity for such high-level consultation, the cases offered here provide readers with excellent examples of how a thoughtful explication of ethical and legal perspectives can be meaningfully incorporated into treatment planning and implementation.

It is important to remember that cases presented in this book are not offered for the purpose of articulating the "right" thing to do. Instead, the purpose is to illustrate the application of a clinical decision-making process that can be used with all cases. In large measure, the value of the model stems from its thoughtful and systematic application. Too often, anxieties about being sued or doing the wrong thing cause clinicians to act precipitously. By faithfully applying the model, clinicians are required to reflect, to consider the possible implications of various actions from multiple perspectives, and to articulate the key considerations on which their actions are based. Such a process not only serves to improve clinical judgment, but when explicated in detailed documentation, it provides a clear intention to act in accordance with the highest standards of the mental health profession. Although such intentions do not guarantee freedom from lawsuits, they do substantially reduce the likelihood that such suits will be successful.

The cases in this book are fictitious, and any scenarios or names that may seem to reflect real-life situations or persons are purely coincidental and unintended by the authors. Any case material that served as inspiration for the development of the fictional vignettes represent composites that are disguised as intended by the APA Ethics Code in Standard 5.08. It is important to note that the authors were asked to develop "messy" scenarios that portrayed clinicians grappling with extremely difficult situations. For example, Sally Jue, the clinical author for chapter 8, was specifically asked by the editors to develop a case scenario in which a clinician breached confidentiality in the context of emotionally charged and ambiguous circumstances. We hope that the "messiness" of the cases presented in this book prepares readers more effectively for the complexities of working with people with HIV/AIDS.

Finally, it is notable that all cases in this book were analyzed in terms of "The Ethical Principles of Psychologists and Code of Conduct" (APA, 1992). The decision to use only the APA Ethics Code primarily had to do with the desire to keep things simple so that readers could focus on learning a systematic decision-making method instead of becoming confused by differences in various professional codes of ethics. However, the decision-making model presented in this book can be used in conjunction with the professional code of ethics associated with any of the major mental health professions. In fact, the beauty of the model presented in this book is that it can be applied so readily across both situations and professions.

REFERENCES

American Psychological Association. (1992). Ethical principles of psychologists and code of conduct. *American Psychologist, 47,* 1597–1611.

Melchert T. P., & Patterson, M. M. (1999). Duty to warn and interventions with HIV-positive clients. *Professional Psychology: Research and Practice, 30*(2), 180–186.

Tarasoff v. Regents of University of California, 551 P.2d 334 (Cal. 1976).

I

CRITICAL FACTORS INFLUENCING CLINICAL DECISION MAKING IN HIV-RELATED PSYCHOTHERAPY

1

HIV-RELATED PSYCHOTHERAPY: PERSONAL AND CAREER INFLUENCES

BOB BARRET

When the history of the HIV epidemic is written, one part of that story will assess the way that this disease changed several professions, especially psychotherapy. In fundamental ways HIV-related psychotherapy has made many of us look very hard at what we are doing. It has challenged us to reexamine the counseling and psychotherapy models that we learned in graduate school and stretched us by its unanticipated complexity and constant changes. For many of us this work has led to introspection about existential concerns such as life and death, suffering and joy and led us toward a keener sense of the dilemmas of ethical practice.

Debates regarding duty to warn, duty to protect, issues of assisted suicide, and end-of-life decisions have become common in HIV-related psychotherapy in all the mental health professions. Although many engage these issues from the safety provided to observers, some of us are down in the trenches trying to sort out ways of finding peace and professional security as we find ourselves involved in struggles that rarely appear in professional publications. In the beginning of the epidemic we had to sort through very bewildering ethical situations without the benefit of more experienced psychologists or a literature to guide us. It is from the proximity of such personal involvement that we emerged changed both as professionals and as human beings. I hope that this chapter will bring readers closer to understanding the ways that these issues have challenged one psychologist who found himself almost by accident in the midst of enormous suffering and confusion.

BACKGROUND

I completed my doctorate in 1979 at the age of 39 after working as a petroleum marketer, a schoolteacher, and a counselor and counselor educator. In the 1980s I was busy beginning my academic and clinical career and focused on being a father to my three daughters. My work and personal lives were flourishing, and I was a respected member of my community, visible through presentations on parenting, adult development, and work with cancer patients. On the outside and, to a large extent, on the inside, my life made sense and was happy. I suppose I looked like the traditional American ideal: a man who was involved with his family and active in career, church, and civic events.

In 1980 I began meeting with individuals and families dealing with the stresses of cancer. I had read Kübler-Ross and attended several training experiences that confronted me with the reality of my own death. I could respond readily to the then popular question of "Have you worked through your own death?" with a confident "Yep." In this work I faced many complex situations. My professional boundaries were challenged in many instances. A 29-year-old woman struggled over leaving her daughter with the stepfamily that treated the young girl cruelly; she refused to discuss this with her family and wanted me to tell her what to do. She died before having made a decision, leaving me to meet with her mother and husband as they tried to find a solution. A 21-year-old man lay dying alone in the hospital because his blended families did not want to deal with him; instead, they wanted me to tell him that he was dying and that they were not going to pay his medical expenses. A man my own age had deteriorated over a 2-year period during which I had become close to his wife and two teenage sons. Being present in his hospital room or home had become a common aspect of my work with his family. Counseling cancer patients was very challenging and certainly did not fit the model that I had learned in graduate school and used in my practice. The role confusion generated by my search for the proper professional boundaries led me to struggle between being both a counselor as well as a friend. I had to learn how to interact with medical personnel, and there was a fairly constant struggle to keep my boundaries clear. I also realized the importance of keeping my personal life vital so that such intense emotions would not burn me out.

Over time many of these issues seemed more routine. I became used to sorting through my own feelings and became more comfortable with the helplessness matrixes that typically presents with dying patients. I was drawn into family matrixes where my role was not always as comfortably clear as in traditional psychotherapy. No longer startled by complex ethical dilemmas, I internalized my awareness of the ethical challenges that accompany counseling and psychotherapy with people who are dying. I began to anticipate these issues and became much more comfortable when they would come up. The work demanded my attention on all levels; at times I felt exhausted by its intensity, but more often I felt energized from the ways death can bring forth greater integrity and a keener appreciation for the richness of life.

After 5 years, I was worn out and decided to take a break. In the summer of 1985, I took my family to England, where I worked in a large mental hospital near London and became totally absorbed in that experience. When I returned to my job in the fall, I was startled by the media attention to a new disease that had put the gay community in the spotlight. I knew something about the psychological experience of terminal illness, and I decided that maybe I could give something to these sick gay men who stirred up the confusion I had felt for years about my own sexual identity. I sought out an opportunity to volunteer and after about 6 months found myself starting the first HIV/AIDS support group in North Carolina.

A CHRONOLOGY OF EVENTS

Starting the HIV group was more complicated than it might seem. Given the hysteria and lack of solid information about HIV transmission, I knew that I might be taking a risk. I was using my private practice office, and I struggled with how public to be about what I was doing. I feared that my other clients would not be comfortable if they knew they were entering a room where people with AIDS had been meeting. Keeping quiet about it seemed necessary, but I also felt torn about what felt like a lie. In those days many were not sure exactly how HIV was transmitted, and there certainly were times when I feared that I might be putting myself at risk. Still, medical professionals assured me that there was no danger. I was not at all convinced that my practice population would agree with them, so at first I did not tell them.

This initial group was composed of Jerry, who you will read about in chapter 7; Bill and his lover Lou, who was in advanced stages of HIV disease, and Marie, Bill's mother; Ruth and Sol, a couple whose son Adam was dying of AIDS in New York; and, occasionally, Sam, a man of uncertain sexual orientation who had contracted HIV from blood transfusions while he was being treated for a rare form of leukemia. It had taken a lot of effort to find these people and even more to convince them that they would be safe talking to me. Ruth and Sol had told no one beyond their family that

Adam was dying. Bill, Lou, and Marie were examples of what I came to call "AIDS on the run" clients. They had moved from San Francisco to Seattle to West Palm Beach before landing in Charlotte. They had come to Charlotte because they knew no one and felt safe even though medical treatment was better elsewhere. Although I knew that my experience with cancer patients would be valuable in this new work, it did not take long for me to realize that issues of prejudice and oppression combined with the absence of medical knowledge about HIV made this work much more complex than working with cancer patients. Still, I was uneasy about my own internal ethical struggle about possibly misleading my other clients by not informing them, and I also worried about the ethics of practicing in an area in which I had received no training.

Soon I was on the founding board of the AIDS service organization, and as the client population increased we created three support groups: one for patients diagnosed with AIDS; one for HIV-positive individuals; and one for friends and family members of HIV/AIDS patients. I began to see a few HIV-positive clients in my practice and to be asked to provide training for others who were becoming involved in this work. Within 2 years I was giving presentations across the state and at national professional meetings, and I even had a paper accepted at the Fifth International AIDS Conference in Stockholm.

In a very short time I had also become a community AIDS activist. I worked to get more resources available to people with HIV disease. I had written a couple of articles for my local newspaper, and I was deeply involved in giving presentations to school and church groups to encourage more acceptance and understanding for people with HIV. Part of my mission included educating the public as well as professionals about the realities of living with AIDS. Once again I had found myself in very unfamiliar waters. All of these public activities were not part of the model of a professional psychology I had learned in graduate school. I realized that I was becoming something like a community psychologist and sometimes worried that I might be demonstrating the worst behavior of psychologists who are active in the media. A number of ethical concerns began to nag at me. My role was often unclear. Was it OK for me to pick up my HIV clients and take them in my car to a university or college where we would give a talk together? Was I being professional when we talked about our personal lives while going to and from events? Did I have any business speaking or training others when I had not been trained myself? I struggled with these questions constantly and felt very alone because there were no other psychologists in my area doing similar work.

At about that time I learned that the American Psychological Association had received a training grant to assist those who wanted to know more about working with HIV clients (National Institute of Mental Health: NIMH-ES-87-008, 1989–1991). I wondered if I might find some help with the ethical questions from other psychologists who were doing this work. I sent a letter (which was an unusual thing for me to do), telling them what I was doing in North Carolina. I was surprised a few weeks later when Walter Batchelor, who was directing the project, invited me to come to Washington to audition for the faculty.

During the 5 days of training, I felt constantly moved by the integrity I experienced in those around me. I realized that I had much to offer in this work and that I wanted to live my life with a similar commitment to being honest and real at all times. I saw other fine psychologists struggling with the same questions that plagued me. Each of us was realizing that there were few experts to guide us. I left Washington affirmed that my knowledge about HIV was solid and that the things we were doing in North Carolina were every bit as creative and on-target as what was happening in New York, Washington, and San Francisco. I was asked to join the faculty, and I returned home excited, liberated from some very old fears.

This focus on professional ethics paralleled my internal desire to express more integrity in my personal life. After that week in 1987 I began the process that led to leaving my family, coming out as a gay man, immersing myself in HIV-related psychotherapy by living for 2 years in San Francisco, and recreating myself both professionally and personally. HIV called me to a higher level of personal accountability. My clients lived with such suffering but maintained a kind of realness that I knew had been missing in my own life. No longer was I content to hide behind the professional mask that psychology had given me. I knew I wanted to integrate more fully who I was as a human being with what I did as a counselor. I resolved to live without letting fear cause me to hide or to deny who I was.

PROFESSIONAL IMPACT

Reflecting on my professional development as a result of working with HIV-positive clients reveals four specific areas that seem most significant. I have had to learn more about ethical decision making and the various models that would fit the kind of work I was doing. I have had to develop knowledge about many cultures I had not been close to before. I have been challenged to understand more fully my own beliefs about life and death and the kinds of end-of-life decisions that accompany HIV. And I have had to keep my eye on a developing legal climate that impacts and informs my work with HIV-positive clients. The challenge has been to explore each of these areas with the most integrity and intelligence that I could muster.

Ethical Decision Making

While in graduate school I learned the importance of ethical practice. I knew, of course, that I should discuss with my clients the limits of confidentiality and that I should rely on the *Tarasoff* (1976) case to define parameters when breaking confidentiality seemed necessary. Prior to working with people with HIV disease, I faced duty-to-protect dilemmas that seemed complex. For example, I struggled to find the limits of confidentiality when confronting circumstances in which an adolescent was seeking an abortion or a client's parent was concerned about her child's substance abuse. On the whole I think I managed them successfully. Still, these experiences left me unprepared for the intensity of HIV-related ethical dilemmas.

In chapter 7 you will read about my client Jerry, who admitted to having unsafe sex with anonymous partners without informing them of his HIV status. When I first listened to Jerry speak about his activity, I was shocked and did not have a clue about what I should do. I was offended that he was so cavalier about spreading HIV infection to others and also placing himself in danger of opportunistic infections. Clearly he was a threat to himself and others. At first, I wanted to call someone, to report him to the authorities or at least to refuse to treat him unless he promised to give up his irresponsible behavior. However, as I reflected about whom to call and what to say, none of the options that came up made any sense. The police might send him to our local mental health clinic, but I knew more about HIV work than they did and, anyway, he could not be held in the hospital until he died.

I wondered whom I might consult with about Jerry. I found myself pretty much without professional resources because there were no other mental health professionals in my community doing this work, and I was not aware of how I might contact people in other communities. I worried that if the public learned that I was seeing Jerry and had not reported him, my own practice might be in danger. I scrambled to find models that might help me. Finally I realized that I was alone with him and that my best approach would be to keep him in treatment in the hope that I could get him to change his behavior.

At first I tried to master the medical background about HIV. It did not take me long to realize that I am a psychologist, not a physician, and that my HIV-positive clients were excellent teachers. Although I did learn about medical aspects of HIV, I learned much more about my clients' bewilderment before a medical system that was as mystified as they were about the kinds of ailments they were experiencing. One of the mysteries of working with HIV-positive patients was that the medical diagnosis was so tentative. Physicians were frequently stumped in determining the causes of the immediate symptoms. Often I was the first to hear about symptoms and felt significant confusion as I encouraged my clients to let their physicians know what was happening to them. I became acutely aware of the tension that many patients feel in trying to hold their physicians' attention, and there were many times when I alerted a physician to the need for careful exploration of a patient's situation.

One client, Mike, came in because of his depression as a result of a diagnosis of Epstein–Barr mononucleosis. As I worked with him I observed many symptoms of HIV and encouraged him to ask his physician for additional testing. Alarmed as time was passing and he continued to trust his physician's statement ("Mike, you do not have HIV"), I worried about the ethics of calling his physician or of giving Mike the funds to get a second opinion. As his symptoms became more obvious, his HIV diagnosis was confirmed by anonymous testing. I had to practice patience to contain my own emotions as he decided not to report the physician or to file a malpractice suit.

Many psychologists work in settings where they are in and out of hospital rooms, often conducting sessions in constantly changing environments. Prior to HIV most of my work had been done in the relative safety of my office. Clients would call to arrange an appointment and arrive on schedule, and we would spend our 50 minutes together at the same time, same day, and same place each week. The "vessel" of time and place provided the context for our work together. HIV work, at least in the early days, did not allow such predictability. Today's more effective treatment has enabled me to return to an office-based practice, but there are still occasions when I might make a hospital or house call.

Aaron called me from jail. HIV-positive and incarcerated because of public drunkenness, he was referred to me by a corrections chaplain who did not have a clue what to do with a person who was HIV-positive. I went to the jail and arranged to see him. Prior to this I had not seen a client in jail, and I struggled with my own anxiety as I went to see him. What might he ask me? What are the limits of confidentiality when I am in the prison system? Might I be placing myself in a role in which I am vulnerable to litigation? Do I have the ethical right to be working in a system I do not know? Doing psychotherapy through a glass window and microphones was new to me and not something with which I was totally comfortable. Still, I was the best that Aaron could find, and I was making myself available, knowing there was not going to be a way for me to charge for my time. What Aaron really wanted was some money for a bus ticket so he could get to his family home in Georgia. Recognizing that being in jail and HIV-positive could be a brutal experience, I handed over the money from my own pocket without hesitation. Over time, I came to recognize that I was a kind of pioneer, exploring unknown territory as I helped people with HIV. I became more comfortable with entering unique environments.

Tom was more typical of the changing challenges I encountered. He contacted me at my office, and for 6 months he came for regular appointments that were billed to his health insurance company. As his health deteriorated, and he was forced to stay at home alone, I began to make home visits on a regular basis. Learning ways to deal with his offers of food and drink and the many familiarities that went beyond the usual boundary between psychologist and client, I found myself worrying about maintaining my professional distance. Trying to decide how to charge for what seemed like a mixture of a counseling session and a home visit was not the only difficulty. One day I found Tom stoned along with the home health care assistant, who gave him dope to keep him quiet! There was no one else other than me to try to straighten out this situation. I stepped into what felt like case management rather than ongoing psychotherapy with much trepidation; I did not want to become a case manager but could see no other alternative.

Months later, I found Tom sick in bed without food. The immediate action required was to go to the grocery, buy some food, return to Tom's, and fix him something to eat. I knew that I had done the right thing; I could not figure out at first whether this was a "billable" hour or exactly what my role was with him. By the time he approached death, still alone, I no longer worried so much about the role I was in. I made him a cake for what I knew would be his last birthday celebration and sat with him as he died because neither of us wanted him to die alone.

Stepping beyond the traditional psychotherapy relationship is not something to be done casually. I had learned to be very careful when the issue of dual relationships emerged. In the past I had carefully protected my boundaries and never had a client who had another role in my life. When I began to make hospital and home visits I was suddenly faced with my client and his support system, and I was aware that I was confronting aspects of my client's life that had been distant before. At first, I kept my interactions within the safe boundary of the client's psychological issues. But later as I found myself struggling with the confining limits of this professional role opposite more human needs, I would step forward hesitantly. When I bought food for Tom or sat down for a cup of coffee with a client's lover, I was careful to comment that we were in a new relationship, one that was not going to be billed and one that had different limits in terms of confidentiality.

Changing hats often became complex at times, but I used that metaphor to keep the client, his support system, and myself aware of what was going on. I have never been sure how an ethics board would evaluate my behavior, and at times I have been anxious about that. I have consistently tried to keep the best interests of my client in the foreground and to carefully evaluate how my behavior affects our professional relationship. Over time, I developed a list of colleagues who serve as reference points when I am particularly concerned. In the early days of HIV we lived with what often felt like a siege mentality. Drawn closer because of the fear and rejection of so many, the support system became intimate in our joint effort to ease the suffering of the person we had come to honor. Nurses, physicians, social workers, psychologists, and even funeral home personnel often became companions to the one who was dying. In many instances I knew that my role as a professional merely brought me to a place so I could fulfill more completely my role as a human being.

The models of ethical decision making that I had learned failed to give me much direction with clients like these. I was learning that HIV required creativity before ethical situations that I would have to resolve on my own. Fortunately, today there is a literature devoted to these situations, and chapters 2 and 3 of this book give background and direction based on research findings about ethics and HIV.

The Cultures of HIV Disease

Prior to working with HIV-positive individuals, most of my clients were pretty much like me—educated, professional, and largely White. I had gay clients before but understood little about gay culture. I had even seen a few people with drug problems, but most of them involved alcohol rather than injected drugs. I had an occasional African American client, but most were professionals. I entered the world of HIV psychotherapy totally unprepared for what I found.

For example, a couple of years after I had started working with people with HIV, I was attending a professional meeting in New York to give a paper on some aspect of my work. Mark Winiarski, a psychologist in Manhattan who worked with clients with HIV, contacted me and asked if I would like to visit the hospital where he worked to see an HIV unit in operation. I accepted eagerly, feeling fortunate that he had called me even though we had never met.

When I entered St. Vincent's Hospital that gloomy Saturday, I was a bit anxious, not sure how he and I would get along, somewhat worried that I was too much of a novice at this work to have much to say to someone working in New York City, and tense about being close to so much illness. As we walked through the hall, my anxieties lessened, and I responded favorably to his offer to let me talk with one of the patients. I was not prepared when asked what kind of patient I would like to see, but I had noticed many Latina women in the unit (few HIV-positive women had been seen in North Carolina in 1988), so I asked if I could talk with an HIV-positive woman who was an IV drug user. He went into a room to speak with the patient and ask if she was willing to speak with me, and then he invited me in. I walked past the suicide watch posted at her door confident that I would be able to understand her.

Dolores clearly was near death. Thin and emaciated, she was turned toward the window, but she spoke with me quite openly. She told me that she had been a prostitute and an IV drug user. She spoke of how she had alienated her family, and she was pretty much alone as she was getting sicker. I was learning from her about the kinds of resources available in New York and her sadness about being so sick and alone. As I listened she seemed to fit the stereotype of a prostitute. I was seeing her only through my own negative lens, and even today I am ashamed of my own smugness as I recall the time with her. As I stood up to leave, I asked about her suicide attempt. What she said startled me and changed my awareness of the work that I needed to do to understand the cultures of HIV. Dolores told me a part of her story I had not anticipated.

> I have been a terrible mother to my three children. They deserved a better mother than I have been. Fortunately for them, DSS [the Department of Social Services] stepped in and took them away from me several years ago, and I have not seen them since. My parents and brothers and sisters gradually gave up on me. I am about to die, and I asked my caseworker to contact DSS so I might meet with my children and apologize to them for letting them down so badly. My request was turned down, and I was told once again that I could have no contact with them for the rest of my life. There is nothing left for me to live for, and I tried to jump out the window. Right now I just want to die. I failed in the most important job that I had. There is no hope for me.

As I have worked in many unfamiliar cultures I have been constantly reminded to leave my stereotypes at the door and to proceed slowly lest I be offensive and ineffective. Dolores taught me one of the more valuable lessons in my life about the error of judging others from my own preconceptions or on the basis of what they do or even who they might appear to be. There is an adage from Eastern culture, "When the student is ready, the teacher will appear." We are surrounded by teachers if we can just slow ourselves down long enough and suspend our belief systems long enough to let them change us. Chapter 4 is devoted to developing an understanding of the various cultures in the HIV community.

Death and End-of-Life Issues

From my experiences with cancer patients I had learned to sit close to people who were dying. Providing support at the end of life is not an easy task. I grappled with my own sense of helplessness and wondered if I was contributing anything. As a kid I had been told many times "Don't just stand there, do something." In working with HIV patients, however, I changed that statement to "Don't just do something, stand there!" I came to realize that just being willing to feel the helplessness of the situation was a contribution. The work inevitably brought up thoughts about my own death, and sometimes I knew what to do from imagining what I might want others to do for me. As difficult as death from cancer can be, it was small stuff compared to the ravages of HIV, particularly in the 1980s and early 1990s.

In those days, HIV clients presented with a level of fear I had not seen before. They were dealing with unfamiliar illnesses that often had no known treatment. These young men were leaving jobs that were secure and giving up dreams of an adult life. They faced the stigma of being gay and HIV-positive and had to interact with a medical and social services system that did not understand them. Many of them faced death without the comfort of family, and they lived in communities where death became almost a daily event.

Death became a constant companion. Too frequently I would be in the early stages of a relationship with a client only to lose him to an unanticipated illness. I found myself resisting getting close to some new clients who were HIV-positive. My own anger about the situations faced by many clients was intense at times. I worried that my whole professional career was going to be dominated by sickness and death. At times I felt just totally empty. At other times I felt like I had never appreciated life so intensely, that I had never worked in an atmosphere so charged with emotion, that I had never learned so much. I encountered so many men and women like Dolores, who were looking down a dark and painful road and just wanted to be in charge of how and when they died.

Saying goodbye to many who had taught me so much was not just a professional activity. Letting my tears flow from more than empathy became a more normal occurrence. Providing a kind of support that might include arranging for an attorney or a religious figure to come to the home or hospital to make particular arrangements or assisting in the planning or speaking at a funeral never became routine for me. But I reached a level of comfort where I did not back away from responding to these kinds of personal needs and requests. There were certainly times when I worried that those who had taught me how to be a psychotherapist would be alarmed to see what I was doing.

The challenge posed by assisted suicide forced me to reexamine my own personal beliefs about death on both a personal and professional level. Like all psychologists I had been trained to act to preserve life, a process that posed no internal conflict for me. Prior to HIV I had found myself in situations in which clients had to be hospitalized, sometimes against their will, in order to keep them from harming themselves. Although I was familiar with the discussion about withholding life support when death seemed certain, I had not encountered situations in which suicide seemed like an acceptable and rational behavior.

Before I had seen 10 HIV-positive clients, I had come to expect to hear thoughts about suicide. People like Mike and Dolores taught me that these thoughts are logical. As I listened to them talk about taking their own lives, I found myself wondering whether they might be right, that ending one's life when there were no treatment options and death was inevitable is a decision that properly falls to the one who is sick. However, I also knew that, like cancer patients, HIV-positive people could appear near death one day and hardly look sick at all 2 days later. Today the incidence of death is vastly lower; in the late 1980s, it was routine. Many people had exhausted all of their resources as they struggled with HIV/AIDS. Some faced their deaths alone, having watched all of their friends die and having no family support. Many worried about the various kinds of debilitating illnesses that might render them unable to be in control of any facet of their lives. Their desire to hoard pills or to acquire other means to end their lives began to seem reasonable. In some instances, their medical support team assisted them in this effort.

Watching an epidemic happen has been a very curious event. Professionals working with HIV/AIDS have had to live in a constantly changing environment. We have watched and assisted as the medical profession and our clients sought and found many experimental treatments that raised our hopes. The lessons that we learned during the days when HIV was seen as inevitably fatal continue to be valuable as we discuss assisted suicide and other end-of-life issues. Today the challenge is not so much one that centers on death. As people return to health, the focus shifts toward acknowledging the many losses that accompany all chronic illness. Chapter 5 gives a flavor of that ongoing dilemma.

HIV and the Law

As medical and psychological treatment matured, there has been a corresponding development of the law as it applies to HIV. Prior to 1988 there were few laws that directly dealt with HIV. At first, the case law that developed dealt with issues of confidentiality. Because of the stigma and an often hysterical public response, the courts began to protect the privacy rights of those who were infected. Later, as more knowledge developed, laws began to direct medical and mental health professionals to break confidentiality in certain instances. Although there have been few lawsuits against mental health professionals, knowledge of the law has become even more essential.

Over the past 15 years I have had to know more about the law than I would wish. At one time I believed that consultations with attorneys were only useful in extreme situations. I remember thinking that rather than have a legal consultation, I would just think of the most conservative course of action possible and act as if that was the advice I would get. In many instances that was true. The attorney would tell me to act in a way that minimized both our risks. Today I know that legal officials can provide useful information. Although HIV law has become as complex as HIV medical treatment, knowledge of some of the basics is essential. Chapter 6 provides at least entry-level information about HIV and the law.

PERSONAL IMPACT

I do this work for reasons that are definitely as complex as the situations that I have faced. I have never been involved in work that seems so vital. It demands a kind of creativity that constantly challenges me, and it places me closer to very real life issues that many communities struggle to understand. Watching individuals, families, and systems deal with stigma, an emerging scientific understanding, limited resources, enormous need, and the many other facets of HIV teaches me about myself and about humanity. It is ironic that in the midst of so much pain and darkness there is often such abundant love and light. I am no longer startled when I hear people who are dying say that their lives have been enriched by HIV disease. They report that the disease has enabled them to know something fundamental and vital about love and acceptance. That is true for me as well.

As I am close to others facing HIV, I have come to see my own life in a new perspective. The integrity of many of my patients has led me to a renewed commitment to live out my own truth more fully. As they struggle to find meaning in their changed circumstances, I also find myself conscious of the ways that I seek meaning and adventure. Over and over I am reminded about the preciousness of love and the importance of intimate relationships. I find myself more ready to let those who are important in my life know my feelings toward them.

The personal impact that flows from my work with HIV clients has been enormous. Living as an out gay professional seems like the backdrop to so many other changes. Naturally it is impossible to separate the influence of HIV work as a distinct cause of a particular change. But the intensity of the work has been totally absorbing at times. I recall the time that my department chair chastised me for being impatient and disengaged from a faculty issue. As we discussed my feelings she suddenly said, "I guess spending so much time with people who are dying puts these struggles at the university at the bottom of the list of what seems important to you." She was right about that, but the work has also placed many things ahead of my career or even of my security. For example, I make a conscious effort to let people know when I am caring about them. Saying "I love you" when I feel it has become almost routine for me today. I also tend to keep my relationships cleaner than before. I do not just walk away from a dispute thinking that I will get back to it later. I have seen far too many instances when there was no later opportunity to work things out.

Across my life I have had an off-and-on dialogue with the church. Raised Presbyterian, I found early on that the simple answers offered in many Christian denominations did not work for me. Encountering the ravages of HIV led me into a new spiritual life. Before such suffering, I am challenged to understand the meaning of existence for both the patient and myself. I wrestle with a crushing cruelty that comes from many so-called Christian groups. I find myself drawn toward Buddhism and eastern forms of meditation. I know that I am a deeply spiritual person and that I have a faith that does not require me to worry about the afterlife but instead calls me to give more fully from a well of love and respect for all peoples. That I often fail in this undertaking is not such a major tragedy. It is important that I continue to try and that I learn to accept my own imperfections. Today I do this outside of any formal religious institution. Still, I yearn for a kind of spiritual community I have not found.

Fears do not immobilize me as they did in the past. As I have watched many people take risks that humbled me, I have come to see that the courage I used to seek is found only in being with my fear. I know I am telling a truth when I say courage is not the absence of fear; rather, courage is being afraid and doing the task anyway. I have grown fond of a statement attributed to Eleanor Roosevelt: "You must do that which you most fear." Truly facing one's fears is the only path to true liberation. For me, this means confronting my supervisor when I learned that I was being underpaid, and even telling the chancellor of my university that his prejudices against homosexual people were showing when we were working on a diversity project. It has also meant continuing to tell two of my daughters that I love them even when they condemn and reject aspects of my life as a gay man.

Ethical situations do not seem nearly as distressing as they did at first. I believe that my whole psychotherapy practice is characterized by a much keener awareness of ethical challenges and an enhanced ability to confront them without such high anxiety. I have learned several ethical decision-making models and read more about ethics than I might have otherwise. My participation in this book stands as a testament to my concern about and interest in ethics and HIV.

Today I can cry more easily than before, but I can also be moved by the sunlight on a tree or by someone taking my hand on a walk, or even by the communion from a meal with friends and relatives. Work is about more than money or power, and I have a deeper sense of an incredible wealth that can be experienced in simple moments. My spiritual life is fuller than before, and I go about my days carrying precious memories of men and women who gifted me with a kind of wisdom that enables me to understand my life more fully.

CONCLUSION

The culture of HIV has changed over the years. Today more people are available to serve as resources. There is a burgeoning literature that informs those new to the work. Still, last summer when a dying client asked me to speak with his lawyer and dictate the terms of his will, I felt a familiar sense of uneasiness. Is this what a psychologist is supposed to do? What liability am I incurring as I tell the lawyer how to disperse the client's property? The problem was that I was the only one who knew how he wanted his property divided, and he no longer had the energy to concentrate on the details. Of course, I had urged him to make a will months before, and I continually brought it up until I realized that the will had become symbolic of his death. By not having a will, he could continue to live. He did die the day after he signed his will, and I left his life knowing that I had enabled him to have at least some of his wishes followed. Would I do something like this again? I don't know. But I do hope that I will continue to explore questions like these with all of my clients. I do not want to hide behind the safety of the limits ethical and legal principles seem to offer when faced with a human being asking for something that seems humane.

There are no easy answers to the ethical dilemmas posed in HIV-related psychotherapy. Using the models presented in this book will help, but ultimately I will have to decide for myself a course of action, and I will have to live the consequences of those decisions. As a psychologist I am prepared to take on this responsibility and to assist my clients in their desire to live and die with the utmost integrity. I hope that I do not sound like I am making myself some sort of supreme judge who is above the limits that exist in most of our work. I particularly dislike that notion. Neither do I want to be the kind of psychologist who lives solely by the rules, who takes no risks or who is unwilling to step outside of the box and wrestle with a situation that generates professional anxiety. As much as we hope that laws and ethical codes give us absolute rules, we must recognize that these are guidelines and do not exempt us from the often-tortuous effort in sorting through options that may be clearly in the best interests of our clients but that also place us in varying degrees of professional peril. Naturally the line between professional and unprofessional conduct has to be drawn somewhere. I hope that I will continue to approach that line with the utmost respect, to honor the wisdom of those who have come before me and who created these rules. At the same time, I hope that my human qualities will be present to remind me that I am working with people, not objects, and that my humane response might just be the most appropriate given the uniqueness of a situation.

Thirty years ago I had no idea that the profession of psychology would offer me so many rich experiences. I have learned more than I could have ever dreamed, found myself in situations that demanded more than I thought I had to give, been touched and enriched by virtually every person I have been privileged to sit with, and can look back on a life of immense richness and complexity. I am more competent in all aspects of my work as a result of the time I have spent with HIV-related issues. I am also a better person as a result, and I believe I have also been at least a cog in the process that leads people to a fuller appreciation and expression of their own humanity. One could hardly ask for more in life.

REFERENCE

Tarasoff v. Board of Regents of the University of California, 17 Cal. 3d 425, 551 P.2d 334 (1976).

2

ETHICAL ISSUES IN THE PRACTICE OF PSYCHOLOGY WITH CLIENTS WITH HIV/AIDS

SARA R. STEVENSON AND KAREN STROHM KITCHENER

What ethical issues have been identified in mental health practice with clients with HIV/AIDS? Does the available research enlighten one's understanding of these issues or how mental health workers act when faced with them? What conclusions have been drawn about these ethical issues that might be of help to those who are faced with ethical dilemmas in everyday practice? What issues have received little or no attention? We address these questions in this chapter.

Pope and Vetter (1992) discussed general ethical areas that have been identified by psychologists as troublesome: confidentiality; blurred, dual, or multiple relationships; competence when working with new populations or with unfamiliar client issues; using and responding to payment providers; testifying in legal cases; and responding to the needs of those who have limited financial resources. We suspect that most of these concerns have parallels in work with HIV-positive clients. Many of the confidentiality issues about which psychologists reported difficulty were those involving potential risk to a third party, an issue that plagues those who work with individuals who have HIV or AIDS. Boundary issues arise when clients are dying or can no longer travel to the therapists' office, and the issue becomes whether therapy should be offered in the client's home. If so, what are the implications for the boundaries of the therapeutic relationship, and how can the relationship be handled ethically? The cases discussed in this book give an indication of the breadth and depth of other issues that need thoughtful attention. One that seems particularly important is that surrounding the perinatal transmission of the virus and its implications for therapists working with women who wish to become pregnant or are engaging in high-risk behaviors.

By contrast, the scope of the ethics literature in this area is narrow. The vast majority of articles are theoretical and concentrate on the question of whether psychologists have a responsibility to break confidentiality in order to protect the partners of HIV-infected clients when clients refuse to inform them about their infection. More recently, issues such as rational suicide and confidentiality, the duty to treat infected patients, HIV-related issues in the treatment of adolescents, and the management of infected psychiatric patients have received some attention in the literature. Each of these is discussed in the following pages.

The AIDS epidemic presents a complex set of ethical dilemmas for psychologists and other mental health professionals. Despite the far-reaching professional, ethical, and legal considerations associated with the AIDS epidemic, the American Psychological Association's "Ethical Principles for Psychologists and Code of Conduct" (Ethics Code; see appendix) does not explicitly address professional decision making in AIDS-related psychological practice. Furthermore, it is often unclear how state laws regarding confidentiality and HIV, written for physicians, generalize to the mental health practitioner. As yet there have been no court cases concerning confidentiality that have interpreted *Tarasoff* with regard to HIV practice. Consequently, in order to clarify this issue, we review the literature in HIV-related mental health care practice. In the absence of clear guidelines for approaching complex ethical issues in AIDS-related practice, it is important for the profession to conceptually examine the challenging ethical decisions that might face psychologists. We hope this chapter helps in that process.

CONFIDENTIALITY VERSUS THE DUTY TO PROTECT

In the mental health literature focused on HIV-positive clients, the ethical issue considered with the greatest frequency focuses on the conflict between the obligation to maintain client confidentiality versus the responsibility to society to prevent the spread of the disease when clients are putting third parties at risk for contracting HIV. To a great extent, the discussion has been dominated by the question of whether the rulings from the *Tarasoff* case (*Tarasoff v. Board of Regents of the University of California*, 1976) regarding the duty to warn or otherwise protect third parties applies to clients with HIV. Although this is, in fact, a legal question, embedded in the discussion are important ethical considerations (see chapter 6 for a discussion of the legal issues).

In *Tarasoff*, the family of a murdered woman sued her killer's therapist, and the Board of Regents of the University of California, for failing to take the steps that might have prevented her death. The majority opinion reached by the California supreme court justices in the *Tarasoff* case concluded that confidentiality in the therapeutic relationship is not absolute. The justices argued that when a therapist determines, on the basis of reasonable standards of the profession, that a client is engaging in, or intends to engage in, behavior that presents a serious danger of violence to a third party, the mental health professional is obligated to exercise reasonable care to protect the potential victim. Here, Justice Tobriner, the author of the majority opinion, offered three alternatives: Therapists might warn the victim, notify the police, or take other steps that might reasonably be necessary to protect the intended victim from danger.

Authors have differed in their beliefs about the applicability of the *Tarasoff* ruling to AIDS clients. Some have viewed the *Tarasoff* decision as indicating that professionals are required to warn endangered third parties of clients' HIV status (Gray & Harding, 1988), whereas others have argued that the application of *Tarasoff* to AIDS-related practice is problematic because HIV involves the transmission of a deadly virus, not the use of violence (Knapp & VandeCreek, 1990; Lamb, Clark, Drumheller, Frizzell, & Surrey, 1989; Melton, 1988b). Because there are no legal precedents related to HIV-positive clients who are endangering others, conclusions are at best reasoned speculation.

In general, the *Tarasoff* ruling has highlighted four elements that must be considered when deciding whether to break confidentiality: the existence of a special relationship, the foreseeability of harm, the identifiability of one or more victims, and the appropriate course of action for the mental health professional. These elements have been examined by numerous authors and are often used as the ethical framework for evaluating confidentiality issues in HIV-related practice.

Special Relationship

The justices in the *Tarasoff* case argued that a special relationship exists between the client and the therapist. The court determined that by engaging in a therapeutic relationship, the therapist assumes some responsibility for the actions of the client. Consequently, the therapist then bears some obligation to protect the safety of the client and those who may be harmed by the client (Lamb et al., 1989). Some assume that the special relationship as defined in the *Tarasoff* decision applies to every therapeutic relationship and therefore would be relevant in the treatment of HIV-related disease (Lamb et al., 1989). This implies that the therapist maintains some culpability for the safety of clients who are HIV-positive and also has some responsibility to respond if they pose a danger to another person.

Foreseeability of Harm

In the *Tarasoff* case justices recognized the difficulty that faces a therapist in determining whether clients pose a danger of violence; therefore, a therapist is not expected to predict clients' dangerousness with perfect accuracy. However, it is expected that therapists will use a level of care and skill in assessing clients commensurate to that possessed by members of their profession under similar circumstances (Fulero, 1988). Assessing the dangerousness of a violent client or an HIV-positive client is fraught with uncertainty (Lamb et al., 1989).

Assessing dangerousness in a case involving an HIV-positive individual may be contingent on a number of factors, including whether the client engages in high-risk behaviors or uses safer sex practices and the stage of the illness. Although there is some medical uncertainty about transmission and progression of HIV and AIDS, some sexual acts imply greater risk than others (Lamb et al., 1989). Safer sex practices and certain types of sexual activity may reduce the risk of transmission (Kain, 1988). For example, engaging in anal intercourse without a condom carries a higher risk of infection than does oral sex without a condom. Breaching confidentiality might be appropriate in the first case, but not in the second because there is less risk of transmission.

The assessment of dangerousness is complicated by two facts: HIV involves a communicable disease, and the determination of a client's HIV status is based on a medical diagnosis (Kain, 1988). Determining behaviors that constitute a serious risk or imminent danger in the transmission of a deadly virus may exceed the boundaries of competence of a psychologist or mental health professional (Kain, 1988; Lamb et al., 1989). In fact, several authors have concluded that the foreseeability of harm is the most ambiguous consideration in applying *Tarasoff* to AIDS cases. Because of the biological variability of the disease, as well as the lack of medical certainty about modes of transmission and the likelihood of the transmission of HIV, it is difficult to identify and predict behaviors that involve an imminent danger (Knapp & VandeCreek, 1990; Lamb et al., 1989). By contrast, Melton (1988b) argued that when a psychologist knows that a client is HIV-positive there is no reason to believe that the prediction of dangerousness is beyond the boundaries of professional competence. He suggested that the determination of foreseeability of risk be mainly based on assessing the behavioral practices of the client, which is a task within the realm of therapeutic practice.

The National Institutes of Health (NIH, 1997) identified unprotected anal and vaginal intercourse and use of nonsterile drug injection equipment as high-risk behaviors. Although there is some indication of oral–genital transmission, the level of risk is unclear, but it is considered to carry less risk than vaginal or anal sexual intercourse. Some authors have concluded that because high-risk behaviors are more likely to transmit HIV, they are more likely to invoke a psychotherapist's duty to protect a third party (Knapp & VandeCreek, 1990).

Contextual factors also influence the likelihood of engaging in high-risk behavior and the risk associated with such behaviors. These include drug and alcohol abuse, level of commitment in a relationship, the existence of untreated sexually transmitted diseases, social norms and values, availability of condoms or sterile needles, the ability to negotiate safe sex practices, age and developmental stage, and political and economic factors (NIH, 1997). Among gay men social support, levels of self-efficacy, and knowledge of seropositive status are additional factors that influence risk-taking behaviors (Martin, in press). Psychologists should understand and consider these issues as they evaluate both the risks clients pose to others and how to manage clinical situations with clients.

Identifiability of the Victim

Identifying third parties who are at risk for contracting HIV is complicated by lack of certainty about HIV transmission (Lamb et al., 1989). Because the disease may lie dormant for several years, the question arises as to whether therapists might be obligated to protect or notify past contacts. However, it has been argued that notification, if warranted, should not extend beyond immediate individuals at risk, because to do otherwise would involve assigning to psychologists "what is essentially a public health burden" (Appelbaum & Appelbaum, 1990, p. 134).

It has also been suggested that HIV-related disease is not subject to the legal conclusions drawn in *Tarasoff* because individuals who participate in high-risk behavior are willingly engaging in activities that put them at risk. In contrast with victims of violence, Kain (1988) argued, needle and sexual partners are complicit in their fate because they freely choose to engage in risky behavior. However, the assumption that individuals are sufficiently knowledgeable to protect themselves is questionable. Members of subcultures that are at high risk, as well as the general population, are prone to ignorance, denial, and misinformation about the transmission of HIV (Appelbaum & Appelbaum, 1990). Moreover, individuals involved in relationships that they perceive to be monogamous are unlikely to take precautions to reduce the risk of contracting a sexually transmitted disease (M. A. Hoffman, 1991).

Course of Action

The *Tarasoff* court maintained that if the danger a client presents is foreseeable and a victim is identified, the therapist should act to protect the victim. The notification of victims is not the only alternative, however. In fact, *Tarasoff* does not necessarily mandate a breach of confidentiality and the warning of a third party. Instead, as already noted, the court also suggested the possibility of informing the police or taking alternative actions that might be required to protect a potential victim.

When considering the management of confidentiality beyond *Tarasoff*, several writers have approached the problems from the perspective of a consequentialist. In other words, the ethical appropriateness of psychologists' behavior should be evaluated according to the consequences that follow from the actions (Appelbaum & Appelbaum, 1990). Authors who are more conservative about breaking confidentiality have argued that there is potential for harm to the client, to the profession, and ultimately to society at large if confidentiality were breached and doing so became the accepted standard of practice. Breaching of confidentiality also creates the potential for the erosion of public trust in therapists (Reamer, 1991). Historically, the relationship between health professionals and the gay community, the group most affected by AIDS, has been strained (Melton, 1988b). Therefore, breaches in confidentiality may create greater tensions and mistrust, discourage individuals from seeking services or disclosing important information, or lead to premature termination (Knapp & VandeCreek, 1990; Melton, 1988b). In addition, reporting clients may lead to an increase in discrimination against gays and others with HIV. For example, reporting clients to county health officials may make them subject to housing, employment, and insurance discrimination (Kain, 1988).

It also is important to recognize the influence that attitudes toward HIV and those who are infected may have on resolving issues of confidentiality. Research has revealed that health professionals harbor negative attitudes toward individuals with HIV and view them as more responsible for their illness than people with other diseases. People with HIV are also perceived as deserving of less sympathy and as less competent and less moral than other groups (Royse & Birge, 1987; Young, Henderson, & Marx, 1990). Studies have also revealed that there is an inverse relationship between health professionals' level of empathy toward AIDS patients and homophobia, as well as less empathy toward gay men with AIDS than toward individuals who contracted the disease through a blood transfusion (Kelly et al.,

1992; Royse & Birge, 1987). Furthermore, psychologists' bias and attitudes toward certain populations may independently influence their clinical decision making (McGuire, Nieri, Abbot, Sheridan, & Fisher, 1995; Totten, Lamb, & Reeder, 1990).

Reporting clients may prevent therapists from working in ways in which they may be the most effective in preventing the spread of AIDS. If psychologists reveal information about behaviors that endanger third parties, clients are liable to be reticent to disclose irresponsible practices. In the absence of client disclosure psychologists cannot intervene therapeutically or educationally to prevent behaviors that place others at risk (Kain, 1988). Therapeutic interventions are particularly critical when the client is endangering anonymous or not easily identifiable individuals.

On the other hand, several have argued (Appelbaum & Appelbaum, 1990; Erickson, 1993; Gray & Harding, 1988) that because HIV is ultimately life threatening and the long-term consequences to the public and the individual are so dire, breaching confidentiality is ethically justified. According to this argument, the rights of the endangered person override the rights of the client to confidentiality because of the fatal nature of untreated HIV. It should be noted that Standard 5.05 of the Ethics Code allows for disclosure of confidential information "only as mandated by law, or where permitted by law for a valid purpose" (APA, 1992).

Attempts to alter client behaviors through clinical management should always be made before breaching confidentiality (Kain, 1988; Knapp & VandeCreek, 1990; Reamer, 1991). These include educating clients, using the therapeutic process to promote more responsible behaviors, assisting clients to obtain condoms or sterile needles, addressing interpersonal or psychological issues that may prevent clients from informing sexual partners of their HIV status, and addressing social or cultural values or norms that inhibit either safe practices or communication of HIV status. If clients are unresponsive to interventions used within the therapeutic process, psychiatric commitment might be considered (Lamb et al., 1989). The use of commitment must be based on a mental condition that creates dangerousness to others, however, not on the diagnosis of HIV (Zonana, Norko, & Stier, 1988). Furthermore, the use of civil commitment with HIV clients who are potentially dangerous to others is unusual and problematic because civil commitment laws were written for the detention of the severely mentally ill and for the treatment of mental illness (D. J. Martin, personal communication, November 15, 1999).

Two additional questions regarding the breach of confidentiality have been raised. First, what is a reasonable amount of time to attempt clinical interventions before considering more extreme measures to protect another person from HIV infection? Second, how should a therapist respond if clients initially discontinue reckless behavior, but then have periodic lapses during which time they endanger others? These unresolved issues are likely to be a central aspect of working with HIV-positive clients.

The Decision to Breach Confidentiality

The APA has not taken a professional stance regarding confidentiality in HIV-related clinical practice. However, APA (1991) has drafted recommendations for legislation (see appendix at end of chapter). The legislative recommendations assert that if state laws are drafted to address the parameters of confidentiality in the treatment of individuals with HIV, they should include several premises: that psychologists should only undertake third-party notification if an identifiable third party is at significant risk, the third party is unaware of the risk, and the patient refuses to inform that person of the risk. Several authors have suggested sequences that therapists might follow if they decide they have a responsibility to protect either needle or sexual partners. Although each model is slightly different, they are all generally consistent with APA legislative recommendations and involve five conditions that must be present.

1. All clients (whether HIV-positive or not) should be informed of the limits of confidentiality (Erickson, 1993; Reamer, 1991). Such statements should include information that confidentiality is limited if a third party is at risk.
2. Therapists should have medical evidence that the client is HIV-positive.
3. There must be an indication that the client is placing a third party at risk for HIV infection and that the client has not informed or is not likely to inform the third party (Cohen, 1990). Because data on HIV transmission are evolving, the conclusion that the client is placing others at risk must be based on current medical authority (which may imply consulting a physician knowledgeable about HIV transmission).
4. The therapist should attempt to educate the client, encourage and support disclosure by the client to the partner, or use other therapeutic methods such as therapy groups to address denial and provide support (Erickson, 1993). Moreover, it may be beneficial to consult with colleagues to identify a community standard.
5. Disclosure must be done in a timely fashion, and the client should be informed of the therapist's intention (Cohen, 1990; Erickson, 1993). Information should be disclosed only to par-

ties at risk and should include only information relevant to the client's medical diagnosis (Cohen, 1990; however, Erickson has also argued that public health officials and the police should be notified).

Some have also argued that therapists are ethically obligated to extend support to those notified by offering professional services or referral (Cohen, 1990) and that documenting decisions in these cases is important (Reamer, 1991). It is also important to recognize laws that may influence the course of action the psychologist takes. For example, in California physicians are the only health care providers permitted to notify a third party at risk for contracting HIV. Therefore, in California psychologists who undertake notification of a third party would be violating the law (Martin, in press), and therefore, Standard 5.05 of the Ethics Code (APA, 1992).

RATIONAL SUICIDE

For clinical psychologists, the responsibility for the prevention of suicide is preeminent (Werth, 1992). Individuals who harm themselves are perceived as irrational or incompetent, and extreme measures are thereby justified to prevent such action. Professional norms regarding the impermissibility of suicide have been influenced by Christian doctrine, which regards suicide as immoral, and a medical conception of suicide as reflecting mental instability (Mayo, 1993). Furthermore, the implicit difficulty in discriminating between rational and irrational suicidal ideation and behavior creates an additional barrier to the acceptance of the notion that suicide may, at times, be a rationally exercised choice. In light of the tremendous responsibility placed on professionals to predict whether clients are likely to kill themselves, an even greater burden would face psychologists in assessing rationality (Mayo, 1993). In failing to acknowledge that suicide may be considered and carried out by a reasonable individual, psychologists may be restrained from exercising professional judgment on a case-by-case basis. However, despite social mores, the implicit moral burden, and the complexity attached to the concept of rational suicide, the mental health profession is currently being challenged to reconsider its absolutist stance toward suicide (Mayo, 1993).

In their survey of APA Division 29 members, Werth and Liddle (1994) found that psychologists were less negative toward suicide ideators who were terminally ill than those who were suffering from physical or psychological pain and advocated less coercive intervention in such cases. Moreover, 80% of the respondents responded affirmatively to the question "do you believe in the idea of rational suicide?" (Werth & Liddle, 1994, p. 447). The belief that under some circumstances suicide may be justified implies an incongruence between psychologists' personal beliefs and current standards of professional practice.

Historically, the profession of psychology has acknowledged that suicide might be a rational option in rare situations (Werth, 1992), but such a conclusion has been questioned with the emergence of the AIDS epidemic. Individuals who are suffering with AIDS are "young, intelligent and educated, and many have already made independent choices about their lives which do not always conform to social conventions" (Boyd, 1989, p. 309). Suicide among the HIV population has been reported to be significantly larger than for demographically similar individuals (Cote, Bigger, & Dannenberg, 1992; Kalichman & Sikkema, 1994; Marzuk et al., 1988). A comprehensive review of empirical findings suggests that individuals are likely to report higher rates of suicidal ideation and attempts early in the disease process (when they first learn they are HIV-positive or when they begin to experience early symptoms of the disease). Moreover, as with suicide in the general population, people with HIV are at greater risk for suicide when they maintain cognitive or affective disturbance, lack social support, have a previous history of suicide attempts, and are substance abusers (Kalichman & Sikkema, 1994). Later in the disease process consideration of suicide appears to be a product of despair, concerns about dependency, fear of physical deterioration, and watching others around them die from AIDS (Kalichman & Sikkema, 1994; Rabkin, Remien, Katoff, & Williams, 1993).

It is important to differentiate depression from normal grief and loss associated with facing a serious illness. Although some may construe suicidal thoughts as normal consequences of HIV illness, the consequences of physical decline do not necessarily lead to such feelings, and such feelings may well be the effects of a treatable clinical depression (Faberman, 1997). Furthermore, because an individual's lifelong temperament and behavior are better indicators of suicidal ideation during a serious illness than pain and physical decline, a careful individual assessment must be conducted in order to realistically determine the source of suicidal ideation and the appropriate clinical response (Faberman, 1997).

Rationality in the AIDS patient is further brought into question because the virus attacks the central nervous system. Rogers and Britton (1994) contended that at this point there is insufficient data on which to base adequate conclusions about the mental competence of individuals with AIDS-related disease. They argued that psychologists have a professional responsibility to assist individuals who suffer with AIDS and HIV in working through developmental issues associated with coping with a terminal illness. Because of the fluctuations in the disease processes associated with AIDS, they suggested that the decision to commit suicide is likely to be transient and that this transience contradicts rationality.

Appropriate intervention involves early treatment to prevent emotional deterioration and efforts to assist the client to cope with the inherent uncertainty of the illness (Rabkin et al., 1993; Rogers & Britton, 1994). Competent intervention should always include the development of a therapeutic alliance, early discussions of suicidal thoughts, instillation of hope, development of social support, encouragement of active participation in treatment and emotional expression, and support for the expression of grief and loss and negative feelings about self and others (Martin, in press). Efforts to offer hospice care, pain management, and psychological support may be appropriate alternatives to suicide (McIntosh, 1993).

Werth (1995) has offered a framework for determining the rationality of suicidal ideation. The first three criteria are drawn from Siegal's (1986) model:

1. The client can make a realistic assessment of the situation.
2. The clients' mental processes are unimpaired by psychological illness or severe emotional distress.
3. The motivation of the client is understandable to a majority of uninvolved community members.
4. The decision must be contemplated and discussed over a period of time.
5. When possible, significant others should actively participate in the decision-making process.

Werth argued that the choice of whether to involve other people should be left to the person who is suicidal and that the wishes of the significant other should not override the decision of the person who meets the first four criteria.

Thus far, there is a paucity of psychological literature, particularly empirical literature, on the rationality of those with AIDS and AIDS-related diseases, as well as on rational suicide, despite the many complex ethical, moral, and legal issues that require addressing. For example, because of the uncertainty of the course of AIDS, as well as the unpredictability of future treatments for the disease, it is difficult to determine at what point a decision could be considered rational and at what point it could not. Furthermore, because the disease is associated with significant depression, loss of social support, and isolation, it is critical to determine how such factors ultimately contribute to individuals' decisions to end their life. These factors may lead psychologists to questions Werth's (1995) criteria for the rationality of suicide because they raise the question of whether such decisions are ever unimpaired by psychological or emotional distress.

ADDITIONAL CONSIDERATIONS

There are a number of areas of professional practice in which one can anticipate the emergence of complex ethical dilemmas related to HIV and AIDS as this epidemic spreads to a broader spectrum of the population. These areas have been minimally addressed in the psychological literature. For example, boundary issues and multiple role issues have been virtually ignored, although in HIV-related practice boundaries sometimes get blurred (see chapter 15). Other areas of concern about which there is a small amount of literature include work with minors, hospitalized psychiatric patients, and issues surrounding perinatal transmission. Furthermore, questions have been raised regarding the professional responsibility of psychologists, if any, to help prevent the spread of AIDS and to provide psychological services to infected individuals (Melton, 1988b).

Adolescent Issues

Because adolescents are known to experiment with both sex and drugs, issues of HIV infection in this population are of particular concern (Olson, Mason, Huszti, & Seibert, 1989). In fact, a significant portion of those who ultimately contract AIDS are likely to have been infected during adolescence (Rotheram-Borus, Reid, & Rosario, 1994; Sobocinski, 1989). There are only a few articles that discuss relevant and distinct ethical issues that recur in the treatment of adolescents in general (Powell, 1984; Sobocinski, 1989) and specifically in the treatment of gay adolescents, a population that is at high risk for HIV infection (Sobocinski, 1989). These articles point to several ethical concerns that emerge in adolescent practice, revolving around confidentiality, competence, and autonomy (Powell, 1984; Sobocinski, 1989). The autonomy allocated to clients in clinical practice bears a direct relationship to their competence to make their own decisions. In fact, adolescence is a period of development that is transitional with respect to individual competence. The age at which adolescents are considered legally competent varies from state to state and is dependent on the context under consideration. Consequently, an adolescent can neither be considered entirely ethically competent nor regarded as completely lacking in competence (Sobocinski, 1989). Furthermore, adolescent competence in decision making is generally associated with the individual's chronological age and intelligence (Powell, 1984). Therefore, the determination of competence will, in part, involve a careful evaluation of the adolescent's chronological age. Powell (1984) and Sobocinski (1989) argued that in situations where the negative consequences of actions are great (e.g., the risk of contracting AIDS through unprotected sexual activity or intravenous drug use), stringent criteria for competence should be applied. Additionally, because adolescents are prone to impulsive behaviors, prevention should be considered standard practice with all adolescents regardless of specific indicators or immediate risk (Melton, 1988a).

In considering issues beyond adolescent competence, research suggests that although adolescents as a group may be prone to impulsive behaviors, they are also responsive to interventions geared toward increasing safe sexual behaviors. Studies document that taking certain measures—using cognitive, social, and behavioral interventions directed at educating adolescents about the risk of HIV infection; assisting them to understand that they are at risk; increasing their sense of self-efficacy; practicing changes in risk-taking behaviors; and decreasing other stresses in their lives—decreases the likelihood of engaging in behaviors that risk HIV transmission (Rotheram-Borus, Mahler, & Rosario, 1995). For example, among inner city African American girls interventions that increased self-efficacy, offer peer support, and encourage the perception that their efforts would lead to positive outcome actually increased their willingness to use condoms during sexual activity (Jemmott, Jemmott, Spears, Hewitt, & Cruz-Collins, 1992). Male bisexual and gay adolescents increased safe sex practices in response to interventions that are educational, that provide models of responding to sexual situations, and that reduce emotional distress (Rotheram-Borus et al., 1994; Rotheram-Borus, Rosario, Reid, & Koopman, 1995). Cumulatively, research suggests that clinical interventions can enhance adolescents' ability to reduce sexual risk behaviors, making more coercive responses less necessary. However, it also suggests that interventions must be tailored to the needs of individual clients.

Professional Responsibility

It has been argued that psychologists carry a heavy burden of responsibility in AIDS prevention because prevention involves psychological intervention (Melton 1988b). However, empirical examination has revealed that mental health professionals, including psychologists, hold prejudicial attitudes toward persons with AIDS (Crawford, Humfleet, Ribordy, Ho, & Vickers, 1991). Mental health professionals reported that they were uncomfortable with being in close proximity with persons with AIDS and taking an individual with AIDS as a client and that they had negative attitudes toward treating gay men and were more likely to refer a gay client than to treat him. Such negative attitudes are liable to interfere with effective intervention. Moreover, evidence suggests that psychologists lack a fundamental knowledge of the treatment of gay male and lesbian clients and that psychologists may be insufficiently trained in HIV-related issues (Graham, Rawlings, Halpern, & Hermes, 1984; Werth & Carney, 1994). On the other hand, health workers with prior education are more comfortable treating and maintaining close proximity with individuals with AIDS, suggesting that bias may be a product of ignorance or general feelings of incompetence with regards to persons with AIDS or gay men and lesbians (Crawford et al., 1991).

Some suggest that insufficient knowledge does not relinquish an ethical responsibility to work with the HIV-infected community. Instead, it becomes the responsibility of the professional to become competent in the provision of services (Melton, 1988b). Psychologists need to remain current in their knowledge of research on how to assist individuals from various populations to reduce behaviors that increase their risk of contracting HIV (NIH, 1997). Furthermore, knowledge of associated mental health issues such as hopelessness and understanding the interpersonal and economic factors affecting those with HIV will allow psychologists to assist those with HIV in more effectively negotiating the many areas of their lives that are affected by the disease, potentially enhancing the quality and length of life.

In fact, psychologists are being approached with a variety of issues regarding HIV clients, including determining whether a client will adhere to the complex combination of drug therapies used in the treatment of HIV (J. A. Anderson, personal communication, September 11, 1997; see Part 2, chapter 14). Because no research suggests guidelines to identify who may or may not adhere to such regimens, this gate-keeping function appears to be a dubious role. A more appropriate role may be to assist patients to comply with this complex course of treatment because noncompliance places them at risk for cross-resistance to other drugs, rendering current and future treatments ineffective (Rabkin & Chesney, 1999). Therefore, it is critical that efforts be directed toward assisting clients in scheduling and planning the implementation of drug therapy. Assisting clients to access and use social and support services may also enhance their adherence (Rabkin & Chesney, 1999).

On the other hand, requiring psychologists to provide services to this population would not necessarily benefit society or those with HIV. Forcing psychologists who are insufficiently trained or biased against populations with AIDS to provide treatment would more than likely undermine the objective of providing adequate services (Melton, 1988b).

Management of Psychiatric Patients With HIV

Individuals with HIV and AIDS may be hospitalized in a psychiatric unit for a variety of reasons, including conditions that limit competence as well as result in behaviors that endanger staff or other patients. Rates of HIV among people who are chronically mentally ill are higher than the general population. Studies have revealed that rates of HIV among patients admitted to psychiatric hospitals in urban areas range from 4% to 23% depending on the location of the study and characteristics of the sample

(Carey, Weinhardt, & Carey, 1995; Cournos, McMinnon, Meyer-Bahlburg, Guido, & Meyer, 1993; Sacks, Dermatis, Looser-Ott, & Perry, 1992). Sexual conduct, although discouraged on psychiatric units, is common among psychiatric patients. However, staff report that they feel ineffective in preventing this conduct and are concerned about their capacity to effectively monitor such behavior (Civic, Walsh, & McBride, 1993; Zonana et al., 1988). Furthermore, psychiatric populations in general appear to be more vulnerable to HIV transmission because they tend to have poor judgment and problem-solving skills, are prone to instability in social and sexual relationships, frequently share living quarters with others who have diminished levels of functioning, and may be more prone to impulsive or indiscriminant sexual activity and more vulnerable to exploitative or transient sexual relationships (Kelly et al., 1992; Sweeman, Lang & Rector, 1990).

Several recommendations have been made for coping with some of the difficulties that may arise when patients with HIV are on a psychiatric ward. Skills-building interventions, such as learning how to use condoms or requesting that a partner use a condom, and education about HIV transmission and safe sex activities should become integral parts of any inpatient program (B. F. Hoffman et al., 1989; Sweeman et al., 1990; Zonana et al., 1988). In fact, research on HIV risk among people who are severely mentally ill reveals that current unsafe heterosexual activity with multiple partners is the most prevalent risk behavior among this population, with past IV drug use or homosexual activity as secondary risk factors (Cournos, McMinnon, Meyer-Bahlburg, Guido, & Meyer, 1993; Kelly et al., 1992). Psychiatric patients reveal a deficient knowledge of the behavioral risks for AIDS transmission; nearly half believe that heterosexual women cannot get AIDS (Kelly et al., 1992). Second, the use of close observation, clinical interventions, or isolation may be used to prevent sexual activity, if the restrictive measures are contingent on specific behaviors that pose a risk to staff or other patients and less restrictive measures are unsuccessful (Appelbaum, 1988; Zonana et al., 1988). Breaching confidentiality to protect those who are at risk may also be warranted (Appelbaum, 1988). However, before doing so psychologists also need to consider ethical standards, particularly Standard 5.05 of the Ethics Code (APA, 1992).

The ethical issues surrounding confidentiality on the inpatient unit are compounded by the dual responsibility to both those who are HIV-positive and other patients who are unaware of the HIV diagnosis. Resolution of this dilemma is likely to depend on a careful case-by-case assessment of patients' capacity to exercise good judgment, the receptivity of HIV-positive patients to educational interventions, and the patients' willingness and ability to participate in a therapeutic contract with regards to discontinuing endangering behavior. Alternatively, the staff may offer to assist the patients in disclosing their HIV status to their partners and offer support to the couple in coping with this issue. Ultimately, the staff must carefully evaluate the level of paternalism that is required. Intrusion into the private relational domain of two individuals must be based on careful assessment of both patients' capacity to exercise independent decisions and actions. Furthermore, it is important to note that a psychiatric patient, who is confused and disoriented on admission, may be quite capable of independent and clear decision making upon discharge and thus be capable of engaging in safer sex practices.

Refusal of Treatment for HIV

Mental health professionals treating people who are seriously mentally ill may also have to deal with patients whose refusal to receive treatment for HIV is related to thought processes impaired by delusions or disorganization or limited insight into their illness. Noncompliance with psychiatric medications can place the patient at serious risk of harm or death. For example, unpleasant medication side effects, socioeconomic factors, and problems in the patient–doctor relationship may all interfere with psychotropic medication compliance (Torrey, 1995). These factors may also influence compliance with treatment for HIV and must be addressed accordingly. Therefore, refusal to participate in HIV treatment might be approached with methods that are similar to those typically used to address psychiatric medication noncompliance.

Although it is ethically questionable whether patients should be left to suffer progression in HIV illness and AIDS, because compromised mental capacity interferes with treatment compliance, imposing coercive methods to persuade them to receive medical treatment is also questionable. The first step should involve addressing underlying psychiatric illness in order to facilitate treatment compliance, followed by a careful consideration of noncoercive alternatives that may encourage participation in HIV treatment, including education, therapeutic intervention, encouragement, and psychosocial support. If these approaches fail, more coercive methods may be justified in order to preserve the health of the patient. However, these issues have not been considered carefully in the literature, and a professional discussion should thoroughly evaluate their ethical implications.

Perinatal Transmission

The primary mode of HIV transmission to children is perinatal transmission; more than 80% of pediatric AIDS and HIV patients were infected as a result of perinatal exposure (Centers for Disease Control and Prevention [CDC], 1995). Among the majority of children with AIDS and HIV, the mothers were at risk for HIV infection either as a result of injecting drug use or heterosexual contact with bisexual men or injecting drug users (CDC, 1995). Given these statistics, psychologists who come in contact with women who are HIV-positive and plan to conceive a child, take inadequate precautions to prevent pregnancy, are HIV-positive and pregnant, or engage in activities during pregnancy that place them at risk for HIV infection are faced with ethical dilemmas in balancing their respect of an individual woman's right to reproductive freedom and the protection of the interest of the fetus.

The primary source of ethical debate is how a mental health professional should approach the counseling relationship (Arras, 1990; Bayer, 1990; Ybarra, 1991). Questions arise as to whether the therapist should take a neutral stance with regard to the decision to conceive a child or abort a pregnancy, providing the client with support in reaching an independent and personal decision. Although psychologists generally advocate respect for client autonomy, particularly in such private matters as reproduction, some view pregnancy among women who are HIV-positive as an exception to this stance because of the potentially life-threatening consequences of HIV to the child. Therefore, some believe that therapists should discourage an HIV-positive woman from having a child (Arras, 1990). This latter approach may involve a degree of coercion from the therapist. Less coercive intervention may require the therapist to educate the client as to the realities of HIV infection to children, providing the client with facts about HIV transmission and carefully challenging the client to consider her decision regarding pregnancy. More coercive methods involve deliberately and forcefully recommending that the client avoid pregnancy or have an abortion (Arras, 1990).

Several medical and contextual issues are relevant. First, medical uncertainty exists about the rate or likelihood of transmission of HIV to a fetus during the course of pregnancy. A child born to an HIV-positive woman who receives no medical treatment for her HIV maintains approximately a 30–50% chance of being HIV-positive (James, 1988). Of these children, 25% are likely to be acutely ill from early infancy and die of AIDS during early childhood. Without treatment, the other 75% percent will remain HIV-positive throughout their childhood and face a shortened life of diminished but not necessarily poor quality (Arras, 1990). However, pharmacotherapies decrease the transmission and lethality of HIV with children, reducing the likelihood and risk associated with HIV transmission. With increased use of ziduvine (AZT or ZDV) during and pregnancy and administered to the child after birth, rates of perinatal transmission have dropped as low as 6.2%–11% (CDC, 1997)

Moreover, there are several routes for transmission of HIV from mother to infant. Transmission may occur in utero, during delivery, or through breast-feeding. The risk may be effected by the stage of the mother's HIV disease and certain obstetric interventions (CDC, 1997). Therefore, appropriate medical attention and education may reduce some of the risk of mother–child viral transfer. Consulting with knowledgeable physicians or becoming more educated about transmission routes may help therapists understand the complexity of the ethical issues.

Several broader issues are also relevant to this discussion. Reproductive interference in the case of HIV may be disproportionately directed at individuals who are ethnically and economically disadvantaged. Because poor women from ethnic minority groups are overrepresented in HIV cases, one may legitimately question whether dissuading reproduction among HIV-positive women would disproportionately discourage reproduction among members of these groups. Because of their lack of power these women are more likely to be vulnerable to undue influence by the therapist (Bayer, 1990).

CONCLUSIONS

Although psychologists have had to face ethical issues surrounding death and dying prior to the AIDS epidemic, dealing with the ethical dilemmas surrounding the treatment of clients who have the HIV infection may force psychology to profoundly reexamine many of its fundamental ethical assumptions. Cases involving clients who engage in unsafe sexual activity with uninformed partners, adolescents who participate in high-risk behaviors, and women with HIV who gamble that pregnancy does not lead to infected fetuses all force psychologists to face their dual obligations to uphold the trust involved in the therapeutic contract and break that trust for the welfare of society at large or for the long-term benefit of the individual involved. Furthermore, the issue of rational suicide, which was seldom discussed in the psychological literature prior to the 1990s (Snipe, 1988), has seen a burst of interest in the last few years. Because the majority of individuals who acquire AIDS are in the age group that frequently seeks psychological services, the issue of rational suicide may become more than an abstract philosophical issue for many psychologists; yet our training and our literature seldom broach the issue. Similarly, there is a need to examine the ethical issues in working with minority populations, who are disproportionately represented among the HIV population (CDC, 1997). An enlarged professional understanding of the different cultures in which clients live becomes more than an academic activity when trying to decide between alternative ethical choices that may harm clients or benefit society. Although ethical issues related to multiple roles and boundary issues are certainly relevant to HIV-related practice, thus far the literature has not examined these issues (see chapters 3 and 15).

Despite the critical nature of many of these ethical issues, there is little discussion in the literature about them. When discussion occurs, there is little consensus about how they should be resolved. On the other hand, there does seem to be a rising consensus about a few issues that need to be considered. For example, authors have recognized that the ability of individuals to make competent decisions free from controlling influences is relevant in several situations including those involving adolescents engaged in risky behaviors and clients contemplating suicide (Mayo, 1993; Sobocinski, 1989; Werth, 1995). Second, breaking confidentiality requires compelling evidence that there is a high risk to a third party and that alternative interventions have been tried and are unsuccessful or that the psychologist has good reason to believe that they would be unsuccessful (Kain, 1988; Knapp & VandeCreek, 1990; Reamer, 1991). These arguments may be generalized to other situations such as those involving attempts to get pregnant when infected with the HIV virus.

Researchers have yet to consider, however, how a psychologist might define confidentiality at the outset of a clinical relationship with an HIV-positive client and how long psychologists should use clinical interventions before using more coercive interventions. The bottom line is that at times ethical responsibilities must be balanced with each other and psychologists may have to break one ethical duty in order to comply with a higher one. If they are to do so, however, all reasonable alternatives should be considered and exhausted and the solution should be one designed to do the least amount of harm avoidable.

Finally, it is important to appreciate how rapidly the underlying ethical issues regarding HIV will continue to change with advances in the treatment of HIV. Given the rapid biomedical advances in HIV, it is essential that psychologists treating clients with HIV remain current with the literature in this area in order to practice competently.

REFERENCES

American Psychological Association. (1991). *Legal liability related to confidentiality and the prevention of HIV transmission.* Washington, DC: Author.

American Psychological Association. (1992). Ethical principles of psychologists and code of conduct. *American Psychologist, 47,* 1597–1611.

Appelbaum, K., & Appelbaum, P. S. (1990). The HIV antibody patient. In J. C. Beck (Ed.), *Confidentiality versus the duty to protect: Foreseeable harm in the practice of psychiatry* (pp. 121–140). Washington, DC: American Psychiatric Press.

Appelbaum, P. S. (1988). AIDS, psychiatry, and the law. *Hospital and Community Psychiatry, 39,* 13–14.

Arras, J. D. (1990). AIDS and reproductive decisions: Having children in fear and trembling. *The Milbank Quarterly, 68,* 353–380.

Bayer, R. (1990). AIDS and the future of reproductive freedom. *The Milbank Quarterly, 68,* 179–202.

Boyd, K. (1989). Ethical questions. In J. Green & A. McCreaner (Eds.), *Counseling in HIV infection and AIDS* (pp. 301–313). Oxford, England: Blackwell Scientific Publications.

Carey, M. P., Weinhardt, L. S., & Carey, K. B. (1995). Prevalence of infections with HIV among the seriously mentally ill: Review of research and implications for practice. *Professional Psychology: Research and Practice, 26,* 262–268.

Centers for Disease Control and Prevention. (1995). *HIV/AIDS surveillance report mid-year edition* (Vol. 7, No. 1). Atlanta, GA: Author.

Centers for Disease Control and Prevention. (1997). *Perinatal HIV prevention update: Evidence of progress and challenges for the future.* Atlanta, GA: Author.

Civic, D., Walsh, G., & McBride, D. (1993). Staff perspective on sexual behavior of patients in a state psychiatric hospital. *Hospital and Community Psychiatry, 44,* 887–889.

Cohen, E. D. (1990). Confidentiality, counseling and clients who have AIDS: Ethical foundations of a model rule. *Journal of Counseling & Development, 68,* 282–286.

Cote, T. R., Bigger, R. J., & Dannenberg, A. L. (1992). Risk of suicide among persons with AIDS: A national assessment. *JAMA, 268,* 2066–2068.

Cournos, F., McMinnon, K., Meyer-Bahlburg, H., Guido, J. R., & Meyer, I. (1993). HIV risk activity among persons with severe mental illness: Preliminary findings. *Hospital and Community Psychiatry, 44,* 1104–1106.

Crawford, I., Humfleet, G., Ribordy, S. C., Ho, F. C., & Vickers, V. L. (1991). Stigmatization of AIDS patients by mental health professionals. *Professional Psychology: Research and Practice, 22,* 357–361.

Erickson, S. H. (1993). Ethics and confidentiality in AIDS counseling: A professional dilemma. *Journal of Mental Health Counseling, 15*(2), 118–131.

Faberman, R. K. (1997). Terminal illness and hastened death requests: The important role of the mental health professional. *Professional Psychology: Research and Practice, 28,* 544–547.

Fulero, S. (1988). *Tarasoff:* 10 years later. *Professional Psychology: Research and Practice, 19,* 184–190.

Graham, D. L. R., Rawlings, E. I., Halpern, H. S., & Hermes, J. (1984). Therapists' needs for training in counseling lesbian and gay men. *Professional Psychology: Research and Practice, 15,* 482–496.

Gray, L. A., & Harding, A. K. (1988). Confidentiality limits with clients who have the AIDS virus. *Journal of Counseling & Development, 66,* 219–223.

Hoffman, B. F., Arthurs, K., Lunn, S., Meyers, L., Trimnell, A., & Farcnik, K. (1989). AIDS: Clinical and ethical issues on a psychiatric unit. *Canadian Journal of Psychiatry, 34,* 847–851.

Hoffman, M. A. (1991). Counseling the HIV-infected client: A psychosocial model for assessment and intervention. *The Counseling Psychologist, 19,* 467–542.

James, M. E. (1988). HIV seropositivity diagnosed during pregnancy: Psychosocial characterization of patients and their adaptation. *General Hospital Psychiatry, 10,* 309–316.

Jemmott, J. B., Jemmott, L. S., Spears, H., Hewitt, N., & Cruz-Collins, M. (1992). Self-efficacy, hedonistic expectancies, and condom-use intentions among inner-city black adolescent women: A social cognitive approach to AIDS risk behavior. *Journal of Adolescent Health, 13,* 512–518.

Kain, C. D. (1988). To breach or not to breach: Is that the question? A response to Gray and Harding. *Journal of Counseling and Development, 66,* 224–225.

Kalichman, S. C., & Sikkema, K. J. (1994). Psychological sequella of HIV infection and AIDS: Review of empirical findings. *Clinical Psychology Review, 14,* 611–632.

Kelly, J., Murphy, D. A., Bahr, G. R., Brasfield, T. L., Davis, D. R., Hauth, A. C., Morgan, M. G., Stevenson, L. Y., & Eilers, M. K. (1992). AIDS/HIV risk behavior among the chronic mentally ill. *American Journal of Psychiatry, 149,* 886–890.

Knapp, S., & VandeCreek, L. (1990). Application of the duty to protect to HIV-positive patients. *Professional Psychology: Research and Practice, 21,* 161–166.

Lamb, D. H., Clark, C., Drumheller, P., Frizzell, K., & Surrey, L. (1989). Applying *Tarasoff* to AIDS related psychotherapy issues. *Professional Psychology: Research and Practice, 20,* 37–43.

Martin, D. J. (in press). Ethics in the treatment of human immunodeficiency virus infection and acquired immunodeficiency syndrome. In S. F. Bucky (Ed.), *The comprehensive textbook of ethics and law in the practice of psychology.* New York: Plenum Press.

Marzuk, P. M., Tierney, H., Tardiff, K., Gross, E. M., Morgan, E. B., Hsu, M., & Mann, J. J. (1988). Increased risk of suicide in persons with AIDS. *JAMA, 259,* 1333–1337.

Mayo, D. (1993, August). *The case for rational suicide.* Presented at the 101st Annual Convention of the American Psychological Association, Toronto, Canada.

McGuire, J., Nieri, D., Abbot, D., Sheridan, K., & Fisher, R. (1995). Do *Tarasoff* principles apply in AIDS-related psychotherapy? Ethical decision making and the role of therapist homophobia and perceived client dangerousness. *Professional Psychology: Research and Practice, 26,* 608–611.

McIntosh, J. L. (1993, August). *Arguments against rational and assisted suicide.* Presented at the 101st Annual Convention of the American Psychological Association, Toronto, Canada.

Melton, G. B. (1988a). Adolescents and prevention of AIDS. *Professional Psychology: Research and Practice, 19,* 403–408.

Melton, G. B. (1988b). Ethical and legal issues in AIDS–related practice. *American Psychologist, 43,* 941–947.

National Institutes of Health. (1997) *Consensus development statement: Interventions to prevent HIV risk behaviors*. Bethesda, MD: Author.

Olson, R. A., Mason, P. J., Huszti, H. C., & Seibert, J. M. (1989). Pediatric AIDS/HIV infection: An emerging challenge to pediatric psychology. *Journal of Pediatric Psychology, 4*(1), 1–21.

Pope, K. S., & Vetter, V. A. (1992). Ethical dilemmas encountered by members of the American Psychological Association: A national survey. *American Psychologist, 47*, 397–411.

Powell, C. J. (1984). Ethical principles and issues of competence in counseling adolescents. *The Counseling Psychologist, 12*(3), 171–177.

Rabkin, J. G., & Chesney, M. (1999). Treatment adherence to HIV medications: The Achilles heel of the new therapeutics. In D. G. Ostrow & S. C. Kalichman (Eds.), *Psychosocial and public health aspects of new HIV therapies* (pp. 68–82). New York: Kluwer Academic/Plenum Press.

Rabkin, J. G., Remien, R., Katoff, L., & Williams, J. B. W. (1993). Suicidality in AIDS long-term survivors: What is the evidence? *AIDS Care, 5*, 401–410.

Reamer, F. G. (1991). AIDS, social work and the "duty to protect." *Social Work, 39*, 56–60.

Rogers, J. R., & Britton, P. J. (1994). Aids and rational suicide: A counseling psychology perspective or a slide on a slippery slope. *The Counseling Psychologist, 22*(1), 171–178.

Rotheram-Borus, M. J., Mahler, K. A., & Rosario, M. (1995). AIDS prevention with adolescents. *AIDS Education and Prevention, 4*, 320–336.

Rotheram-Borus, M. J., Reid, H., & Rosario, M. (1994). Factors mediating changes in sexual HIV risk behaviors among gay and bisexual male adolescents. *American Journal of Public Health, 84*, 1938–1946.

Rotheram-Borus, M. J., Rosario, M., Reid, H., & Koopman, C. (1995). Predicting patterns of sexual acts among homosexual and bisexual youths. *American Journal of Psychiatry, 152*, 588–595.

Royse, D., & Birge, B. (1987). Homophobia and attitudes towards AIDS patients among medical, nursing, and paramedical students. *Psychological Reports, 61*, 867–870.

Sacks, M., Dermatis, H., Looser-Ott, S., & Perry, S. (1992). Seroprevalence of HIV and risk factors for AIDS in psychiatric inpatients. *Hospital and Community Psychiatry, 43*, 736–737.

Siegal, K. (1986). Psychosocial aspects of rational suicide. *American Journal of Psychotherapy, 40*, 405–418.

Snipe, R. M. (1988). Ethical issues in the assessment and treatment of a rational suicide client. *The Counseling Psychologist, 16*(1), 128–138.

Sobocinski, M. (1989). Ethical principles in the counseling of gay and lesbian adolescents: Issues of autonomy, competence, and confidentiality. *Professional Psychology: Research and Practice, 21*, 240–247.

Sweeman, M. V., Lang, M., & Rector, N. (1990). Chronic schizophrenia: A risk factor for HIV? *Canadian Journal of Psychiatry, 35,* 765–767.

Tarasoff v. Board of Regents of the University of California, 17 Cal.3d 425, 551 P.2d 334 (1976).

Torrey, E. F. (1995). *Surviving schizophrenia: A manual for families, consumers and providers.* New York: Harper Perennial.

Totten, G., Lamb, D. H., & Reeder, G. D. (1990). *Tarasoff* and confidentiality in AIDS-related psychotherapy. *Professional Psychology: Research and Practice, 21,* 155–160.

Werth, J. L., Jr. (1992). Rational suicide and AIDS: Considerations for the psychotherapist. *The Counseling Psychologist, 20*(4), 645–659.

Werth, J. L., Jr. (1995). Rational suicide reconsidered: AIDS as an impetus for change. *Death Studies, 19*(1), 65–80.

Werth, J. L., Jr., & Carney, J. (1994). Incorporating HIV-related issues into graduate student training. *Professional Psychology: Research and Practice, 25,* 458–465.

Werth, J. L., Jr., & Liddle, B. J. (1994). Psychotherapists' attitudes towards suicide. *Psychotherapy: Theory, Research and Practice, 31,* 440–448.

Ybarra, S. (1991). Women and AIDS: Implications for counseling. *Journal of Counseling and Development, 69,* 285–287.

Young, M., Henderson, M. M., & Marx, D. (1990). Attitudes of nursing students towards patients with AIDS. *Psychological Reports, 67,* 491–497.

Zonana, H., Norko, M., & Stier, D. (1988). The AIDS patient on the psychiatric unit: Ethical and legal issues. *Psychiatric Annals, 18*(10), 587–592.

APPENDIX
Legal Liability Related to Confidentiality and the Prevention of HIV Transmission

WHEREAS the status of privileged communication between psychologist and client is legally protected; WHEREAS information regarding an individual's HIV status may be particularly sensitive given the personal nature of such information and the potential for discrimination involved; WHEREAS providers of psychological services are also concerned about the prevention of HIV transmission and promotion of the public health; WHEREAS respect for personal dignity, protection of clients/patients from harm, and promotion of access to mental health services demand protection of confidentiality in all but the most extraordinary circumstances;

WHEREAS psychological services to HIV-infected individuals make an important contribution to the reduction of risk behaviors that spread such infection; WHEREAS legislatures considering exceptions to privileged communications in cases involving HIV infection may benefit from the APA position on the issue;

THEREFORE, BE IT RESOLVED that APA's position on legislation regarding confidentiality and the prevention of HIV transmission is as follows:

1. A legal duty to protect third parties from HIV infection should not be imposed.
2. If, however, specific legislation is considered, then it should permit disclosure only when (a) the provider knows an identifiable third party who the provider has compelling reason to believe is at significant risk for infection; (b) the provider has a reasonable belief that the third party has no reason to suspect that he or she is at risk; and (c) the client/patient has been urged to inform the party and has either refused or is considered unreliable in his/her willingness to notify the third party.
3. If such legislation is adopted, it should include immunity from civil and criminal liability for providers who, in good faith, make decisions to disclose or not to disclose information about HIV infection to third parties.

Note: From Fox, R. E. (1992). Proceedings of the American Psychological Association, Incorporated, for the year 1991; Minutes of the annual meeting of the Council of Representatives August 14 and 17, 1991 San Francisco, and February 24–March 1, 1992, Washington, DC. *American Psychologist, 47,* 893–954.

3

THINKING WELL ABOUT DOING GOOD IN HIV-RELATED PRACTICE: A MODEL OF ETHICAL ANALYSIS

KAREN STROHM KITCHENER AND BOB BARRET

People who work in an HIV-related practice typically have an unusually strong commitment to doing good, and doing good is what being ethical is all about. Unfortunately, it is sometimes difficult to do good, because the most ethical course of action is not always clear, particularly for psychologists in an HIV-related practice. Rarely does the mental health professional find a more complex set of ethical issues, especially in relation to multiple-role relationships and confidentiality. Because of the complex ethical dilemmas involved in HIV-related practice, mental health professionals must become adept at thinking well about the ethical issues that they face.

When faced with tough ethical choices, people sometimes hold out the hope that someone has the "right" answer. Mental health professionals may call state boards, their national associations, HIV/AIDS service organizations, or other resources with the expectation that they can provide a clear solution. Similarly, they may look to legal cases such as *Tarasoff v. Board of Regents of the University of California* (1976), which focused on the therapist's responsibility to break confidentiality when an unknown third party is threatened by a patient, because they assume that the law may provide clear direction. However, court case decisions are sometimes contradictory, and precedents relevant to a particular situation are lacking (Burris, chapter 6, this volume; Stevenson & Kitchener, chapter 2, this volume). Even the direction provided by state boards or ethics committees may seem vague or ambiguous, especially when practitioners want comprehensive guidance out of fear that what they are doing may not be right. In fact, in the Ethical Principles for Psychologists and Code of Conduct (Ethics Code; APA, 1992a; see appendix) and in the commentary written on it (Canter, Bennett, Jones, & Nagy, 1994), no mention is made of most of the special issues that surround treatment of people with the HIV infection. Although the Ethics Code provides much guidance about HIV-related issues such as when and under what conditions confidentiality may be broken, codes cannot address all specific situations.

Take, for example, psychologists who work with clients whose health deteriorates to the point that death is imminent. Home and hospital visits are common in these situations, and sometimes psychologists face requests to assist with care or help arrange a funeral. Here, psychologists are confronted with a series of ethical questions: Do the ethical standards on multiple-role relationships (APA, 1992a) prohibit such interventions, or is assisting with care in this situation responsive to the aspirational principles of Social Responsibility and Concern for Others' Welfare from the APA Ethics Code? What is in the best welfare of the client? The Ethics Code tacitly suggests that multiple-role relationships are potentially harmful, but how should this possibility be balanced with the potential to provide solace and comfort to someone at the end of life? Similarly, when a psychologist is working with an HIV-positive client who reports having unsafe sex with an identifiable partner, what is the psychologist's ethical responsibility? Should he or she terminate treatment or break confidentiality and inform the partner? What is the therapist's responsibility when a client thoughtfully plans to terminate life as health deteriorates? Each of these situations presents an ethical dilemma that requires an astute analysis of the ethical issues involved.

When faced with ethical problems, mental health providers are usually taught to consult their profession's ethical standards. Typically, professional ethics codes fulfill the function of both defining how professionals ought to behave toward others and identifying when they should be criticized or punished for their behavior. For example, the American Psychological Association's Ethics Code (see appendix) indicates that psychologists should not have sexual relationships with clients. Consequently, the APA Ethics Committee (APA, 1992b) is responsible for punishing psychologists when they break this standard by reprimanding them, censuring them, or recommending they be expelled from the association. However, the ethics codes cannot address every specific set of facts. As a consequence, the decisions that face psychologists who work with HIV-infected patients or their relatives are not easily resolved by consulting the Ethics Code, and for many of the ethical issues that arise, no choice seems completely satisfactory. In other words, the ethical issues involve an ethical dilemma.

We continue to struggle with such situations, even though one of us (Karen Strohm Kitchener) served as chairperson of the APA Ethics Committee and was involved in drafting an early version of the 1992 Ethics Code, and the other (Robert Barret) taught workshops on ethical decision making and has been involved in HIV-related practice for several years. Sometimes it is hard to understand how the Ethics Code applies in a particular case. In other cases, where the Ethics Code recommends operating in the "best" interests of the client, it is very difficult to determine what action would best serve the client's welfare. Furthermore, because the Ethics Code also requires that psychologists operate out of a concern for the welfare of their clients as well as with an awareness of their responsibility to society, it may be difficult to decide whether the responsibility to society or to the client ought to take precedence. In other words, deciding what it means to "do good" is not an easy task. Consequently, professionals must have a decision-making system available to them.

Mental health providers can find guidance in both their profession's code of ethics and in foundational ethical assumptions, and that guidance is the focus of this chapter. Both provide a consistent framework that has helped us think well about the ethical decisions we are making. In the following pages we use the APA Ethics Code and foundational ethical principles to analyze the tough ethical decisions surrounding the HIV epidemic in hopes that mental health providers from a variety of professions will find it useful as well. The same framework is used to analyze the ethical issues surrounding specific cases drawn from HIV-related practice in part 2 of this book.

The model for ethical decision making presented here can be considered in two different stages (Kitchener, 1984, 2000). In the first stage, mental health providers ought to consult their professional code of ethics. However, when a code of ethics is silent, is difficult to interpret, or offers ambiguous advice, psychologists can seek guidance from five foundational ethical principles. It is sometimes necessary to balance even these foundational assumptions, and we suggest a way to do so. Although the 1992 APA Code of Ethics is used in the following analysis, it is important to note that other professional codes of ethics can be substituted for use with mental health providers who are not psychologists.

PROFESSIONAL ETHICAL CODES

The first stage in ethical decision making involves consulting the ethical rules of the profession, in this case the Ethics Code (APA, 1992a). In fact, psychologists who become members of the APA agree to operate in a way that is consistent with the code. Despite the occasional case on which the code is silent or suggests contradictory courses of action, it offers very explicit advice on many more. Consequently, the Ethics Code often provides solid guidance that can help psychologists define an ethical course of action with clients.

The Ethics Code contains two parts, an aspirational section and a sanctionable section. The aspirational section contains two parts, the preamble and the general principles. There are six general principles: Competence, Integrity, Professional and Social Responsibility, Respect for People's Rights and Dignity, Concern for Others' Welfare, and Social Responsibility. Although these principles are not enforceable by the Ethics Committee, they can be used to interpret the specific standards that follow. For example, Principle B: Integrity suggests that psychologists' professional relationships should be respectful of others as well as honest and fair. This obviously applies to their relationships with HIV-positive clients as well.

The sanctionable section of the code includes standards that describe the specific rules that should guide the conduct of psychologists. The standards are organized into eight sections: General Standards; Evaluation, Assessment, or Intervention; Advertising and Other Public Statements; Therapy; Privacy and Confidentiality; Teaching, Training, Supervision, Research, and Publishing; Forensic Activities; and Resolving Ethical Issues. The standards are sanctionable, that is, they are enforceable by the association. When a complaint is filed against a member, the APA Ethics Committee has the responsibility of evaluating whether the psychologist has violated the standards (APA, 1992b). The standards are sometimes also used by state ethics committees, state grievance or licensing boards, and the courts to help establish standards of practice or care against which psychologists' behavior can be judged.

For example, Standard 1.17, Multiple Relationships, acknowledges that avoiding all extratherapy contacts with clients may not be feasible, but when participating in extratherapy contacts psychologists must always consider whether the new relationship is likely to harm the client or others. Furthermore, it stipulates that psychologists should not enter such relationships if it is likely that the relationships might cloud their objectivity, exploit the other person, or in some other way interfere with their effectiveness. In other words, it requires that psychologists estimate the likelihood of one of these potential events occurring. For example, a dying current client might ask his therapist for help in making his funeral arrangements. In this case, the therapist would need to ask whether compliance with the request might lead to one or more of the following: clouded objectivity, exploitation of the client, harm to the client or others, or some other unintended consequence. If such things were likely to occur, the new relationship would be prohibited by the code. This standard should lead psychologists who are faced with such decisions to ask the following questions: Could an agreement to aid in funeral preparations cause boundary problems for other patients with whom I am working? How will I handle the confidentiality of the client? Will I be identified as the deceased client's therapist, and what are the implications of that? If the APA Ethics Committee were reviewing a complaint regarding such a situation, it is helpful for the psychologist to be able to describe the process by which he or she considered answering these kinds of questions. Even if the committee finds a violation, the thoughtful approach may be a mitigating factor considered in adjudication.

When faced with an ethical problem, psychologists should first consult the Ethics Code (APA, 1992a) to identify whether there is an explicit standard that addresses the issue or whether any advice can be gleaned from the general principles about what course of action may be best. In order to do so, psychologists need to become familiar with the Ethics Code. Many psychologists currently practicing were trained prior to the publication of the most recent code and may not be familiar with some of the changes in it. For example, the 1992 Ethics Code is more explicit about requiring psychologists to discuss possible limitations on confidentiality with clients or others at the outset of a relationship. Familiarity with the standards may help psychologists avoid problems before they occur.

Next, one should consult the literature. Articles regarding the implications of the APA Ethics Code for HIV-related practice are beginning to appear in the literature. Martin (in press), for example, has suggested ways in which the Ethics Code gives explicit advice regarding the treatment of those with HIV.

FOUNDATIONAL ETHICAL PRINCIPLES

Although ethics codes should be the first documents to consult when making an ethical decision, there are times when codes are silent or give ambiguous advice. Consider the AIDS patient who is in late stages of the disease, is contemplating suicide, and appears to be fully rational as he articulates the reasons for wanting to end his life. Here, several standards from the APA Ethics Code could be relevant, including the one requiring psychologists to be competent (Standard 1.04). This standard would suggest that, at a minimum, psychologists working with such patients should be competent to assess for suicidal ideology, knowledgeable about the literature on the circumstances surrounding suicidal ideology in AIDS patients, and familiar with the legal issues involved. Furthermore, Standard 5.02 indicates that psychologists have a "primary" responsibility to maintain confidentiality, suggesting the importance of maintaining the client's confidence regarding the decision. On the other hand, Standard 5.05 indicates that psychologists may disclose confidential information when "mandated" or "permitted" by law for a valid purpose. One of those purposes is protecting a patient or client from harm. At the same time, the standard does not require psychologists to break confidentiality in all cases when patients or clients pose a danger to themselves. In other words, the Ethics Code does not tell the psychologist whether to break confidentiality or not in cases like the one described above. Consequently, it is important for professionals to have the tools to think further about the issues involved. (See part 2, chapter 16 for an elaboration of the issues involved with suicidal ideation in terminal AIDS patients.)

Mental health professionals sometimes must move to a second stage in order to think clearly about their ethical decisions. Here, five foundational ethical principles can help clarify the ethical issues involved and guide decision making. These principles are respect for autonomy, beneficence (do good), do no harm (nonmaleficence), fidelity (be faithful or trustworthy), and justice. They are central to ethical discussions in psychology (Bersoff & Koeppl, 1993; Kitchener, 1984, 2000) as well as other professions (Beauchamp & Childress, 1994), and they can provide a common vocabulary to use when discussing ethical issues with other health or mental health professionals who are not bound to follow the APA Ethics Code. By describing the principles and clarifying their usefulness, we hope that mental health providers find them meaningful when conceptualizing the ethical dilemmas they face when dealing with HIV-related issues. Although the five principles will not be relevant in every case, the relevance of each should be considered before making an ethical decision.

Respect for Autonomy

Respect for autonomy refers to respecting the unconditional worth of each individual, especially his or her right to make life decisions if competent to do so. This concept is both fundamental to any ethical system and the foundation of a therapeutic relationship. Most therapists would be hard pressed to imagine any therapeutic relationship in which the client's worth and dignity were not respected. However, the principle of autonomy should remind practitioners that respecting others includes respecting their choices and desires and implies that mental health providers should not impose their opinions or beliefs on clients by force or coercion (Engelhardt, 1986). In the Ethics Code (APA, 1992a), Principle D: Respect for People's Rights and Dignity and ethical standards involving informed consent, confidentiality, and the rights to privacy can be understood as deriving from the rights accorded to autonomous persons.

Beauchamp and Childress (1994) suggested that the core idea of autonomy derives from the concept of self-rule or living according to a plan that the person has chosen for himself or herself. It is generally understood to include two aspects: freedom of action and freedom of thoughts and beliefs.

Neither freedom is absolute; both are limited by the understanding that people are free to do and act as they wish as long as they do not restrict similar freedoms of others.

On the other hand, acting as an autonomous person is dependent on being able to make autonomous choices. Such choices have three character-istics. They must be intentional, they must be based on adequate understand-ing, and they must not result from controlling influences (Beauchamp & Childress, 1994). *Understanding* in this case means having both adequate knowledge as well as the competence to comprehend the information and its implications. For example, to make an autonomous choice to enter therapy, a prospective client must understand clearly what the parameters of the relationship are going to include. For the person with HIV disease, the social stigma surrounding the disease is such that one of those parameters is knowing both the extent of and limits on confidentiality. In other words, one of the fundamental ways for therapists to respect a client's autonomy is to provide the client with real informed consent to treatment. In the spirit of respecting autonomy, this would include providing clients with enough information to make a reasonable decision and ensuring that they understand that information.

Similarly, a therapist can exert a "controlling influence" on a client because of the power differential between them. To the extent that a therapist does so the client's decisions are not autonomous. Obviously, clients may have others in their lives, such as mothers, brothers, aunts, uncles, and partners, who also exert controlling influences on their decisions. The question the therapist must ask is, Do these influences substantially decrease the client's ability to make reasonable decisions? When clients' choices are substantially nonautonomous because others are controlling them or because they lack understanding or intentionality, there may be good ethical reasons (related to other ethical principles, such as beneficence or doing good) not to comply with their choices.

As an example of how this principle may affect practice, consider that mental health providers in HIV-related work sometimes deal with clients who are unable to make rational decisions because of immaturity, depression, the influence of drugs or alcohol, dementia, or other conditions that cloud their thinking. On one hand, it would be equally unethical to restrict clients' decision making when they are capable of autonomous choice and to allow them to make choices that are harmful if, in fact, their understanding of the situation and its consequences is limited or inaccurate. This is especially true in cases where the decisions are life-threatening and irrevocable. More specifically, client competence is one of the difficult issues that mental health providers must consider when deciding whether or not to intervene if a client in the final stages of AIDS is contemplating suicide. Many have argued on the basis of the principle of autonomy that if suicide is rational then clients have the right to take their own lives (Siegel, 1986; Werth, 1992, 1995). If on the other hand, the client is not competent, then mental health providers would have a responsibility to protect them from the harm that would result from their own actions.

This is not to say that clients are either autonomous or nonautonomous. Rather, autonomy is best conceptualized as a continuum, with some clients capable of autonomous choice under some conditions and not others. The most challenging HIV-positive clients are those who are neither fully competent nor totally incompetent to make autonomous choices such as might be the case in the final stages of the disease or with adolescents. Under these circumstances mental health providers should evaluate whether clients' decisions are substantially reasonable given the circumstances of their lives.

In HIV-related psychotherapy the issue of autonomy is also relevant when considering the actions of HIV-positive clients who are having anonymous unprotected intercourse without disclosing their HIV status. Although such clients have the right to make their own decisions, unprotected intercourse with an HIV-negative partner, who does not know he or she is at risk, threatens the autonomy of that partner; thus, some may argue it is ethically justifiable under this circumstance to break confidentiality. By contrast, take an HIV-negative client who reports sharing needles or having unprotected intercourse with known HIV-positive partners. If the client is capable of making rational decisions, is fully informed, and is not being coerced, the principle of autonomy suggests that mental health providers should respect the confidentiality of the relationship and not limit the client's actions even if the mental health providers believe they are mistaken and potentially life-threatening. Under both these circumstances, however, the psychologist must consider not just issues of autonomy, but other ethical responsibilities as well.

Beneficence

Being beneficent means acting in a way that benefits or helps other people. In short, it means to "do good." The principle seems so self-evident that sometimes it hardly seems worth repeating. In addition to doing good, however, it involves preventing harm like intervening when a client who is clearly not autonomous is attempting suicide. Beneficence underlies much of the Ethics Code (APA, 1992a), particularly Principle E: Concern for Others' Welfare and Principle F: Social Responsibility.

Although it is easy to say that mental health providers should "do good," it is much more difficult to determine what course of action is good for the client and to decide the limits of beneficence. For example, providing money for food or medical care to an indigent client with HIV disease clearly is beneficial, but such an action clashes with the traditional notion of the limits of the therapeutic relationship. For example, does beneficence mean that psychologists should assist with funeral planning or help the client obtain Medicare benefits? Even more important in light of the AIDS epidemic is the question of whether the profession of psychology has a responsibility to train psychologists who are competent to treat individuals infected with the virus (Melton, 1988). Each of these questions revolves around the issue of what it means to "do good."

Other difficult decisions arise when clients cannot be helped without harming them in other ways. For example, take the patient who becomes suicidal upon learning about a positive HIV test result. Breaking confidentiality and arranging emergency treatment may help the client, but it may also harm the client's sense of trust in others and violate his or her autonomy. As already noted, it is difficult to justify forcing clients who are capable of making autonomous decisions to do what mental health professionals believe is in their best interests, simply because the professional thinks their decisions are mistaken. In fact, forcing a client or patient to comply with a health care professional's wishes when the client does not concur with them has sometimes been labeled *paternalism*. On the other hand, it would be equally difficult to justify not intervening in clients' lives when their ability to make autonomous choices is limited because their ability to make rational choices is clouded as it may be in the case of most suicidal clients. At a minimum, beneficence requires that psychologists balance the goods that will result from their actions against the harms. In fact, the majority decision in the *Tarasoff* case (*Tarasoff v. Board of Regents of the University of California*, 1976) argued that there was a duty to protect others based on balancing the social goods that come from taking steps to protect the victim against the harms that might arise from breaking confidentiality.

The issues raised in the *Tarasoff* case help identify a third area that often poses difficult decisions for mental health providers. It involves the question of how to balance doing good and acting in the best interests of individual clients against the welfare of society. Historically, psychology in general and therapists in particular have focused primarily on the good of the individual. In fact, the therapeutic contract is with a particular individual or a group of individuals (in the case of family or group therapy). As a result, psychologists have a *prima facie* obligation to make the client's best interests their primary concern. On the other hand, psychology is conducted in a social system. Thus, psychologists have some ethical obligation to that system and to prevent harm from occurring to others in that system, particularly when that harm is life-threatening.

Beauchamp and Childress (1994) suggested that when dealing with potentially life-threatening situations, health care professionals should consider both the magnitude as well as the probability of harm to others. As both the magnitude and the probability of harm increase, the ethical obligation

TABLE 3.1
Balancing the Magnitude and Probability of Harm

TABLE 3.1
Balancing the Magnitude and Probability of Harm

Probability of harm	Magnitude of harm	
	Major	Minor
High	1	2
Low	3	4

Note: From *Principles of Biomedical Ethics* (4th ed., p. 297), by T. L. Beauchamp and J. F. Childress, 1994, Oxford, England: Oxford University Press. Copyright 1994 by Oxford University Press. Reprinted with permission.

to intervene becomes stronger (see Table 3.1). The magnitude of harm encompasses both the severity of harm as well as the numbers of people involved. Harm that is life-threatening is more severe than the harm involved in hurting someone's feelings. Clearly, the more potentially severe the harm, the greater the responsibility to take action to protect society. Harm that affects large numbers of people (as was the case in the Oklahoma City bombing) involves a great ethical responsibility to intervene. If the harm is minor or the probability of harm is low, there may be no ethical obligation to intervene. In other words, as the risk approaches 1 (i.e., near certainty with severe harm; see Table 3.1), the responsibility to intervene increases. This model may be useful when considering how to balance a responsibility to individual clients with the harm to society or individuals in society who are not clients.

Do No Harm

The third principle that should help guide ethical decisions is non-maleficence, the responsibility to not harm or damage those whom we have contracted to help. This idea is articulated in the Ethics Code in Standard 1.14 (APA, 1992a): "Psychologists take reasonable steps to avoid harming their patients or clients, research participants, students, and others with whom they work, and to minimize harm where it is foreseeable and unavoidable." In general, *do no harm* means not inflicting either psychological or physical harm on consumers, and this principle must be balanced against the responsibility to do good. Defining what constitutes harm is a complex task, however. No one would argue that the therapist whose client suffered the typical stress and discomfort associated with therapy is unethical or that deliberately harming clients without a reasonable treatment related reason is ethical. For example, if an HIV-positive client revealed that he had changed a prescription for tranquilizers to 200 tablets rather than the 20 intended by the physician so he could sell the extras, the harm caused by reporting the client to the authorities and breaking confidentiality would need to be balanced with the social responsibility to prevent harm to those to whom he intended to sell the drugs. The ethical responsibility of fidelity illuminates the decision in this and similar cases.

Fidelity

The principle of fidelity (Ramsey, 1970; Ross, 1930) is the one that often seems most familiar to many therapists because it involves promise keeping, truthfulness, and loyalty, all of which are central to building trust. Lying, deception, and failure to be trustworthy would have devastating consequences for mental health providers who are working with those who have HIV-related diseases. They would destroy clients' faith in the therapist to be helpful as well as in the mutuality of human relationships in general (Kitchener, 1984).

Issues of fidelity arise when people enter into some kind of voluntary relationship such as the one between therapists and clients. When professionals accept clients into therapy, they enter into a fiduciary relationship, meaning obligations to clients are incurred that take precedence over obligations to others who are not clients. In other words, the obligation to a client is stronger, other things being equal, than to others in society at large. One of the obligations incurred in therapy is to keep information confidential. Thus, when mental health providers consider breaking confidentiality they need to balance not harming others with respect for their client's autonomy and fidelity to the relationship.

Even when clients give up their rights to act as autonomous agents because their actions may threaten the life or liberty of others, therapists still must consider their promise to keep information confidential. If therapists were known to lie to their clients about such issues and regularly to break promises, no meaningful therapeutic relationships could exist. If lying and deceit were perceived as the norm for professional relationships, clients would ultimately be suspicious of the therapist's motives and would feel no obligation to be truthful in turn. Furthermore, such actions might also breech the responsibility to do no harm by destroying the client's faith in the mutuality of relationships in general.

Issues of fidelity are particularly sensitive in HIV-related practice because discussions about HIV transmission typically involve the most private aspects of a person's life. Clients must have deep trust in their therapists in order to reveal such information. Similarly, those facing death are among the most vulnerable in society; thus, the loyalty and truthfulness of therapists may be essential to helping them die with dignity. In addition, the relationship between those infected with AIDS and mental health professionals has sometimes been a tenuous one. Breaking promises can further destroy trust in therapists and may deter HIV-positive individuals from seeking help (Dardick & Grady, 1980; Melton, 1988).

Justice

Justice is related to the fair distribution of goods and services and the fair treatment of others (Benn, 1967). In the realm of psychotherapy, justice sometimes involves deciding who should receive the benefits of treatment. This is a particularly difficult issue with the HIV population because many of those infected have limited resources to pay for psychotherapy even in the early phases of the disease, and resources are often diminished by the costs associated with medical care. Justice also implies that therapists act impartially in deciding whom to treat and how to treat them. It suggests that characteristics that are irrelevant to people's need for treatment or the type of treatment they receive such as age, gender, and ethnicity should not be considered in allocating services. This aspect of justice is highlighted in the Ethics Code in Standard 1.10, Nondiscrimination (APA, 1992a).

Issues of justice sometimes do not seem particularly relevant for psychologists when they already engage in HIV-related practice. They are, however, more compelling when considering the treatment of those with HIV-related disease in general. This is especially true when considering that data suggest that many psychologists and social workers hold biased and negative attitudes toward those who are infected with AIDS and do not want to work with them in a therapeutic setting (Crawford, Humfleet, Ribordy, Ho, & Vickers, 1991). The same study indicated that a negative bias toward gay men and lesbians continues to exist in the mental health community and exacerbates negative feelings toward those with HIV-related disease. These data raise the question of whether those infected with HIV can receive fair and unbiased treatment in the wider psychological community and whether the profession has adequately addressed negative stereotypes. Clearly, these are important issues of justice.

DO ETHICAL PRINCIPLES OFFER ABSOLUTE GUIDANCE?

Some people believe that moral principles are absolute and must be followed without exception to circumstance. In some ways, this idea is seductively appealing. If moral principles were absolute, there would be clear recipes to follow when therapists are faced with an ethical dilemma. For example, there would be no exceptions to keeping a client's confidentiality because keeping promises would be absolutely binding. On the other hand, many modern philosophers (e.g., Abelson & Nielsen, 1967; Hospers, 1961) have pointed out that following such dictums absolutely would lead to immoral decisions. An example would be maintaining confidentiality even when a client threatens to deliberately infect as many other people with the HIV virus as possible. Under such circumstances, most would think it justifiable to break confidentiality even though a professional had promised to keep it. Bok (1983) has argued that no one should expect professionals to maintain confidentiality under such circumstances because to do so would make them complicitous in the acts.

On the other end of the continuum, some people believe that if there are no moral absolutes then everything is relative to the particular time, place, or circumstance. This point of view leads to that position that an action is right if someone thinks it is. If this were so, however, then there would be no way to evaluate actions as morally wrong. Yet professionals clearly do so when other professionals act maliciously or engage in thoughtless actions that harm their clients. In fact, professional ethics committees make such decisions on a routine basis.

Many contemporary ethicists take a third position, which holds ethical principles to be *prima facie* valid (Ross, 1930). The legal concept of *prima facie* means that a contract is binding unless there are stronger obligations or the particular facts of the case suggest it is no longer relevant. In ethics, *prima facie* suggests that the five ethical principles just described are always relevant. In other words, they should always be considered when moral issues arise, but one may be overridden if the facts of the case make others more meaningful. Thus, the duties of respecting autonomy, benefiting others, doing no harm, being faithful, and being just give consistent guidance about how to treat clients. If they are overturned, the reasons for doing so must be morally relevant ones.

HOW SHOULD ETHICAL RESPONSIBILITIES BE BALANCED?

If ethical principles are *prima facie* binding, then some way must be found to strike a balance between them. As a result, sometimes ethical responsibility is not clear because the principles themselves may offer conflicting advice. As clinicians, we (the authors of this chapter) also struggle with this issue. What follows are some guidelines we have found helpful as we have tried to identify the best ethical road to follow with our clients.

Before turning to those guidelines, however, it is important to remember that debates over ethical issues sometimes can be reduced to a debate over the facts of the case. In HIV/AIDS work this is particularly important because the information base is growing. What appears to be a fact about the transmission of the HIV virus this year may be proven wrong next year. Facts sometimes enter into ethical decisions in central ways. For example, the debate about breaking confidentiality when an infected person is engaging in unprotected sex may be reduced to a disagreement about how probable it is to transmit the disease under these circumstances. In other words, before interpreting the Ethics Code or considering ethical principles, practitioners should be sure they have the correct facts—both about the disease and the client.

On occasion, however, there is a fundamental conflict among ethical obligations rather than a disagreement about facts. When that happens a way must be found to balance them. One perspective that we have found helpful is contained in the APA Ethics Code (APA, 1992a) in Principle E: Concern for Others' Welfare, which suggests that when conflicts occur psychologists should "perform their roles in a responsible fashion that avoids or minimizes harm." Toulmin (1950) similarly suggested that when there are conflicts between ethical obligations, individuals should act in a way that does the least amount of avoidable harm. In other words, other things being equal, there is a stronger obligation to avoid hurting people than to help them. That seems particularly important in work with people who have HIV disease. Hurting those people we have agreed to help, particularly those who are so vulnerable, would be ethically troublesome. (As discussed previously, however, sometimes practitioners may have to balance harming clients with the potential harm they may do to others.) What these perspectives suggest is that we need to think carefully about the effects of our actions on our clients as well as others. After balancing all of our ethical obligations we must choose the path that is both responsible and does the least amount of long-term harm that is possible to foresee.

Engelhardt (1986) suggested a slightly different approach to balancing ethical obligations. He noted that when tough ethical decisions must be made, the best way to do so is "to act so as to lose as few goods as possible and to violate as few rights as possible" (p. 99). His position seems helpful to us because it suggests that when balancing ethical obligations, clients' rights to respect, privacy, and autonomous decision making are always important considerations.

What is implied by the above is that when tough ethical decisions have to be made, sometimes one moral responsibility may be compromised to uphold another, stronger, ethical obligation. Such is the case when therapists make the decision to break the promise to maintain confidentiality in order to prevent life-threatening harm from occurring to someone else. Others (Nozic, 1968; Ross, 1930) have noted that such actions may leave the decision maker with feelings of moral regret. Furthermore, being ethical sometimes needs to be balanced with legal requirements. When faced with sorting out ethical and legal responsibilities, consulting with colleagues may be immeasurably helpful.

Behaving ethically is not easy, and sometimes even the most ethical choice may result in disappointment. Perhaps psychologists who do not feel some regret or guilt in such situations end up callused and less concerned with harming others. The idea of moral regret should never be used, however, as an excuse for not taking the most moral course of action possible.

BEYOND CODES AND PRINCIPLES

No procedure can guarantee a correct ethical decision, especially in those situations that involve making choices between two potentially ethical courses of action. Deciding on a course of action may be a lonely experience. Although the above discussion is designed to help with the process, in the end the individual therapist must face his or her HIV-positive client or the client's friends and family. Furthermore, moral rules and moral principles may help define what is morally required in a particular situation, but they do not completely capture what it is to be a moral professional (Kitchener, 2000; Meara, Schmidt, & Day, 1996). We all know therapists who treat others in a mean-spirited manner or follow the rules to the extent that it is necessary to get by but cut ethical corners when they do not think they will get caught. Although sometimes it is difficult to pinpoint what is wrong with their actions, they seem to lack what is commonly called good *moral character*. Defining what it means to have good character (also known as *virtue ethics*; see, e.g., MacIntyre, 1984; Mayo, 1993; Meara et al., 1996) is beyond the scope of this chapter. However, we note that practitioners cannot begin to act in a moral fashion without having integrity, responsibility, and a deep and abiding concern for the well-being of others—what might be labeled *benevolence*.

Nel Noddings, the feminist ethicist, argued that principles do not indicate how people ought to act in their relationships with others or (as she put it) "how we meet the other morally" (1984, p. 5). She contended that to reach the ethical ideal, an attitude toward others that sustains caring must be maintained by considering how rules and principles affect the real client in the real situation. Others have called this *compassion* (Beauchamp & Childress, 1994). Being with and developing a human bond with a client who has AIDS may be the greatest gift that a mental health provider can give. Noddings's work should remind therapists working in an HIV-related practice that ethics codes, ethical principles, and legal requirements should not be applied without compassion. In the end, she argued that being ethical depends on remaining "in caring relation to the other" (Noddings, 1984, p. 103).

CONCLUSION

Therapists who work in HIV-related practice cannot avoid ethical dilemmas. Sometimes professionals who have good moral character and who care deeply about their clients still have difficulty identifying the most ethical course of action. Ethical codes and the principles of respecting autonomy, beneficence, doing no harm, fidelity, and justice can provide ways to sort out the issues involved and to choose an ethical course of action. In other words, they can help us think well about doing good as we work with our clients who have HIV-related disease.

REFERENCES

Abelson, R., & Nielsen, K. (1967). History of ethics. In P. Edwards (Ed.), *The encyclopedia of philosophy* (Vol. 3, pp. 81–117). New York: Macmillan.

American Psychological Association. (1992a). Ethical principles of psychologists and code of conduct. *American Psychologist, 47,* 1597–1611.

American Psychological Association, Ethics Committee. (1992b). Rules and procedures. *American Psychologist, 47,* 1612–1628.

Beauchamp, T. L., & Childress, J. F. (1994). *Principles of biomedical ethics* (4th ed.). Oxford, England: Oxford University Press.

Benn, S. I. (1967). Justice. In P. Edwards (Ed.), *The encyclopedia of philosophy* (Vol. 4, pp. 298–301). New York: Macmillan.

Bersoff, D. N., & Koeppl, P. M. (1993). The relation between ethical codes and moral principles. *Ethics & Behavior, 3,* 345–357.

Bok, S. (1983). *Secrets: The ethics of concealment and revelation.* New York: Random House.

Canter, M. B., Bennett, B. E., Jones, S. E., & Nagy, T. F. (1994). *Ethics for psychologists: A commentary on the APA Ethics Code.* Washington, DC: American Psychological Association.

Crawford, I., Humfleet, G., Ribordy, S. C., Ho, F. C., & Vickers, V. L. (1991). Sigmatization of AIDS patients by mental health professionals. *Professional Psychology: Research and Practice, 22,* 357–361.

Dardick, L., & Grady, K. E. (1980). Openness between gay persons and health professionals. *Annals of Internal Medicine, 93,* 115–119.

Engelhardt, H. T., Jr. (1986). *The foundations of bioethics.* Oxford, England: Oxford University Press.

Hospers, J. (1961). *Human conduct: An introduction to the problems of ethics.* New York: Harcourt, Brace & World.

Kitchener, K. S. (1984). Intuition, critical evaluation and ethical principles: The foundation for ethical decisions in counseling psychology. *The Counseling Psychologist, 12*(3), 43–55.

Kitchener, K. S. (2000). *Foundations of ethical practice, research and teaching in psychology*. Mahwah, NJ: Erlbaum.

MacIntyre, A. (1984). *After virtue* (2nd ed.). Notre Dame, IN: Notre Dame Press.

Martin, D. J. (in press). Ethics in the treatment of human immunodeficiency virus infection and acquired immunodeficiency syndrome. In S. F. Bucky (Ed.), *The comprehensive textbook of ethics and law in the practice of psychology*. New York: Plenum Press.

Mayo, B. (1993). Virtue or duty? In C. Sommers & F. Sommers (Eds.), *Vice and virtue in everyday life* (pp. 231–236). New York: Harcourt Brace Jovanovich.

Meara, N. M., Schmidt, L., & Day, J. D. (1996). Principles and virtues: A foundation for ethical decisions, policies, and character. *The Counseling Psychologist, 24*, 4–77.

Melton, G. B. (1988). Ethical and legal issues in AIDS related practice. *American Psychologist, 43*, 941–947.

Noddings, N. (1984). *Caring: A feminine approach to ethics and moral education*. Berkeley: University of California Press.

Nozic, R. (1968). Moral complications and moral structures. *Natural Law Forum, 13*, 1–50.

Ramsey, P. (1970). *The patient as person*. New Haven, CT: Yale University Press.

Ross, W. D. (1930). *The right and the good*. Oxford, England: Clarendon Press.

Siegel, K. (1986). Psycho-social aspects of rational suicide. *American Journal of Psychotherapy, 40*, 405–418.

Tarasoff v. Board of Regents of the University of California, 529 P.2d 553 (Cal. 1974), aff'd, 551 P.2d 334, 331 (Cal. 1976).

Toulmin, S. (1950). *An examination of the place of reason in ethics*. Cambridge, England: Cambridge University Press.

Werth, J. L., Jr. (1992). Rational suicide and AIDS: Considerations for the psychotherapist. *The Counseling Psychologist, 20*, 645–659.

Werth, J. L., Jr. (1995). Rational suicide reconsidered: AIDS as an impetus for change. *Death Studies, 19*, 65–80.

4

CULTURAL CONSIDERATIONS IN HIV ETHICAL DECISION MAKING: A GUIDE FOR MENTAL HEALTH PRACTITIONERS

SALLY JUE AND SANDRA Y. LEWIS

Unlike most other chronic illnesses, HIV/AIDS forces us to look at social issues and issues of difference. HIV/AIDS pushes every social button: race, ethnicity, sex, reproductive choices, sexual orientation, death and dying, drug use, and relationships. Winiarski (1997) noted that HIV/AIDS "holds a mirror to the face of America and is not concerned about flattery" (p. 83). Since the beginning of the epidemic, HIV/AIDS has forced us to examine how our biases affect our work with people living with and affected by the disease.

As the HIV pandemic has evolved, mental health practitioners are likely to be working with clients diverse not only in sexuality but in ethnicity. Between July 1997 and June 1998, 51% of male adults and adolescents with AIDS, 77% of female adults and adolescents with AIDS, and 85% of all children with AIDS in the United States were African Americans, Hispanics, Asian Pacific Islanders, and Native Americans. In 1998, African Americans and Hispanics represented 84% of all pediatric AIDS cases and the majority of adult minority AIDS cases (Centers for Disease Control and Prevention [CDC], 1998).

Although the impact of HIV/AIDS on ethnic minorities increases the racial ethnic diversity of HIV clients, culture is not limited to one's race, ethnicity, or minority status. We define *culture* as the attitudes, values, and beliefs shared by a group of people that provide them with a framework for interpreting and interacting with their environment. According to this broader definition, individuals are a product of several cultural influences, including race, ethnicity, nationality, socioeconomic class, community, profession, and other affiliations. As such, culture is a factor of human experience with both practitioner and client bringing their unique cultural perspectives to the therapeutic relationship.

Working with culturally diverse clients living with HIV/AIDS presents challenges over and above those with a life-threatening illness. As mental health practitioners providing HIV/AIDS-related psychotherapy we must develop a keen awareness of our core values, feelings about difference, our biases or preferences, and those events that stimulate anxiety or that "sinking feeling in the pit of our stomach" commonly known as *countertransference* (see chapter 5 in this volume). As early as 1988, Macks found countertransference reactions in professionals working with HIV-positive women. These reactions included fear of contagion; discomfort with sex, sexuality, and sexual behavior change; anger; victim blaming; and fear of professional inadequacy. Boyd-Franklin and Boland (1995) reconfirmed that providers experienced anger toward women and blamed them for infecting their children. Hunter and Ross (1991) found that health professionals perceived clients who acquired HIV through sex or drug use as having less moral integrity than those infected by transfusion. Jemmott, Freleicher, and Jemmott (1992) found that individuals who expressed more negative attitudes toward intravenous drug users or homosexuals were more likely to report intentions to avoid caring for AIDS clients. Others (McGuire, Nieri, Abbott, Sheridan, & Fisher, 1995) investigated the relationship between a therapist's beliefs and ethical decision making in AIDS-related psychotherapy and found a significant relationship between a therapist's homophobia and likelihood of breaching confidentiality, concluding that personal bias may affect ethical decision making. Boyd-Franklin and Boland (1995) also reported overidentification, blurring of boundaries, and feelings of inadequacy and grief related to a client's death.

Bernstein and Klein (1995) explored countertransference issues of group psychotherapists working with primarily Black and Hispanic HIV-positive clients. Specific countertransference issues included reactions to clients' cultural backgrounds, drug abuse, and lifestyles, including homosexuality. Other research has shown that ethnic minority individuals tend to underutilize and prematurely terminate therapy services because they view them as culturally inappropriate, insensitive, and sometimes oppressive and antagonistic (Boyd-Franklin, 1989; Sue & Sue, 1990).

When countertransference issues and cultural differences converge, we may very well experience discomfort, value conflicts, and uncertainty in our work. When specific ethical issues arise, decision making becomes even more complex. How much do we expect our culturally different clients to adjust to our cultural and professional norms and values? How much should we accommodate their cultural needs? How might our biases affect our clinical judgment and decision making? What degree of cultural accommodation from both client and therapist constitutes ethically and clinically sound practice? This chapter highlights the issues most likely to create cultural and ethical dilemmas when working with HIV-affected clients from various cultures, raises critical questions, and provides suggestions on how to integrate cultural considerations into clinical ethical decision making.

ISSUES MOST LIKELY TO CREATE ETHICAL AND CULTURAL DILEMMAS

Helping Relationships

Many cultures, including some within the United States, are unfamiliar with psychotherapy and counseling as it is taught in American universities and professional schools. Clients from other cultures often define helping or helpful relationships differently. Their viewpoints influence their expectations of counselors and therapists, yet because many clients cannot clearly articulate their expectations, therapists may misinterpret client behaviors and make clinical decisions on the basis of inaccurate assumptions. For example, clients from cultures that do not have psychotherapy may have no idea how "talk therapy" can be helpful. They may push the therapist for concrete advice, information, and assistance rather than discuss their feelings. A therapist's interpretation of this behavior as resistance could be detrimental to forming a therapeutic alliance, whereas assisting clients with concrete needs or "real-life problems" can be a means of connecting with them (Boyd-Franklin, 1989).

For any client, but particularly for clients who are unfamiliar with psychotherapy and counseling, it is helpful to explore their expectations of us as clinicians and to explain what expectations we can fulfill and how we intend to work with them. This dialogue opens the door for both client and clinician to negotiate how to best set up the therapeutic relationship and begin the process of learning more about each other's cultures.

For example, talking about feelings is one of the cornerstones of psychotherapy, yet many Asian Pacific Islanders and Native Americans would consider this to be unacceptable behavior (Williams & Ellison, 1996; Yamashiro & Matsuoka, 1997). With these clients, the therapist or "listener" should be able to infer or interpret the feelings when listening to a description of events or actions. This of course, requires being able to put the client, actions, and events within a cultural context that may be quite different and foreign to the therapist's own experience. Latino clients tend to respond to the personal connection they make with the therapist rather than the institution of psychotherapy. They may not disclose personal feelings until they feel the therapist is a "member of the family" (Medrano & Klopner, 1992, p. 121).

Client reactions to the structure of psychotherapy often reflect their cultural norms about information sharing. For example, many clinicians conduct intakes during their first meeting with new clients. At that time, they usually request information that many cultural groups consider private and perhaps irrelevant to their presenting problems. Such information may include client sexual orientation and mental health, substance use, and family and sexual history. African American clients may approach this aspect of therapy with "healthy cultural paranoia" (Grier & Cobbs, 1968, p. 135), a response to generations of racism and discrimination in the United States. Clients may also come from cultures in which it would be considered ludicrous for individuals to make numerous personal self-disclosures to someone they have just met. African Americans, Latinos, Asian Pacific Islanders, Native Americans, and working-class gay men could easily view such history taking as intrusive and inappropriate with strangers, especially those who refuse to make similar self-disclosures (Boyd-Franklin, 1989; Chersky & Siever, 1994; Everett, Proctor, & Cortmell, 1983; Laval, Gomez, & Ruiz, 1983; Sue & Sue, 1990).

Clients from cultures where psychotherapy is nonexistent may also define the boundaries between personal and professional relationships differently (Medrano & Klopner, 1992; Williams & Ellison, 1996; Yamashiro & Matsuoka, 1997). Clients may want to give gifts, especially if the therapist works for an agency that does not charge clients for counseling services. A client with HIV may also leave the therapist something in his or her will, and the therapist may not find out until after the client has died. Are some gifts more acceptable than others? Would it depend on how personal or expensive the gift was? Might the client view refusal to accept a gift as a personal rejection? How might this affect our relationship with the client? One must evaluate the client's motives and cultural context for gift giving as well as how refusal or acceptance of the gift might affect treatment (Haas & Malouf, 1995).

In addition to these cultural differences regarding therapy in general, there are other differences associated with an HIV or AIDS diagnosis. Given the stigma attached to HIV and its associated risk behaviors and, in many cases, the repeated rejections experienced by people with HIV (especially those from already stigmatized groups), people with HIV tend to be wary mental health consumers. Many clients with HIV want information about their therapist's sexual orientation, HIV status and experience, or personal life to help them determine his or her ability to suspend judgment (Curtis & Hodge, 1995). If the client asks for specific information about our families or sexual orientation, should we reveal it? How comfortable are we sharing this information? What are the potential consequences of not making personal self-disclosures with clients clearly uncomfortable with the "rules" of psychotherapy?

Native American, Asian, Hispanic, and gay clients may feel more comfortable making their own self-disclosures and trusting us if we answer their inquiries about our sexual orientation or experience with a particular cultural group (Boyd-Franklin & Garcia-Preto, 1994; LaFramboise, Saks-Berman, & Sohi, 1994; Larkin, 1994; Lau-Chin, 1994). In these situations, it is helpful to assess what personal self-disclosures are vital to building connections with clients of different cultural norms and the therapeutic value such disclosures may have for the client.

The home visit presents another challenge. For many immigrant cultures, sharing meals is a source of bonding and a sign of accepting the host's hospitality. For clients with HIV, sharing a meal also shows we do not fear transmission from meal sharing and gives us the opportunity to alleviate anxieties that a client's family may have about HIV transmission through casual contact. Clients may not discuss business until we are introduced to the family and share a meal or at least a beverage. If we arrive at the client's home and refuse an offer of food, how might the client react? What message might our refusal unintentionally convey about HIV transmission? Sharing a meal, then moving on to the "business" reasons for our visit often takes longer than the 50–60 minutes we allot for a standard counseling session. Should we bill for the extra time? If so, what effect might that have on our relationship with the client?

Other situations that present cultural and ethical challenges are client requests that we be the executors for their will, exercise durable power of attorney, or speak at their memorial service. Some cultures might view such requests as appropriate, especially if the client has not disclosed his or her HIV status to anyone else and is uncomfortable doing so. Would cultural considerations affect our decision for some clients but not others? If so, could this be construed as favoritism or discrimination? How might our refusal affect our relationship with our HIV-positive clients? How might we seek to explain our position, or our agency's, as we attempt to negotiate a workable solution with our clients?

Culture can also affect clients' views on confidentiality. Confidentiality is based on the right to privacy, derived in part from the Bill of Rights of the United States. According to the Ethical Principles of Psychologists and Code of Conduct (American Psychological Association, 1992),

"Psychologists have a primary obligation and take reasonable precautions to respect the confidentiality rights of those with whom they work or consult, recognizing that confidentiality may be established by law, institutional rules, or professional or scientific relationships" (Standard 5.02). Confidentiality also "protects the public trust in the mental health professions more generally" (Haas & Malouf, 1995, p. 35).

Culturally diverse clients who come from small towns or from countries with very oppressive governments may believe confidentiality is impossible, which makes trust harder to build. However, the therapist who is able to win their trust may face a whole set of ethical dilemmas: What information should be shared and with whom, and what must be kept confidential? If the client is an HIV-positive girl who does not know her HIV status and whose parents have forbidden disclosure of the diagnosis, how does one respond to her repeated questions regarding why she feels ill or has to take so many medications? If the client is a child who asks whether her parents are HIV-positive, how does one respond if one knows they are but has been instructed not to discuss this with her? What do you do if you run into clients while you are out shopping with family or friends?

Many Asian Pacific Islander, Latino, Caribbean, and Native American cultures have their own healing traditions that are often viewed as ineffective by Western practitioners (Gock, 1994; Medrano & Klopner, 1992; Williams & Ellison, 1996). Clients from these cultures may choose to forgo Western medicine in favor of their own cultural healing methods or combine traditional and Western treatments. If they do, their physicians may ask for a mental health or psychiatric evaluation, especially because the advent of Highly Active Anti-retroviral Treatment (HAART) requires clients to adhere to complex treatment regimens in order to reduce HIV viral load and prevent developing treatment resistant viral strains. Health care providers are also likely to call on us to provide interventions that increase treatment adherence. However, successful treatment adherence requires us to acknowledge and incorporate the client's social and cultural background. We must assess its potential effect on our clients' perspective about disease process, medical interventions, and ability and willingness to comply with treatment regimens (Crespo-Fierro, 1997; Langer, 1999, p. 24). What do we do if we do not believe that the client's traditional methods are helpful or could prevent him or her from accessing HAART? Would challenging the client's decision negate client autonomy in the interest of our own beliefs? Would supporting traditional healing over Western medicine not benefit the client and possibly cause harm? Would supporting traditional healing be of benefit to the client emotionally or physically or both? How might we support traditional methods that could benefit clients? Would it be appropriate for us to consult with traditional healers from the client's culture?

When clinicians and clients have different cultural norms for helping relationships, clinicians who cannot accommodate some of these cultural differences will be unable to form a therapeutic relationship with their clients. Despite the guidance provided by legal parameters, professional standards, and codes of ethics, there remains a great deal of ambiguity and lack of clear direction in how to resolve cultural dilemmas that render the standard psychotherapeutic relationship ineffective. How can we set up an effective therapeutic relationship with a client whose cultural expectations differ from standard practice? To answer this question, we examine other key cultural issues likely to arise in HIV-related psychotherapy and offer some suggestions for developing a culturally competent ethical practice.

Communication Styles

For effective counseling to take place, the therapist and client must be able to accurately and appropriately send and receive verbal and nonverbal messages to each other (Sue & Sue, 1990). Communication styles have a significant impact on face-to-face encounters, and culture is a powerful determinant of communication style, especially nonverbal communication. Because we often look to nonverbal communication to support, negate, or give nuance to the verbal message, it is crucial that therapists try to discern the possible cultural meanings of nonverbal messages. It is also difficult to distinguish between personal style and cultural norms. For example, depending on the observer's culture and personal style, a client's lack of eye contact with the therapist may be interpreted as shyness, intimidation, respect for authority or an elder, submission, hiding information, avoidance, or resistance. To remain true to the ethical principle of justice, which requires that we treat others equally and afford all clients their due portion, we must try to discern how cultural factors (ours and theirs) influence our interpretations of client nonverbal communication.

Written, mail, and telephone communications and home or office visits may also have different meanings to clients from other cultures. Some may view written communications as impersonal and distant and home visits as more social than office visits. If HIV-positive clients have not told family members with whom they live about their HIV status, or if they do not want family members to know that they are receiving psychotherapy, it is important to ask them how they want to handle mailings and telephone messages.

To better understand our clients' communication styles, we can seek information from cultural consultants, the literature, and the client (if the client is able to articulate the cultural differences). However, it is equally important to examine our own counseling and communication styles and their impact on the therapeutic relationship. Boyd-Franklin (1989) discussed the concept of "vibes" referring to clients' attention not only to our words but also to our body language and other subtle messages we communicate. How might our nonverbal messages reveal our personal and cultural biases? How might clients from other cultures interpret our style? Could our helping styles hinder our ability to work effectively with culturally different clients, thus violating the ethical principle of nonmaleficence? How much are we willing to shift our counseling style and techniques to accommodate culturally different clients? Acknowledging and sharing our limitations with our clients, their possible impact on the client, and our willingness to learn and be flexible are important first steps in bridging the communication style gap.

Client Support Systems

When assessing our clients' support systems, we should always explore what, if any, support our clients might receive from their families. Because many people with HIV have experienced or fear rejection by their families of origin, they often "create" new families from friends and community groups. Friends and same-sex partners are usually the primary source of support for HIV-positive gay clients (Hays, Chauncey, & Tobey, 1990), whereas friends are often the primary source of support for drug-using clients (Stowe, Ross, Wodak, Thomas, & Larson, 1993). Homeless youth are more likely to consider as "family" their peers on the street than their family of origin.

Other cultural groups also have their own definitions of family. Among many African Americans and Latinos, family includes nonblood kin such as godparents, close friends, neighbors, and fellow church members (Boyd-Franklin, 1989; Boyd-Franklin & Garcia-Preto, 1994). For Native Americans, family may include all tribe or clan members (LaFramboise et al., 1994), and Asian and Pacific Island cultures have highly interdependent family networks consisting of multiple generations of extended family that share child rearing and support functions (Bradshaw, 1994). Clients from racial–ethnic groups may refer to individuals with whom they have no blood, marriage, or legal ties as their parents, aunts, uncles, or cousins. In such cases it is helpful to determine how clients define the term *family* and what family relationships are most significant to them. Boyd-Franklin, Aleman, Steiner, Drelich, and Norford (1995) suggested that once trust is established, a genogram (diagram of family and relationships) should be developed with the client to identify key support.

To work effectively with HIV-positive people from different cultures, we must also understand culturally defined family member roles and functions, including spousal, parent–child, sibling, extended family, and nonblood kin relationships. In some cultures, for example, the client may defer to his or her partner, spouse, or family member because of that person's culturally determined higher status. Higher status might be based on age, gender, or traditional family role. It is important to determine whether this is the case before assuming that such behavior is symptomatic of a problem in the relationship.

In some cultures, deferring decision making to a family member is the norm. In these cases, the client may refer the therapist to a family member to make decisions about treatment or other needed services. In some Eastern European and Asian cultures, physicians never inform the patient of a poor prognosis or a highly stigmatized diagnosis. That information goes to family members, who assume responsibility for treatment decisions and what information is shared with the patient (Gordon, 1996). The patient and family may also prefer to defer decision making to the physician (Gordon, 1996). This would seem to violate the principle of client autonomy, yet these patients may view delegating some of their decision-making power to others as an appropriate way to exercise their autonomy. Once we have obtained information about our clients' culturally determined family roles, it is helpful to explore how they feel about current family relationships and what if any changes they want to make. This helps us engage clients in clarifying their desires and identify other family members who might be included in the therapy process (Boyd-Franklin & Garcia-Preto, 1994).

Individual self-fulfillment is a strong American value. However, other cultures value group harmony over individual desires, which often means that group needs supersede an individual's (Bradshaw, 1994; LaFramboise et al., 1994; Vasquez, 1994). In more traditional cultures, this has meant that the family, rather than the government or peer group, is the primary socializing force in an individual's life. Clients from more family-dominant cultures tend to make decisions on the basis of what is best for the family, even when those decisions may exact personal costs to the individual. When this happens to our clients, what would be the most beneficent and nonmaleficent course of action to take? Should our views of what is best for our clients be based on our cultural norms or the clients'? Making a clinically beneficent decision requires that we support client autonomy within our clients' cultural comfort zone, something we cannot do without first understanding their cultural values and norms.

Many HIV-positive clients may decide not to disclose their risk factors or HIV diagnosis to protect their family from disappointment or to protect themselves from family rejection and disapproval. If we impose Western views valuing individualism and freedom from the "emotional field of the family" (Sue & Sue, 1990, p. 122) onto clients whose views favor family harmony, we could easily do harm to our clients. A more effective approach would be to help the client make the most of existing family and other support networks. To do this, we need to learn what those networks are and how they function, as well as perhaps letting go of our own preconceived notions of family.

Sexuality and Gender Roles

According to the 1998 Centers for Disease Control and Prevention *HIV/AIDS Surveillance Report*, men who have sex with men represent 40% of AIDS cases in the United States. Men who have sex with men and who are also injection drug users make up 4% of reported AIDS cases. In addition to these men, there are HIV–positive people who identify themselves as gay, bisexual, and transgender but who are not included in the surveillance report. It is therefore important to be aware of our own cultural and religious beliefs toward transgender, gay, and bisexual people. If our cultural and religious beliefs have strong biases against people who engage in same-sex behavior or who are transgender, can we work effectively with them? Working effectively and ethically with these clients means being able to set aside one's own beliefs if they interfere with the client's autonomy and the ethical principles of justice, beneficence, and nonmaleficence.

Cultural definitions of homosexual behavior vary. There have been several studies documenting a wide range of same-sex behaviors for men who do not identify themselves as gay (Carrier & Magana, 1991; Carrier, Nguyen, & Su, 1992; Gant & Ostrow, 1995; Jue, 1987; Peterson & Marin, 1988). Many of these men are married and have children, and others who know of their same-sex behaviors do not necessarily consider them to be gay or their behavior to be abnormal. Carrier et al. (1992) reported that Vietnamese men who identified themselves as gay often "restrict their sexual behaviors to the passive role of fellating 'masculine' men" who are not considered gay because of the Vietnamese societal belief that equates homosexuality with feminine sexual behaviors (p. 553). Carrier and Magana (1991) reported that in Mexican culture, there are at least two different male groups with same-sex contacts. Mexican society would consider the man taking the anal-receptive role as gay, but not necessarily the man taking on the anal insertive role (p. 198). Gant and Ostrow (1995) found that some African American men who have sex with other men often "reject the gay or bisexual indicator of self expression in favor of the behavioral description" because they feel the terms *gay* and *bisexual* imply lifestyles different from their own (p. 222).

For the clinician, it is more useful to collect information on specific behaviors than to ask clients to identify themselves as gay, bisexual, or heterosexual. For some clients, their native languages may have only pejorative terms for these groups, and the client may perceive the question as an insult. It is also helpful to ask for the client's perception of his behaviors and their significance to self, family, and community.

In the United States, children become adults at the age of 18, yet laws vary on the age at which young people are "capable" of consensual sexual relations with an adult or other minor. Cultural norms also influence the "acceptable" age for sexual activity for young people as well as specific sexual practices such as the use of anal penetration to prevent pregnancy or maintain virginity. Our cultural norms and personal beliefs about sexual activity for minors may not coincide with our clients' reality or their cultural belief systems. This has led to debate on the content of HIV prevention programs and the age groups targeted by prevention programs. How might culture influence how we provide HIV prevention information to underage clients? How might the sexual orientation, sex, or age of their partners influence our choice of interventions? How do we balance our legal reporting responsibilities with cultural ethical considerations?

Most cultures also have strong beliefs and norms for male and female roles and relationships. Many of these values contradict Western feminist or more egalitarian perspectives. However, many HIV prevention programs have encouraged women to insist that their male partners use condoms and to negotiate safer sex practices. Where it is culturally acceptable for women to do this, therapists encouraging such behavior would not be violating ethical principles. In Latino and Asian Pacific cultures, however, these behaviors may be viewed as insulting or inappropriate and could lead to verbal or physical abuse of the woman (Amaro, 1995; Land, 1994; Medrano & Klopner, 1992), resulting in the unintentional violation of the beneficence and nonmaleficence ethical principles. Reframing interventions within the client's cultural context is effective, but to do so we must first have an understanding of that culture and its interface with the client's personal values. Clinicians can obtain information by exploring the client's perspective, reviewing the literature, and seeking cultural consultation.

Recent policy changes in some states now require that the names of HIV-positive individuals be reported and that their partners be notified. For clients who have a history of domestic violence with their current partner, parents, or other adults in their household, we must evaluate the potential harm to clients if we report their HIV status and their partners to the authorities (North & Rothenberg, 1993). Careful evaluation of cultural factors is especially important given recent court cases of men killing their wives when their wives transgressed culturally determined sex roles as well as cases of women committing suicide after killing their children when they felt they had either failed or shamed their husbands and families (Coleman, 1996; Sacks, 1996).

Reproductive Issues

Although the use of anti-retroviral treatments has reduced the risk of HIV-positive women transmitting the virus to their unborn babies, the long-term effect of these drugs on infants remains unknown (Levine, 1994), and pregnancy in HIV-positive women still carries some risk to both mother and child. Women also need to consider long-term planning for their children should their health eventually deteriorate. Despite the risks and possible complications, some women still desire children with their HIV-positive partners to fulfill culturally defined marital obligations and personal desires, even at the risk of becoming infected with HIV. In such cases, how do we handle conflicts we may have over the client's right to autonomy and our obligation to uphold beneficence and nonmaleficence when what we feel to be in the client's best interests and the interests of relevant third parties differs from the client's point of view?

Cultural and religious or spiritual beliefs may contribute to a woman's denial about the possible consequences to herself and her child should she continue a pregnancy without receiving HIV testing, relevant medical information, and good prenatal and postnatal care. Other cultural and ethical dilemmas arise when pregnancy might seriously compromise the health of a woman with AIDS. These dilemmas become more acute when the client's views and those of her therapist differ on abortion, how her health status could affect her parenting abilities, and the advisability of forgoing Western medicine in favor of traditional or religious healing. Underlying these differences is the fundamental issue of whether a woman's procreative autonomy is more important than the effect that decision has on others, including the child who could be born with HIV (Nolan, 1989). The stronger our emotional reactions are to clients and their situations, the more crucial it is to evaluate whether our personal views interfere with our ability to uphold the ethical principles of justice and client autonomy.

Culturally based contraceptive choices also affect HIV risk reduction. Although barrier methods such as male and female condoms and diaphragms and cervical caps used with male condoms provide more protection against HIV infection, some cultures teach women that it is inappropriate to touch their genitals. For these women, oral or injection contraceptives or intrauterine devices (IUDs) are the methods of choice. Unfortunately, these methods do not prevent HIV transmission, and IUDs can increase the risk of vaginal and pelvic infections in HIV-positive women (Kelly, 1992).

The cultural and ethical challenges raised by reproductive and contraceptive issues increase when our clients are minors from cultures whose beliefs differ significantly from our own. These challenges are made even more complex by possible legal issues concerned with confidentiality, contraceptive options for minors, and newer laws in most states that mandate HIV counseling and voluntary testing for all pregnant women.

Drug Use

Many mental health providers refuse to see clients with a history of substance abuse if the client has not abstained from substance use for at least 6 to 12 months. However, HIV community providers may make exceptions depending on the reasons for using certain drugs. For example, many people with AIDS find marijuana more effective than prescription drugs for relieving nausea and the side effects of chemotherapy and stimulating appetite to combat wasting syndrome, and some Native American clients may use peyote for spiritual purposes. These practices may be acceptable to some clinicians and not others. It is also important to examine whether we find some drugs more acceptable to use than others and whether we are therefore more accepting of clients who use these drugs rather than drugs we view less tolerantly. To forgo such self-examination could lead us to violate the ethical principle of justice by not treating all clients fairly.

Contrary to the total abstinence model favored by Alcoholics Anonymous and other 12 Step programs, the HIV community has developed its own cultural norms for treating drug users. Rather than deny services to clients still actively using drugs, many HIV providers offer services along with risk reduction information (Friedman, 1991; Shernoff, 1992). The goal is to modify the drug-using behavior in ways that reduce the risk of HIV transmission and enable the therapist to begin building a relationship with the client that could eventually lead to abstinence or significantly reduced drug use. A risk reduction approach acknowledges that relapse could occur and is part of the recovery process.

Perhaps one of the most controversial aspects of a risk reduction approach to drug use is whether it conveys an implicit approval of drug use. These opposing views make it difficult to integrate substance abuse treatment with HIV prevention. Any attempt by the clinician to refer drug-using clients to a needle exchange program, teach and encourage them to clean their works or not share needles, and provide safer sex information could be and has been viewed as undermining substance abuse treatment and prevention by condoning drug use (Hagan, 1991). A practitioner's personal views about appropriate treatment intervention may also contradict his or her agency's policies and procedures.

Regardless of our approach, it is important to examine our personal views toward drug users. How might age, HIV status, sex, race, and socioeconomic class affect our perceptions of drug-using clients? How might our actions differ if our needle-sharing clients were members of the local high school football team shooting steroids? How might we feel about HIV-positive clients who cannot support themselves or their children on social security and sell drugs to make ends meet or to pay for their expensive HIV treatments? What about clients who say they cannot give up drug use after learning of their HIV diagnosis because it is the only coping mechanism they feel they have? What if drug treatment centers refuse to take them because they have AIDS-related health problems? The quality, quantity, and availability of services to HIV-positive drug users tends to be influenced by a belief that they are irresponsible, antisocial, and thus more "undeserving" of services than other clients (Stein, 1992). Might we also carry a similar bias that translates into expending less effort and energy for HIV-positive drug users so that we can give more to clients we perceive as more deserving?

Death and Dying

Some of the greatest ethical challenges associated with HIV treatment concern questions related to death and dying. Questions regarding quality of life versus longevity and control over the amount of pain and suffering the client endures can lead to intimate discussions about living with and dying of HIV-related illnesses.

Clients' coping mechanisms are often culturally shaped and may not always be compatible with the clinician's beliefs. Many Asian Pacific people view illness as the fate they were dealt or their karma (Yamashiro & Matsuoka, 1997, p. 178). Their quieter acceptance of their HIV status is often misinterpreted as "giving up" or "giving in." Traditional Navajo Indians do not talk about death, believing that discussion of it may attract it (Mercer, 1996). This could be perceived as denial and avoidance. Dealing with illness, death, and grief through cultural and spiritual rituals rather than verbal discussion is another common coping mechanism in many cultures.

Different cultures also have varying views on suicide and assisted suicide. Western culture has traditionally valued life over death, viewing life as sacred, whereas many Eastern cultures often view release from life as a goal to be sought (Albright & Hazler, 1995). Suicide can be an honorable way to die. For some clients, it is an acceptable option that spares one's family from the shame of HIV and the undue burden of caring for the client in the later stages of illness. Clients who blame themselves for acquiring HIV and putting such a burden on their families may also contemplate suicide out of guilt.

For many clients with AIDS, when the quality of life becomes intolerable and the medical prognosis is terminal, rational suicide becomes a viable option. Rational suicide is one in which clients, being of sound mind, make an informed and well-planned decision to end their lives. Cultural factors may play a major part in this decision-making process. Our own personal biases as clinicians could easily influence our choice of interventions as we struggle to reconcile our views, our clients' views, professional ethics, and the law.

Euthanasia or assisted suicide presents additional dilemmas. A friend or family member may feel that honoring the client's dying request to assist with a suicide is a sacred promise or a familial obligation. In The Netherlands, physician-assisted euthanasia is generally accepted when strict conditions are met (Albright & Hazler, 1995). Clients sometimes want to discuss their experience of witnessing or assisting the suicide of a friend or relative with AIDS. Although society has yet to resolve its dilemmas over suicide and assisted suicide for people with terminal illnesses, clinicians who are trying to decide how to intervene should be guided by the ethical principles of client autonomy, nonmaleficence, and beneficence.

Spirituality

Different spiritual beliefs lead to different interpretations of high-risk behaviors and their connection to HIV infection as well as one's ideas about death, dying, and what might happen to people with AIDS after death. Dealing with spiritual and religious beliefs that we feel are detrimental to our clients' well being presents unique challenges. For example, how do we respond when clients say that they will trust God or traditional spiritual healers and rituals to cure them rather than seek conventional Western medical treatment? What if some practices they choose (such as the use of hallucinogenic drugs or animal sacrifice) are illegal? Unlike most other issues clients bring to us, spirituality is based on faith and does not readily respond to logic or reality testing. Clients could question such interventions as religious intolerance or a direct challenge to their beliefs.

Clients' spiritual and religious beliefs can also influence their perception of why they acquired HIV and the amount of guilt and shame they experience. Gay clients who were raised in religions that forbid or condemn homosexuality sometimes feel that HIV is a punishment for being gay. Other clients have viewed HIV as punishment for other perceived transgressions such as sexual relations outside of marriage, drug use, or leaving the church. These perceptions can lead to depression, guilt, and low self-esteem, causing clients to seek various ways to do penance. Some bargain for a cure in exchange for going back to the church or giving up the behaviors or relationships that they feel led them to acquire HIV.

On the other hand, clients and caregivers may use their spiritual beliefs to reframe more positive reasons for their illness. For example, based on spiritual beliefs, a family caregiver might tell the child with HIV that she is one of God's special angels who has come to earth to help us deal with the HIV crisis. If the child responds with an increased but not unrealistic sense of hope and a stronger will to live, what harm might a therapist create by openly challenging this family's way of coping with HIV? Holaday (1984) observed that assigning meaning to illness is an essential strategy for enhancing coping.

It is especially important to suspend judgment when working with clients whose spiritual beliefs differ from our own. Although clients bring their religious views to counseling, psychotherapy is generally a secular service and must remain free of religious judgment in order to be effective. What is most helpful is learning as much as possible about the client's religious and spiritual beliefs and trying to frame interventions within the context of those belief systems. We also need to remember that we could do more harm and violate the client's autonomy by directly challenging or minimizing the validity of spiritual beliefs alien to our own.

BECOMING A CULTURALLY COMPETENT ETHICAL CLINICIAN

Ethical clinicians comply with their profession's ethics codes and uphold and balance the principles of autonomy, beneficence, nonmaleficence, justice, and fidelity. Adhering to these principles when working with HIV-affected clients from other cultures also requires us to develop cultural competence. If we ignore, minimize, or in any way judge our clients' cultural differences, we will not have the empathy, trust, and understanding necessary for building the therapeutic relationship. If we allow ourselves to remain blind to our cultural biases and unreceptive to exploring alternate explanations for client behavior, our work with culturally different clients invariably becomes unethical and ineffective.

Becoming culturally competent forces us out of the comfort zone of our own worldview, but it does not require us to abandon our values and beliefs or to become immediate experts on other cultures and how best to work with them. Sue and Sue (1990) defined *culturally competent counselors* as those who are actively developing awareness of their own cultural assumptions, actively attempting to understand their clients' worldviews, and then actively developing and practicing appropriate, relevant, and sensitive intervention strategies and skills. According to Langer (1999), cultural competence within the context of managing a therapeutic alliance requires "developing awareness, sensitivity, knowledge and skills that encourage interaction that is enhanced rather than hindered by differences" (p. 22).

Self-assessment, then, is the first step to becoming culturally competent (Boyd-Franklin, 1989; Carter & Orfanidis, 1976; Jacobson, 1988). An honest self-assessment also requires us to set aside our assumptions about ourselves as well as others, because our assumptions about ourselves influence how we view our clients (Marks, 1998). How do we really feel about the cultural differences our clients present? Do we even view cultural differences as a way to explain behavior that makes us uncomfortable or perplexed? Because we cannot always know the meaning of the behaviors to which we react, we must train ourselves to constantly ask, "Did that mean what I thought it did?" (Fullilove, 1998, p. 3). Do clients present cultural differences that violate values we hold in high esteem? If so, how might that affect our ability to be fair or empathetic? How might that affect our diagnosis? What aspects of our clients' culture do we find positive and comfortable? What values might we share? Finding common ground helps prevent differences from becoming barriers to effective treatment and enables clients and clinicians to feel more comfortable with each other and more willing to engage on a deeper level.

Our ability to relate effectively to culturally different clients varies. No matter how skilled or knowledgeable we are, we cannot accommodate everyone, and we should not view this as a weakness. Honestly accepting our limitations and sharing them with our clients while also demonstrating a sincere desire to help, despite our limitations, may be sufficient basis for establishing rapport (Sue & Sue, 1990). Boyd-Franklin (1989) underscored this type of self-exploration as key to maintaining our focus on the human element—the relationship between client and therapist.

Consultation is an invaluable part of self-assessment. Because we all have cultural and personal blind spots, "we must share our work with colleagues from different backgrounds who may act as our eyes and ears, that is, as our interpreters" (Fullilove, 1998, p. 3). Sharing our dilemmas with professional colleagues, especially those having the same cultural background as our clients, also gives us input on current community standards of practice and helps us clarify what cultural information we need to work effectively with our clients.

Where can we learn more about other cultures? Mental health colleagues from our clients' cultures and professional publications can give us cultural information as well as culturally appropriate clinical interventions. If these sources are not available, we need to take the initiative and seek other resources such as professional organizations, ethnic community service or cultural groups, or individuals from the cultural group in question. Sources who do not have a mental health background can still provide valuable information about that culture's values and how they are expressed, acceptable behaviors, family roles, spiritual beliefs, and traditional practices.

Sometimes our clients may be our best resource for obtaining the information we need to more effectively assist them. The LEARN model (Berlin & Fowkes, 1983) is a useful tool for eliciting cultural information from clients while enhancing rather than interfering with the therapeutic process. LEARN is an acronym for listen, elicit, acknowledge, recommend, and negotiate. *Listen* means to hear what our clients tell us without letting our cultural biases interfere and render premature judgment. It means to focus not only on our clients' perception of the problem, but also their related psychosocial and cultural adjustment issues as well as their strengths, including those that are culture based.

We must *elicit* not only general information about clients' worldviews, but also how their cultural values affect their perception of their problems. After hearing from them, we need to share how we view their problems and needs. This dialogue helps us uncover differences early in the relationship and demonstrates our willingness to better understand our clients' perspective.

Acknowledge and discuss our differences and similarities with our clients. Focusing only on differences could create barriers, whereas focusing only on similarities could lead clients to believe we are uninterested, uncomfortable, or oblivious to important differences. Discussing similarities facilitates greater connection with our clients.

Recommend actions and interventions using the information obtained during the first three steps of the LEARN model and any cultural, professional, or legal consultants.

Negotiate actions and interventions. If our clients do not respond favorably to our suggestions, it is important to go back to the first four steps of the model so that we can understand our clients' reactions. During the negotiation process, it is helpful to discuss the possible consequences of each option. For clients who have not been in the United States very long, it is important to inform them of any possible legal consequences of their actions or lack of action. In some jurisdictions, ignorance of the law is no excuse, and pleading cultural differences as a defense has had limited admissibility and inconsistent success in American courts.

The LEARN model teaches us to maintain the position of the learner, which may be contrary to our professional training to be the expert. By being in the learner role, we practice parity in building therapeutic relationships. The model establishes collaboration as a cornerstone of culturally competent mental health service. It helps us to build on our clients' strengths, values, and perspectives. Rather than to see them as obstacles, with the LEARN model we can ask ourselves: What might be the positive intention of my clients' behavior? What values underlie their choices? What good are they attempting to achieve?

CONCLUSION

Ridley (1985) described cultural competence as an "ethical imperative" (p. 613) in the training of psychologists. As mental health practitioners, regardless of our own ethnicity and other cultural influences, we must apply and continually develop our cultural competence skills in order to understand and effectively address the unique needs of diverse clients. The numerous social and value-laden issues arising in HIV-related mental health practice require that we apply our cultural competence skills in ethical decision making.

Ethical issues related to working with culturally different HIV-affected clients force us to make hard choices. If we are to rise to the challenge, we must actively engage in a continuous process of improving and refining our skills and knowledge in both HIV/AIDS and cultural competence. By honestly assessing our biases and taking responsibility for acquiring the input, information, and skills we need to work effectively with our clients, we can be confident that we have done our professional and personal best. We will be able to stand by the hard choices we make with perhaps mixed feelings but a clear conscience.

REFERENCES

Albright, D. E., & Hazler, R. J. (1995). A right to die: Ethical dilemmas of euthanasia. *Counseling & Values, 39*, 177–189.

Amaro, H. (1995). Love, sex and power: Considering women's realities in HIV prevention. *American Psychologist, 50*, 437–447.

American Psychological Association. (1992). Ethical principles of psychologists and code of conduct. *American Psychologist, 44*, 1597–1611.

Berlin, E. A. & Fowkes, W., Jr. (1983). A teaching framework for cross-cultural health care. *Western Journal of Medicine, 139*, 934–938.

Bernstein, E. A., & Klein, R. (1995). Countertransference issues in group psychotherapy with HIV-positive and AIDS patients. *International Journal of Group Psychotherapy, 45*(1), 91–100.

Boyd-Franklin, N. (1989). Black families in therapy: A multisystems approach. New York: Guilford Press.

Boyd-Franklin, N., Aleman, J. del C., Steiner, G. L., Drelich, E. W., & Norford, B. C. (1995). Family systems interventions and family therapy. In N. Boyd-Franklin, G. L. Steiner, and M. G. Boland (Eds.), *Children families and HIV/AIDS: Psychosocial and therapeutic issues* (pp. 115–126). New York: Guilford Press.

Boyd-Franklin, N., & Boland, M. G. (1995). Caring for the professional caregiver. In N. Boyd-Franklin, G. L. Steiner, & M. G. Boland (Eds.), *Children, families and HIV/AIDS: Psychosocial and therapeutic interventions* (pp. 216–232). New York: Guilford Press.

Boyd-Franklin, N., & Garcia-Preto, N. (1994). Family therapy: The cases of African American and Hispanic women. In L. Comas-Diaz & B. Greene (Eds.), *Women of color: Integrating ethnic and gender identities in psychotherapy* (pp. 239–264). New York: Guilford Press.

Bradshaw, C. (1994). Asian and Asian American women: Historical and political considerations in psychotherapy. In L. Comas-Diaz & B. Greene (Eds.), *Women of color: Integrating ethnic and gender identities in psychotherapy* (pp. 72–113). New York: Guilford Press.

Carrier, J., & Magana, R. (1991). Use of ethnosexual data on men of Mexican origins for HIV/AIDS programs. *Journal of Sex Research, 28*(2), 189–202.

Carrier, J., Nguyen, B., & Su, S. (1992). Vietnamese American sexual behaviors and HIV infection. *Journal of Sex Research, 29*, 547–560.

Carter, E., & Orfanidis, M. M. (1976). Family therapy with one person and the family therapist's own family. In P. J. Guerin (Ed.), *Family therapy: Theory and practice* (pp. 193–219). New York: Gardner Press.

Centers for Disease Control and Prevention. (1998). *HIV/AIDS surveillance report: US HIV & AIDS cases reported through June 1998, mid year edition 10(1)*. Atlanta, GA: Author.

Chersky, B., & Siever, M. D. (1994). Counseling working-class gay men. *Focus, 9*(3), 5–6.

Coleman, D. L. (1996). Individualizing justice through multiculturalism: The liberals' dilemma. *Columbia Law Review, 96*, 1093–1167.

Crespo-Fierro, M. (1997). Compliance/adherence and care management in HIV disease. *Journal of Nursing in AIDS Care, 8*, 31–43.

Curtis, L. C., & Hodge, M. (1995). Boundaries and HIV-related case management. *Focus, 10*(2), 5–6.

Everett, F., Proctor, N., & Cortmell, B. (1983). Providing psychological services to American Indian children and families. *Professional Psychology: Research and Practice, 14*, 588–603.

Friedman, S. R. (1991). Organizing drug injectors. *Focus, 6*(11), 1–4.

Fullilove, M. T. (1998). Beyond stereotypes: Stigma and counseling. *Focus, 13*(12), 1–4.

Gant, L. M., & Ostrow, D. G. (1995). Perceptions of social support and psychological adaptation to sexually acquired HIV among White and African American men. *Social Work, 40*(2), 215–223.

Gock, T. S. (1994). Acquired immunodeficiency syndrome. In N. W. S. Zane, D. T. Takeuchi, & K. J. Young (Eds.), *Confronting critical health issues of Asian and Pacific Islander Americans* (pp. 247–265). Thousand Oaks, CA: Sage.

Gordon, E. (1996). Multiculturalism in medical decision: Making the notion of informed waiver. *Fordham Urban Law Journal, 23*, 1321–1362.

Grier, W., & Cobbs, P. (1968). *Black rage*. New York: Basic Books.

Haas, L., & Malouf, J. (1995). *Keeping up the good work: A practitioner's guide to mental health ethics* (2nd ed.). Sarasota, FL: Professional Resource Press.

Hagan, H. (1991). Studies supporting syringe exchange. *Focus, 6*(11), 5–6.

Hays, R. B., Chauncey, S., & Tobey, L. A. (1990). The social support networks of gay men with AIDS. *Journal of Community Psychology, 18,* 374–385.

Holaday, B. (1984). Challenges of rearing a chronically ill child: Caring and coping. *Nursing Clinics of North America, 19,* 361–368.

Hunter, C. E., & Ross, M. W. (1991). Determinants of health-care workers' attitudes toward people with AIDS. *Journal of Applied Social Psychology, 21,* 947–956.

Jacobsen, F. M. (1988). Ethnocultural assessment. In L. Comas-Diaz & E. E. H. Griffith (Eds.), *Clinical guidelines in cross-cultural mental health* (pp. 135–147). New York: John Wiley & Sons.

Jemmott, J. B., Freleicher, J., & Jemmott, L. S. (1992). Perceived risk of infection and attitudes toward risk groups: Determinants of nurses' behavioral intentions regarding AIDS patients. *Research in Nursing & Health, 15*(4), 295–301.

Jue, S. (1987). Identifying and meeting the needs of minority clients with AIDS. In M. Fimbres & C. Leukefeld (Eds.), *Responding to AIDS: Psychosocial initiatives* (pp. 65–79). Silver Spring, MD: National Association of Social Workers.

Kelly, P. (1992). Fertility, menstruation and birth control in HIV. *Treatment Issues: Gay Men's Health Crisis Newsletter of Experimental AIDS Therapies, 6*(7), 10–14.

LaFramboise, T., Saks-Berman, J., & Sohi, B. K. (1994). American Indian women. In L. Comas-Diaz & B. Greene (Eds.), *Women of color: Integrating ethnic and gender identities in psychotherapy* (pp. 30–71). New York: Guilford Press.

Land, H. (1994). AIDS and women of color. *Families in Society: The Journal of Contemporary Human Services, 75*(6), 355–361.

Langer, N. (1999). Culturally competent professionals in therapeutic alliances enhance patient compliance. *Journal of Health Care for the Poor and Underserved, 10*(1), 19–25.

Larkin, M. (1994, March/April). Finding the right balance: Counselors reveal how they set professional boundaries while still extending themselves to clients. *HIV Frontline: An Informational Newsletter for Professionals Who Counsel People Living with HIV, 17,* 4–6.

Lau-Chin, J. (1994). Psychodynamic approaches. In L. Comas-Diaz & B. Greene (Eds.), *Women of color: Integrating ethnic and gender identities in psychotherapy* (pp. 194–222). New York: Guilford Press.

Laval, R. A., Gomez, E. A., & Ruiz, P. (1983). A language minority: Hispanics and mental health care. *American Journal of Social Psychiatry, 3,* 42–49.

Levine, C. (1994, Spring). Commentary on ACTG 076. *The American Foundation for AIDS Research Report,* pp. 4–5.

Macks, J. (1988). Women and AIDS: Countertransference issues [Special issue: AIDS: Bridging the gap between information and practice]. *Social Casework, 69,* 340–347.

Marks, R. (1998). Editorial: Working with culture. *Focus, 13*(12), 2.

McGuire, J., Nieri, D., Abbott, D., Sheridan K., & Fisher, R. (1995). Do *Tarasoff* principles apply in AIDS-related psychotherapy? Ethical decision making and the role of therapist homophobia and perceived client dangerousness. *Professional Psychology: Research and Practice, 26*, 608–611.

Medrano, L., & Klopner, M. C. (1992). AIDS and people of color. In H. Land (Ed.), *AIDS: A complete guide to psychosocial interventions* (pp. 117–139). Milwaukee, WI: Family Service of America.

Mercer, S. (1996). Navajo elderly people in a reservation nursing home: Admission predictors and cultural care practices. *Social Work, 41*(2), 181–189.

Nolan, K. (1989). Ethical issues in caring for pregnant women and newborns at risk for human immunodeficiency virus infection. *Seminars in Perinatology, 13*(1), 55–65.

North, R. L., & Rothenberg, K. (1993). Sounding board: Partner notification and the threat of domestic violence against women with HIV infection. *New England Journal of Medicine, 329*, 1194–1196.

Peterson, J. L., & Marin, G. (1988). Issues in prevention of AIDS among Black and Hispanic men. *American Psychologist, 43*, 871–877.

Ridley, C. R. (1985). Imperatives for ethnic and cultural relevance in psychology training programs. *Professional Psychology: Research and Practice, 16*, 611–622.

Sacks, V. L. (1996). An indefensible defense: On the misuse of culture in criminal law. *Arizona Journal of International and Comparative Law, 13*, 523–550.

Shernoff, M. (Ed.). (1992). *Counseling chemically dependent people with HIV illness.* Binghamton, NY: Harrington Park Press.

Stein, J. (1992). HIV disease and substance abuse: twin epidemics, multiple needs. In H. Land (Ed.), *AIDS: A complete guide to psychosocial interventions* (pp. 107–115). Milwaukee, WI: Family Service of America.

Stowe, A., Ross, M. W., Wodak, A., Thomas, G. V., & Larson, S. A. (1993). Significant relationships and social supports of injecting drug users and their implications for HIV/AIDS services. *AIDS Care, 5*, 23–33.

Sue, D. W., & Sue, D. (1990). *Counseling the culturally different: Theory and practice* (2nd ed.). New York: Wiley.

Vasquez, M. J. T. (1994). Latinas. In L. Comas-Diaz & B. Greene (Eds.), *Women of color: Integrating ethnic and gender identities in psychotherapy* (pp. 114–138). New York: Guilford Press.

Williams, E., & Ellison, F. (1996). Culturally informed social work practice with American Indian clients: Guidelines for non-Indian social workers. *Social Work, 41*(2), 147–151.

Winiarski, M. G. (1997). Cross-cultural mental health care. In M. G. Winiarski (Ed.), *HIV mental health for the 21st century* (pp. 82–115). New York: New York University Press.

Yamashiro, G., & Matsuoka, J. (1997). Help seeking among Asian and Pacific Americans: A multiperspective analysis. *Social Work, 42*(2), 176–186.

5

THE EFFECTS OF GRIEF AND LOSS ON DECISION MAKING IN HIV-RELATED PSYCHOTHERAPY

LYNN BONDE

The face of AIDS and the needs of people living with AIDS have changed dramatically over the past decade and a half. Early on in the history of the epidemic in America, AIDS ravaged whole neighborhoods of White gay men, killing dozens in months or weeks. Today, new therapies and vectors have transformed AIDS from a short-term, dramatically fatal disease affecting predominantly White, gay men to a longer term, more chronic disease for that cohort. In poorer communities, where compliance with the complicated regimens that have been so effective for White gay men is less possible or predictable, and the cost of the drugs may be prohibitive, HIV and AIDS are increasingly devastating realities for heterosexual people of color. In 1998, African Americans, who represent 12% of the total U.S. population, accounted for nearly half of the AIDS cases reported in that year (Centers for Disease Control and Prevention, 1999). HIV-positive women, who are largely poor women of color, face documented barriers in gaining access to health care services (AIDS Legal Referral Panel, 1998).

With these shifts, the nature and types of loss and grief experienced by people with AIDS and the mental health providers who treat them also have changed. Clinicians are less likely to find themselves tracking the

83

devastating physical, and often mental, deterioration of healthy, sexually active gay men over a stunningly brief period. Instead, clients' issues of grief and loss are often subsumed by a much broader, sometimes overwhelmingly complex, blend of concerns, as demonstrated by the cases discussed in the following chapters.

Those who have responded successfully to treatment may be struggling with the consequences and meaning of virtually eradicating evidence of the virus in their bodies. Patients who had been too ill to work had retired with disability benefits, planned funerals, and emotionally positioned themselves for death now confront the psychological impact of a literal "new lease on life." Although this gift of days is precious, it does not come without the burden of adjusting to a changed reality and set of expectations for the future. Instead of helping patients cope with imminent death, clinicians may now be supporting them in contending with the reality of a future that they believed had already been lost.

Clinicians dealing with minority populations must educate themselves about HIV and AIDS and its effects on the often already overburdened family systems of African Americans and Latinos. Lewis and Jue (chapter 4, this volume) skillfully described these considerations in great detail.

Despite all of the advances in treatment, however, AIDS and HIV continue to be synonymous with loss. Even though some patients live longer than they used to, not all do, and none are cured. Thus, clinicians who choose to treat patients with HIV and AIDS must take account of the unique losses associated with the disease. For clients, these losses begin with diagnosis and continue to death, although death itself may not represent the most devastating loss over the course of a patient's illness. For practitioners, facing the death of clients from AIDS creates a singular set of considerations that must be incorporated into the process of making treatment decisions.

People living with AIDS face unique issues of loss compared with those dying of other diseases. HIV and AIDS inflict losses arising out of prejudice, stigma, fear of exposure, and the effects of the disease on the patient's sexual and social identities. These realities generally are not part of the experience of patients dying of other diseases. A woman dying of breast cancer, for example, while grieving the loss of her future with her children, does not also confront the burden of the fact that she may have transmitted the disease to those children. Patients dying of emphysema or lung cancer related to a history of smoking may experience a lack of sympathy or even prejudice based on the view that their own addiction led to their disease. However, these people do not also confront the moral and ethical dilemmas faced by people with HIV or AIDS, who must consider whether and how to notify sexual partners of their status.

Clinicians treating people with HIV likewise face the burden of these unique losses along with challenges to their own feelings about sexuality, sexual activity, and drug use presented by people with HIV. Some clinicians may also have to cope with negative reactions of family, friends, and colleagues outside the AIDS community about their treating patients infected with the virus. These assaults, unique to treating people with HIV, can constitute a threat to clinicians' feelings of therapeutic objectivity and complicate the feelings of loss they may feel contemplating the incapacitation and death of clients. In all, the emotional terrain of treating patients with HIV and AIDS can be uncertain ground for the most confident of mental health providers.

Those experienced in dealing with the grief of others are often surprised when personal losses drive them into rage and depression. The death of a family member or friend can lead to an introspective journey into sometimes frightening and usually painful territory. This is as difficult for a mental health provider as for anyone else. Dealing with death in a professional context is yet another facet of the experience of facing loss. Clinicians whose patients die grieve for those patients. Facing the deaths of those one has come to know as one can only in treatment engenders a complex set of responses. Practitioners who treat significant numbers of dying people deal with a phenomenon of grief that is related not only to the fact of each death of a patient, but also to the impact of facing large numbers of dying people. The sheer magnitude of losses has its own constellation of effects. Acknowledging and confronting the pain and discomfort of these feelings is a significant part of ethical practice.

UNDERSTANDING GRIEF

Definitions help to structure a discussion about grief. Commonly, three terms are conflated, although each refers to a clinically different aspect or orientation of the process. *Grief* refers to the subjective experience of the psychological, behavioral, social, and physical reactions to a specific loss (Rando, 1993). *Bereavement* is the state of having suffered a loss. *Mourning* is variously defined as the public demonstration of grief and the intrapsychic process of resolving loss.

John Bowlby's (1979) work on attachment serves as the conceptual framework in this chapter for understanding the grief response. Bowlby identified attachment as a fundamental and instinctive need observed in virtually every species. Extinction of the attachment elicits a predictable series of responses: numbing, yearning and searching, disorganization and despair, and reorganization. The strength and qualities of the connection between the individual and the object of attachment often determine the intensity of the experience of loss and the difficulties that may arise in the process of reorganization and integration.

Grief can make a bereaved person feel crazy. Normal grief reactions include sleep and somatic disorders; exaggerated or extinguished libido; hallucinations of the visual, aural, tactile or olfactory presence of the deceased; uncontrollable weeping; feelings of shame, guilt, and rage; and suicidal ideation. A man will sleep in his dead lover's shirt for months after the death. A mother will leave her child's room exactly as it was at the time of the child's death, sometimes for years. A young woman will for weeks refuse sex with her partner following the death of her father and then find herself compulsively seeking sex in a series of one-night stands. Bereaved people scream, wail, weep, rail against God, look for someone to sue. They can't move and they can't sit still. They can't sleep and they can't get out of bed. They can't concentrate and they perseverate on the last conversation they had with the deceased. The discomfort of the pain of grief is unavoidable and generates myriad defensive reactions.

A new loss also can generate renewed pain over previous losses, leaving the bereaved person to confront seemingly unrelated reactions to the immediate death that exacerbates his or her confusion and distress. This is especially problematic when the earlier loss is incompletely processed. A client of mine sought treatment to help resolve what he experienced as emotional numbing after the death of his partner from AIDS-related complications. The client had cared for him over the last several months of his life at the home that they shared. The partner had died peacefully at the home surrounded by loved ones. Over time, it became clear that the client's grief over his partner's death literally had been blocked by his unresolved feelings over the death of his father, who had died painfully in the hospital. The client felt that he had failed his father in not having helped him to die more easily, in less pain, with less fear. He experienced flashbacks of his father's face in the moments before his death, twisted in a grimace of agonized confusion. Once the client worked through the shame and guilt that his sense of failure produced, he was able to confront the death of his partner and acknowledge the success of his own efforts to ease his partner's suffering and to prevent a repetition of the circumstances of his father's death.

Faced with symptoms of normal grief, many practitioners would assess a bereaved person as suffering from depression. The differential diagnosis, however, turns on the presence of a significant loss and leads to an important difference in treatment decisions. Although normal grief reactions are sometimes indistinguishable from symptoms of clinical depression, ignoring the work of processing the broken attachment prevents clients from engaging in the tasks necessary to integrate the loss into their lives.

Resolving a loss means working through the pain of the broken attachment. Many models have been developed to describe this process. Worden (1991) and Rando (1993) have developed stage models that delineate steps or tasks through which the bereaved person proceeds to integrate, normalize, and move beyond the acute pain of the loss. These tasks involve a process of recognizing and accepting the reality of the loss; acknowledging and confronting the pain of the grief associated with the loss; reviewing and resolving one's relationship with the deceased; readjusting oneself to live in a world without the deceased; and, finally, establishing a relationship with the deceased and the fact of the loss that allows one to move forward in one's own life. Each step or task must be relatively well-completed for the bereaved to be considered to have integrated the loss effectively. Most people facing the loss of a loved one move back and forth among the tasks, each time consolidating gains and incrementally moving to a point where the pain of the loss, although never completely extinguished, sufficiently abates for the person to reengage with life.

The model is equally applicable to the therapist who loses clients to AIDS. These unique losses must also be processed through the tasks of grief in the context of the therapeutic relationship. Grieving psychotherapists must acknowledge their own grief as a prerequisite to integrating the losses psychologically and emotionally. The model of simple grief is not, however, sufficient to the clinician's task. The psychotherapist who treats large numbers of dying patients also must grapple with the effect of the multitude of these losses. Failure to recognize and deal with the reality of grief can have serious consequences for therapists and their patients.

THE GRIEVING PSYCHOTHERAPIST

The tasks of coping with the clinician's own grief over the death of clients and of incorporating the results of those coping mechanisms into subsequent therapeutic relationships call on the clinician's most deeply felt human impulses and professional skills. How can the practitioner determine whether he or she is being affected by feelings of grief, and what can be done with those feelings? How can a grieving clinician continue to practice without creating risks for clients?

The first step in the model for ethical decision making contained elsewhere in this volume (see chapter 7) is to "pause and identify your personal responses to the case." This step, however, requires that clinicians acknowledge their own grief at the loss of clients, naming the phenomenon and identifying its effects. Clinicians who are distracted, have difficulty focusing during therapy, experience flashes of memories of deceased clients, behave in a short-tempered or disengaged manner in personal relationships, or exhibit other typical grief symptoms are likely to be experiencing grief over the deaths of their clients. Indeed, psychotherapists who treat dying patients cannot avoid this grief.

Psychotherapists' feelings of grief are legitimate responses to the deaths of patients. The therapeutic relationship is an intimate attachment; when broken by death, the result is a loss that requires attention. One barrier against this process is the clinicians' belief that grief for clients is somehow an inappropriate reaction. "Professionals don't cry," reported one psychologist in describing this resistance (Ussher, 1991, p. 284). The clinician's fear of focusing attention on the effects of these losses because the feelings themselves are beyond those the therapist "ought to" experience denies the very reality and substance of the relationship out of which they were born. This belief may arise not only out of a conception of the therapist's role as requiring emotional disengagement from the client, but also out of the absence of social sanction for this manifestation of grief.

Grief specialists identify the perception that one's grief is inappropriate to one's relationship or role in the life of the client as *disenfranchisement*. In his seminal work on the subject, Doka (1989) defined as *disenfranchised* the "grief that persons experience when they incur a loss that is not or cannot be openly acknowledged, publicly mourned, or socially supported" (p. 4). Disenfranchised grief arises if the relationship is not perceived or recognized socially as one that would generate grief. The loss may not be sanctioned as permitting public expression of grief or as a legitimate loss. Disenfranchised grief may be a product of any or all of these disabling conditions, creating a conflict with clinicians' feelings over lost clients. They may not see the therapeutic relationship as one that entitles them to experience grief over the loss, given that their work with the patient often focuses on working through the patient's feelings about his or her impending death. Clinicians may expect that they have "worked through" the reality of the patient's death and dismiss the feelings of grief that follow the event. They may also view their participation in the rituals surrounding the client's death, such as funeral or memorial services, as an inappropriate interposition of their own feelings and needs into the patient's world.

One clinician avoided attending the funerals of the first several clients she lost to AIDS early in the epidemic because she thought that it would be an inappropriate breach of therapeutic boundaries. A decade after their deaths, however, she began to report disturbing flashbacks involving some of these clients that became intrusive in both her work and personal life. Although she began to attend clients' funerals or memorial services in the mid-1990s, her participation in these rituals did not enable her to address her feelings of anger, horror, loss, and inadequacy over those earlier losses. Reentering psychotherapy, she was able to begin to address the multiplicity of losses and her reactions and to begin to process her grief over those earlier deaths.

Disenfranchisement and the conflict that accompanies it can create significant distress for clinicians. Their defenses against such unacknowledged grief can generate feelings of guilt, anger, and despair that can become chronic and immobilizing. Grief can generate a sense of helplessness and despair, anger toward and blaming the victim, blurred ethical and professional boundaries, and fear of professional inadequacy (Dane, 1995). Such conflicts can easily begin to interfere with clinicians' therapeutic persona and their ability to make neutral, ethical decisions in treatment.

For clinicians treating patients with AIDS, grief that is chronically disenfranchised coupled with the complex tasks of processing numerous deaths can create compounded difficulties. These traumatizing effects can easily be overlooked or ascribed to burnout. However, psychotherapists who deal with these feelings as though they were solely burnout realize only partial resolution of the source of their distress. Grief must be addressed on its own terms.

MULTIPLE LOSSES AND THE TRAUMA RESPONSE

Detachment

A clinician's failure to address feelings of grief may cause profound damage to subsequent therapeutic relationships. Grieving clinicians risk becoming disengaged and more detached from clients. They may isolate themselves or avoid, withdraw from, or in other ways restrict their personal involvement with dying patients (Dane, 1995). This reflects clinicians' difficulty in confronting the broken attachment produced by the patient's death and their attempt to deal with the traumatic aspects of multiple losses. It represents a defense against their own fear of abandonment and sense of loss of control.

The sheer volume of the losses takes its toll as well. In the words of one clinician, "You get kind of numb. It's not possible to grieve each person because you see so many" (Sleek, 1996, p. 2). When losses come with abnormal frequency, the process of resolving one's relationship to a single death is halted as loss is piled on loss before the grieving individual has the time, distance, or opportunity to integrate each one and heal. The bereaved person may be left psychically numbed, without self-direction. Clinicians often cope with this type of trauma by disengaging from their current clients rather than confronting the weight of the multiplicity of losses that they have endured.

One therapist experienced in treating patients with AIDS recalls struggling to hide her sense of helplessness and loss as one patient after another succumbed to wasting disease and died. She found herself moving away from her clients, pitying them, unable to engage in the therapeutic empathy she knew that they required. She sought supervision to help her acknowledge her growing discomfort with both her feelings of grief and the defense mechanism that she found herself using to cope with them.

Detachment—an understandable, but ultimately dysfunctional reaction to the overwhelming grief of multiple loss and fear of abandonment—may be difficult for clinicians to acknowledge and even more difficult to overcome. Fear and anger at one's helplessness can damage clinicians' sense of control and identity and impair their ability to engage with clients in the manner required by the therapeutic relationship. The numbness of this detachment inevitably infects the therapeutic relationship and impairs clinicians' ability to cope with future losses.

Overinvolvement

For many working with people with HIV and AIDS, the defensive alternative to disengagement is overinvolvement with patients and their environments. Appropriately permeable boundaries may disappear altogether as practitioners lose themselves and their roles as clinicians. "Bending the frame" in response to the sometimes overwhelming needs of people with AIDS may disable therapists from approaching clients from the necessary perspective of clinical objectivity and empathic neutrality.

Inappropriate engagement can take many forms, from the personal to the material, blurring the therapeutic frame into dissolution. The grieving clinician is drawn too close to the client's psychological experience and physical death. The clinician may become enmeshed in a dying client's impending death, using it to blunt his or her own responses to feelings of helplessness and grief over the death of the client.

Potential overinvolvement with patients is indicated by such clinician behaviors as excessively visiting the patient's home or hospital room, beyond those normally associated with the therapeutic schedule or emergency needs; becoming involved with the patient's family, not normally part of the therapeutic relationship; buying food or supplies for the patient or loaning the patient money; providing transportation to appointments; serving in a case management role; helping the patient and family access other services or helping to arrange financial support or funeral arrangements; helping with the patient's physical needs, including personal care such as changing diapers or linens; and doing laundry or housework. As seen in the cases that follow, the threat of this behavior to ethical practice can be significant.

Clinicians explain the activities by the patient's obvious need and apparent helplessness. Yet, the primary focus of these activities may be clinicians' own feelings of helplessness in the face of the patient's ultimate death. The need to feel useful or helpful in such a situation, to remain active and doing, can often camouflage the clinician's discomfort with feelings of grief.

Overinvolvement risks blurring the psychotherapeutic boundary, leaving both the client and the clinician swamped by the therapeutic experience. Distancing avoids the essential edge where psychotherapeutic magic reveals itself. To avoid these potentially injurious defensive reactions, the psychotherapist must become conscious of their source and begin the process of defining the point of healthy interplay between maintaining the therapeutic frame and willingness to place one's self in awkward, uncharted terrain (Fishman, 1994). This often involves defining new boundaries and roles within which to navigate this new landscape, without sacrificing the clinical posture that will most effectively help to meet the patient's psychological needs.

Anticipatory Grief

One particular risk for practitioners is the phenomenon of anticipatory grief when working with HIV-positive clients. Clinicians may withdraw from their clients, avoiding actively entering into therapeutic relationships as fully as they might with other, healthy clients. They may find themselves thinking about their clients' impending death, unwilling to invest in individuals who may not live long enough to benefit from the work. Clinicians might start to miss clients even while they are in session together. This anticipation of death creates a barrier to the development of a psychotherapeutic relationship.

Rando (1986) identified both cognitive and affective processes in the anticipatory grief of the caregiver of a dying person. Of primary importance among these for the clinician is the acknowledgment of the separation anxiety and fear of permanent loss that are generated by confronting a person one believes may soon be dead. The defensive reactions of withdrawal or disengagement, on the one hand, and overinvolvement or boundary confusion, on the other, also pose a threat to sound practice and must be addressed.

The fundamental challenge of the process and phenomenon of anticipatory grief is to find a manageable balance between the desire to direct increased attention to the patient and the desire to begin to decathect from a person who will no longer be present. The risk of anticipatory grief is that the clinician will become immobilized by these contradictory forces and be unable to engage appropriately in the therapeutic relationship. The emotional or intrapsychic paralysis of this process can produce a profound disconnection with the client. On the other hand, acknowledgment of the sadness of the impending loss, both internally and with the client, can help clinicians cope effectively with anticipatory grief and even to strengthen the relation-ship with the dying patient.

Burnout

Other professional hazards mimic the effects of grief but should be distinguished and addressed independently of the tasks of grief work.

Psychotherapy is inherently stressful work. The therapeutic stance demands unwavering attention to maintaining one's instinctual restraint, balanced attentiveness, patience, confidence, and neutrality (Horner, 1993). The constant stress of sustaining this delicate equilibrium can be exacerbated by the unrealistic expectation that it can be done with absolute consistency. When this unrealizable expectation collides with the unpredictable and uncertain reality of difficult clients with intractable conditions, the thera-pist's ego ideal suffers under the attack. Defenses against frustration, fear of failure, and shame begin to appear.

These defenses produce the experience of a significant discrepancy between the amount of effort clinicians expend in their work and the rewards they receive (Farber, 1990). The resulting fatigue and frustration can produce symptoms of physical and emotional depletion; increased lability or irritabil-ity; and a loss of empathy, respect, and positive feelings for clients (Skorupa & Agresti, 1993; Yiu-Kee & Tang, 1995). Clinicians can experience somatic symptoms including insomnia, ulcers, headaches, and hypertension; begin to engage in alcohol or other substance abuse; and suffer increased interpersonal difficulties and conflicts (Farber, 1990). This is burnout.

The psychotherapist's grief over clients lost to AIDS can amplify and aggravate the potent mix of factors that produce burnout. The steps one might take to ameliorate symptoms of burnout may also help to relieve the pain of grief. However, grief and burnout are not synonymous. Acknowledg-ing the existence of feelings of grief and addressing the ways in which those feelings may affect clinical judgment require a somewhat different approach to the clinician's experience and the resolution of painful feelings.

Horner (1993) identified the perfectionist ego ideal of the therapist as a principal contributing factor of burnout. Other researchers have focused on the externalities of a toxic work situation as the primary cause: burnout as a situationally induced phenomenon (Freudenberger, 1974; Maslach, 1981). Some researchers have suggested that mental health providers work-ing in institutional settings are more likely to experience burnout than those in private practice (Farber 1990). Others attributed burnout to coping style (Thornton, 1992) or personal disposition. However, even those most allied with the theory that personality is the principal determining factor in burnout acknowledge that some situations can be so overwhelming that "even the hardiest individuals can succumb to emotional and physical exhaustion" (Piedmont, 1993, p. 469). Working with people with HIV and AIDS is certainly one of those situations.

Burnout among the medical, mental health, and personal caregivers of those living with HIV infection occurs with unsurprising frequency and is well-documented (Bennett, Kelaher, & Ross, 1994; Davidson & Foster, 1995; Shernoff & Springer, 1992; van Servellen & Leake, 1993). On the Maslach scale (Maslach & Jackson, 1981), frequently used to measure several factors associated with burnout, the scores of those who care for large numbers of people with HIV and AIDS indicate high levels of emotional exhaustion and depersonalization and moderate to low levels of personal achievement.

Caring for oneself, taking time off, learning to reframe the tasks of treating people with HIV and AIDS, receiving additional training and supervision, and finding support among co-workers or others engaged in similar struggles are all palliative steps for the caregiver who experiences burnout (Bennett, 1995; Horner, 1993; Skorupa & Agresti, 1993). These palliatives also are of value in processing feelings of grief, although the latter task requires a specific focus on the facts of the loss being grieved.

Countertransference

Countertransference is generally understood as the clinician's emotional response to the patient (Hamilton, 1990). Traditional theories admonish therapists to avoid any interpolation of their own feelings into the psychotherapeutic process. Psychotherapists are expected to be neutral instruments in the exploration of the patient's unconscious (Giovacchini, 1989). A less traditional approach (Barret, 1997) suggests the unavoidability of the therapist's response to clients and acknowledges that countertransference can be understood to be of service in meeting client needs.

Countertransferential responses may appear when therapists are made anxious by some aspect of the patient's presentation and when their desire to avoid this anxiety forces them into assuming defensive postures (Barret, 1997). These defenses may produce feelings of anger toward the patient that are expressed in overt or covert hostility, annoyance, or inappropriate friendliness.

Working with HIV-positive and AIDS patients provides stimuli that could serve as potential countertransferential triggers. Homophobia, fear of infection, stigma, helplessness and hopelessness, and one's own conflicted or unresolved feelings about death can evoke powerful unconscious forces that challenge the therapist's ability to maintain an appropriate empathic posture. Perhaps the most instinctive defense mechanism for many therapists to these complex assaults is disengagement. The empathic ground falls away and therapists find themselves distanced and distracted. Blaming the patient often follows (e.g., Barret, 1997; Cadwell, 1994; Carmack, 1992; Dane, 1995; Fishman, 1994).

Although countertransference is a powerful force with which the clinician treating people with HIV and AIDS must contend, it is not grief. Rather, the phenomenon of grief, although potentially encompassing countertransferential aspects, reflects a separate facet of the relationship between psychotherapist and patient.

HEALING THE GRIEVING THERAPIST

The therapist's ego identification with the image of a detached, neutral presence can interpose a powerful barrier against his or her ability first to acknowledge and then to process grief. Miller, Wagner, Britton, and Gridley (1998) posited a dichotomy of healing in which clinicians are invested in maintaining the appearance of good mental health while struggling to deny and hide their wounds. The conflict inherent in attempting to sustain such an image in the face of the trauma of disenfranchised grief and multiple loss leaves them seriously vulnerable.

The defensive reactions to grief of disengagement and overinvolvement have obvious consequences for ethical decision making in treatment. These impairments pull psychotherapists away from the balanced stance that allows therapy to proceed in the best interests of the patient. The challenge for clinicians is to address their own grief, process their feelings of loss, resolve the traumatic effects of multiple loss, and reestablish an appropriate relationship with their dying clients.

Worden (1991) suggested three guidelines for those working with dying patients to help confront and resolve their grief: (a) be aware of personal limitations in terms of the number of dying patients with whom you can work intimately at any given time, (b) engage in active grieving, and (c) know how to reach out for help and support. The first of these guidelines requires therapists to acknowledge limits to their ability to deal with continuous loss and to explore this boundary. Most likely this process can be accomplished only with supervision or in the clinician's own therapy. Accepting that multiple losses and unresolved grief can pose such a limitation to one's ability to work with additional dying clients creates an additional vulnerability that requires appropriate support. The very existence of such limits can threaten the psychotherapist's sense of professional competence, forcing a reexamination of the ego ideal that surrounds the therapist role. Acknowledging that one must curtail or suspend one's work with dying patients is not synonymous with failure; rather, it reflects a healthy respect for the depth of one's connections and attachments. At the same time, failing to explore and ultimately integrate these limits can pose a perilous risk to the clinician and his or her patients.

The second step in the psychotherapist's process of addressing his or her grief is to engage in active grieving and demonstrations of mourning behavior. Psychotherapists are well-served by acknowledging themselves as mourners of the deceased and opening themselves to the vulnerability of their feelings of loss. They may attend funerals or memorial services, engage in private memorial rituals, write or speak publicly or privately about their memories and experiences with the deceased, or set aside special moments of recollection of their clients (Cho & Cassidy, 1994; Gabriel, 1991). One clinician reports that "every now and then I go down to my basement, turn on some music and think of the people who died" (Sleek, 1996, p. 2). Active grieving requires that clinicians allow themselves the freedom to use whatever mode of expressing these painful feelings suggests itself, consistent with other ethical responsibilities.

Rando (1993) counseled practitioners to "adjust [their] expectations about the intensity of reactions, pacing, and duration of treatment for these types of mourners" (p. 78). She cautioned that practitioners must be prepared for an extended period of treatment where nothing seems to be happening. Multiple loss or "bereavement overload" is traumatizing, and the clinical course reflects the need to address this additional psychic injury (Elia, 1997).

Rando's cautions apply equally to the clinician experiencing multiple losses of clients to AIDS. How are the processes of grief to be apportioned? How are the grieving person's various broken attachments to be identified and processed? The psychotherapist whose practice includes many clients who die from AIDS-related complications must confront not only personal grief over the broken attachments to these individuals, but the trauma associated with multiple loss. Therapists clearly do not feel the same depth of grief and distress for every client who dies. Each loss assumes its own importance and requires its own process. Facing the weight of multiple losses involves sorting out one's relationship to each person who has died and assigning one's own measure of meaning to it.

One final task in the process of coping with all of the emotional burdens of treating dying patients is to reach out for emotional support and sustenance. This may be among the most difficult steps for clinicians to take, but it is essential to dealing with burnout, countertransference, and especially grief and the trauma of multiple losses. If work with the dying teaches anything, it is that therapists cannot proceed in isolation, and the literature sounds a continuous admonition to psychotherapists to find support in peer supervision, support groups, or their own psychotherapy. This repetition suggests the intractability of psychotherapists' reluctance to open themselves to their own needs.

At the core of clinicians' grief is their own relationship to death. Clinicians working with people infected with HIV confront mortality on a daily basis. Such proximity cannot be ignored. Up close, death demands a response. Clinicians' exploration of the mystery of their own mortality, their anxieties about death, their spiritual orientation to death, their previous losses, and similar material can begin to restore a sense of balance in the face of the seemingly endless deaths associated with AIDS. To continue to engage in sound practice, clinicians must reach a point of congruence where they can experience the emotions attached to their losses without jeopardizing their work with clients (Boniello, 1990).

CONCLUSION

Grief and multiple losses can affect the psychotherapist's ability to make sound decisions in treatment by generating defensive reactions that interfere with the ability to maintain an appropriately neutral and empathic stance. The effects of loss must be addressed on their own terms and not conflated with burnout or confused with countertransference, although all of these phenomena may affect the clinician dealing with large numbers of patients dying from AIDS-related complications.

Facing grief and loss requires psychotherapists to explore their own limits to dealing with dying patients. The grieving therapist is served by actively grieving clients' deaths and seeking support from peers or in psychotherapy to process the effects on these losses.

REFERENCES

AIDS Legal Referral Panel. (1998, September). *Barriers to health care for HIV-positive women: Deadly denial.* San Francisco: AIDS Legal Referral Panel.

Barret, R. L. (1997). Countertransference issues in HIV-related psychotherapy. In M. G. Winiarski (Ed.), *HIV mental health for the 21st century* (pp. 39–51). New York: New York University Press.

Bennett, L. (1995) AIDS health care: Staff stress, loss and bereavement. In L. Sherr (Ed.), *Grief and AIDS* (pp. 87–102). Chichester, England: Wiley.

Bennett, L., Kelaher, M., & Ross, M. W. (1994). Impact of working with HIV/AIDS on health care professionals: Development of the AIDS impact scale. *Psychology and Health, 9*(3), 221–232.

Boniello, M. (1990). Grieving sexual abuse: The therapist's process. *Clinical Social Work Journal, 18,* 367–379.

Bowlby, J. (1979). *The making & breaking of affectional bonds.* London: Routledge.

Cadwell, S. A. (1994). Empathic challenges for gay male therapists working with HIV-infected men. In S. A. Cadwell, R. A. Burnham, Jr., & M. Fornstein (Eds.), *Therapists on the frontline: Psychotherapy with gay men in the age of AIDS* (pp. 475–496). Washington, DC: American Psychiatric Press.

Carmack, B. J. (1992). Balancing engagement/detachment in AIDS-related multiple losses. *IMAGE Journal of Nursing Scholarship, 24*(1), 9–14.

Centers for Disease Control and Prevention. (August, 1999). *Fact sheet: HIV/AIDS among African Americans* (on-line). Available: http://www.cdc.gov/nchstop/hiv_aids/pubs/facts/afam.htm.

Cho, C., & Cassidy, D. F. (1994). Parallel process for workers and their clients in chronic bereavement resulting from HIV. *Death Studies, 18*, 273–292.

Dane, B. O. (1995). Overcoming grief associated with caring for AIDS patients. In W. Odets & M. Shernoff (Eds.), *The second decade of AIDS* (pp. 275–291). New York: Hatherleigh Press.

Davidson, K. W., & Foster, Z. (1995). Social work with dying and bereaved clients: Helping the workers. *Social Work in Health Care, 21*(4), 1–16.

Doka, K. J. (1989). *Disenfranchised grief: Recognizing hidden sorrow.* New York: Lexington Books.

Elia, N. (1997). Grief and loss in HIV/AIDS work. In M. G. Winiarski (Ed.), *HIV mental health for the 21st century* (pp. 67–81). New York: New York University Press.

Farber, B. A. (1990). Burnout in psychotherapists: Incidence, types, and trends. *Psychotherapy in Private Practice, 8*(1), 35–44.

Fishman, J. M. (1994). Countertransference, the therapeutic frame, and AIDS: One therapist's response. In S. A. Cadwell, R. A. Burnham, Jr., & M. Fornstein (Eds.), *Therapists on the frontline: Psychotherapy with gay men in the age of AIDS* (pp. 497–516). Washington, DC: American Psychiatric Press.

Freudenberger, H. J. (1974). Staff burnout. *Journal of Social Sciences, 30*(1), 159–165.

Gabriel, M. A. (1991). Group therapists' countertransference reactions to multiple deaths from AIDS. *Clinical Social Work Journal, 19*(3), 279–292.

Giovacchini, P. L. (1987). *Countertransference triumphs and catastrophes.* Northvale, NJ: James Aronson.

Hamilton, N. G. (1990). *Self and others: Object relations theory in practice.* Northvale, NJ: James Aronson.

Horner, A. J. (1993). Occupational hazards and characterological vulnerability: The problem of "burnout." *American Journal of Psychoanalysts, 53*(2), 137–142.

Maslach, C. (1981). Burnout: A social psychological analysis. In J. Jones (Ed.), *The burnout syndrome: Current research, theory, and interventions* (pp. 142–163). Park Ridge, IL: London House.

Maslach, C., & Jackson, S. E. (1981). *Maslach burnout inventory: Research edition manual.* Palo Alto, CA: Consulting Psychologists Press.

Miller, G., Wagner, A., Britton, T. P., & Gridley, B.E. (1998). A framework for understanding the wounding of healers. *Counseling and Values, 42*, 124–132.

Piedmont, R. L. (1993). A longitudinal analysis of burnout in the health care setting: The role of personal dispositions. *Journal of Personality Assessment, 61*, 457–473.

Rando, T. A. (Ed.). (1986). *Loss and anticipatory grief.* Lexington, MA: Lexington Books.

Rando, T. A. (1993). *Treatment of complicated mourning.* Champaign, IL: Research Press.

Shernoff, M., & Springer, E. (1992). Substance abuse and AIDS: Report from the front lines (The impact on professionals). *Journal of Chemical Dependency Treatment, 5*(1), 35–48.

Skorupa, J., & Agresti, A. (1993). Ethical beliefs about burnout and continued professional practice. *Professional Psychology: Research and Practice, 24*, 281–285.

Sleek, S. (1996, June). AIDS therapy: patchwork of pain, hope. *APA Monitor.* Available: http://www.apa.org/monitor/jun96/practica.html.

Thornton, P. (1992). The relations of coping, appraisal, and burnout in mental health workers. *Journal of Psychology, 126*, 261–271.

Ussher, J. (1991). Professionals don't cry—Death and dying in AIDS psychology. In C. Newnes (Ed.), *Death, dying and society: A special issue of Psychology and Psychotherapy.* Hove, England: Lawrence Erlbaum.

van Servellen, G., & Leake, B. (1993). Burn-out in hospital nurses: A comparison of acquired immunodeficiency syndrome, oncology, general medical, and intensive care unit nurse samples. *Journal of Professional Nursing, 9*(3), 169–177.

Worden, J. W. (1991). *Grief counseling and grief therapy: A handbook for the mental health practitioner.* New York: Springer.

Yiu-Kee, C., & Tang, C. S. (1995). Existential correlates of burnout among mental health professionals in Hong Kong. *Journal of Mental Health Counseling, 17*(2), 220–229.

6

CLINICAL DECISION MAKING IN THE SHADOW OF LAW

SCOTT BURRIS

A client asks you to help him die. Or tells you that he is so weak that he uses his cane to depress the brake pedal in his car. Or states an intention to have unsafe sex despite her HIV infection. At once, and with apparently little time for reflection, you are presented with a demand for clinical judgment. Is this client depressed? Angry? Homicidal? Clinical evaluation is neither straightforward nor mechanical even under the best of circumstances. Diagnosis, and the prediction of future behavior, present numerous opportunities for error. Professional rules of thumb may enhance the chances of mistake (Bersoff, 1992). No ethical rule or professional standard of care provides a specific answer to your questions.

Even if you feel relatively comfortable in your analysis of the client's mental state, dilemmas like these frequently turn on questions of fact that the professional is not trained to answer or whose answer depends on information that simply is not available. How dangerous is my client's driving? What are the chances of my client actually transmitting HIV to another person?

You feel the vaguely disorienting tug of community obligation. Accustomed to a client-centered focus, you are now in a position of protecting third parties or of imposing others' choices on your client. You are being asked to decide moral questions that are of great importance to society and

99

to which society itself has no answer. When does life cease to be worth living? Does the client have a right to die? Who is responsible for preventing HIV transmission? At this point, the shadow of the law becomes apparent. There are rules about protecting third parties, but it is not clear what behavior they dictate here. Moreover, even the clear rules raise questions: Assisting a suicide is against the law, but so what? In many states, so is sodomy. Is this law still "the law," or is it honored only in its breach? Ought it to be honored, or does honor itself require disobedience? At any rate, the law does not enforce itself. Your "legal risk" depends on someone who learns of your choices and wants to sue or prosecute you. You wonder how that all works.

In accepting responsibility for the problem, you face your own limitations. Assuming that you want to act to change the client's intentions, what can you do? The usual tools of therapy work gradually; much depends on the client, and there are no guarantees. The client in your dilemma does not oblige by displaying the conventional markers of courtroom-drama madness. You are still not sure that there is really a problem. You wonder if you are overreacting. Yet the law seems to require of you a decisive act, without telling you what that act should be. Is this a police matter? Are you supposed to bodily confiscate the client's keys? Tack up "unwanted posters" wherever your client seeks sex? What about your own well-being and your fear of being humiliated or ruined by a lawsuit?

In a moment like this, law may loom as a threat, in which form it does not help you make a good decision and may actually impel you into unnecessarily harming your client or yourself. In this chapter, I present more than just the rules that you might think of as "the law." To assess your "legal risk," you need to recognize the social and cultural aspects of the law. Among other things, law is a set of relations among lawyers, clients, police, and judges, relations that are marked by often extreme differences in raw power, professional authority, knowledge, and socioeconomic status. The production and interpretation of legal rules take place on a field of political and social conflict and often mirror rather than resolve major social disputes. It can be helpful to see law operating in this kind of messy complexity, rather than as a coherent, monolithic system producing clear rules. At least it suggests that you are not alone in your uncertainty and that you can use the same tools that you use to navigate the messy channels of your own life to get your bearings in a legal dilemma.

For all its built-in uncertainty, law is also a professional discipline with a well-developed approach to analyzing and making judgments about how rules will be applied to individual disputes. Many of its analytic techniques, although clothed in terms of doctrinal rules, actually concern the values and biases within and beyond the legal culture. The behavior of police, prosecutors, and judges is reasonably predictable within the norms and values prevalent in the legal system in any particular locality, and good lawyers can help their clients make decisions that are both morally sound and legally supportable.

Psychotherapists can be sued when they fail to fulfill their professional duties to clients. Law does provide a set of rules that set meaningful limits on professional behavior in areas including privacy, assisted suicide, and the obligation to protect third parties from a dangerous client. I introduce these rules in this chapter and discuss them in more detail throughout the case studies. But the rules are only part of the story. Social and psychological factors are decisive in determining who is or is not hauled into court. Once there, legal procedure and litigation tactics can be as important as the content of the rules in determining the outcome. I discuss these factors—who sues, who doesn't; what happens in litigation; the influence of socioeconomic and political factors—and then conclude the chapter with a checklist for assessing legal risk within a professional dilemma.

LEGAL RULES

Psychologists (and other practitioners such as psychiatrists and social workers) are licensed by the state and are subject to rules of professional conduct administered by a professional board or licensing agency (e.g., PA. STAT. tit. 63, 2000). Licensing rules usually specify forms of unprofessional conduct and set out procedures for disciplining licensees accused of violating professional norms. *Unprofessional conduct* is sometimes defined to embrace violating a criminal statute or chronically failing to meet professional standards of care. I assume that the reader is familiar with licensing requirements and the rules of professional conduct; they are not addressed in this chapter.

Key Concepts in Tort Law: Duty, Causation, and Breach

Torts is the branch of law that allows one person to sue another for acting carelessly and causing harm. *Professional malpractice* is the tort of harming a client by conduct that does not measure up to the standards of the profession. In essence, it is doing things in care that most of one's peers would not do or failing to do things that most of them would. The professional's conduct is assessed by the judge or jury by reference to testimony about the proper course of professional conduct provided by professionals appearing as expert witnesses (Herman & Burris, 1993).

The most famous, not to say notorious, malpractice case involving psychotherapy is surely *Tarasoff v. Board of Regents of the University of California* (1976), which arose after Tatiana Tarasoff was murdered by Prosenjit Poddar. Poddar was a graduate student at the University of California and a patient of Dr. Lawrence Moore, a university employee. The plaintiffs (Ms. Tarasoff's parents) claimed that Poddar had told Moore that he intended to kill Tatiana and that Moore, his supervisor, and the campus police were negligent for failing either to confine Poddar or warn Tatiana of the danger. The California Supreme Court eventually ruled that it would be malpractice for a psychotherapist to fail to take reasonable steps to warn or otherwise protect a person in Tatiana's situation and sent the case back to the lower court to determine whether or not the defendants had in fact taken reasonable steps. The case was settled before a trial could answer the question.

Tarasoff was a dramatic case, which was unusually well-publicized among psychotherapists and which generated considerable controversy within the mental health professions (Givelber, Bowers, & Blitch, 1984). Its actual significance in law has been far less than its reputation suggests, but it is a good example of a tort case, and I use it to illustrate key legal concepts throughout this chapter.

Lawyers are trained to deal with the social as well as the intellectual complexity of the legal system, and much of the predictability of the system is owed to the uniform training of all lawyers. Phrases like "thinking like a lawyer" or "applying the law to the facts" capture, but unfortunately do little to convey, the essence of legal reasoning, largely because being a lawyer is as much a cultural as an analytic experience. I cannot recreate 3 years of law school acculturation here, but I can at least illustrate the approach law school inculcates by looking at three of the most important concepts in tort law.

Legal rules are divisible by lawyers into distinct "elements." For example, the tort of negligence is usually said to require proof by the plaintiff of the existence of a duty owed by the defendant to the plaintiff, a breach of the duty, and injury to the plaintiff caused by the breach (Herman & Burris, 1993). Lawyers then use these elements to organize the facts of the case, assigning to each fact a degree of relevance according to how it serves to establish the existence or nonexistence of each element. This, in turn, leads to the identification of the "real" issues in the case—the elements most lawyers will find to be questionable or "in dispute." Because plaintiffs must establish all the elements of their cases to prevail, defendants and courts will often concede or assume that some elements have been proven in order to focus more clearly on the most fatally defective one. The practice of categorizing and labeling, often using counter-factual assumptions, is the lawyer's stock in trade and has many benefits. Through this approach, complicated situations can be made coherent (at least to the lawyers), and the process, particularly in its prospective form, promotes close attention to facts.

In the *Tarasoff* case, there was no dispute that there had been an injury, nor, for purposes of the legal argument about the existence of a duty to protect, did the parties argue over whether the psychotherapist in fact breached the duty or whether that breach was the cause of the harm. That is very important to understanding the meaning of *Tarasoff*. No court ever considered the question of whether the defendant psychotherapist had actually failed to live up to professional standards of care. Had not the case been settled after the supreme court's ruling, Dr. Moore would have argued that he satisfied his professional obligations by alerting the campus police of the threats and trying to commit Poddar.

The plaintiff in every tort case must prove not only that the defendant did something wrong, but also that that faulty act or omission was the cause of the plaintiff's injury. This element of the case is referred to as *cause in fact*. People do many negligent things without committing torts, because there is no liability unless the act has caused harm. Perhaps Moore was an incompetent psychotherapist, but most of his student clients were intelligent or resilient enough not to have been harmed by his many professional failures. Under these circumstances, although he had a duty to meet the standard of care of comparably trained therapists, and although he may have breached this duty in case after case, he committed no tort because his breaches caused no harm.

The allegation in *Tarasoff* was that a competent psychotherapist would have warned Tatiana of the danger and that such an action would have prevented her death. Causation is often difficult to assess from the retrospective position of a judge or jury. It can be hard to decide what would have happened if something that was not done had been done. It seems reasonable to assume, however, that if Dr. Moore had succeeded in committing Poddar, or warning Tatiana, Poddar would not have been able to kill her.

Duty in tort law is a relationship with another that creates an obligation to act with reasonable prudence in matters that would affect that individual. It has proven impossible to specify the sort of relationship needed to create a duty, yet the concept is a useful one for lawyers. Whereas causation looks back to what has happened because of an act or omission, the duty analysis looks forward from the moment of action to who was likely to be affected. Had promises been made? Who stood in harm's way? What were their expectations of the actor's conduct? To what consideration and care were they entitled? This, of course, was the issue in *Tarasoff*: If the psychotherapist had no obligation to watch out for nonpatients under any circumstances, then the Tarasoffs' case should be dismissed, even if he failed to meet professional standards and caused Tatiana harm. In thinking through a legal dilemma, the notion of duty helps the lawyer identify the significant stakeholders whose concerns need to be considered.

Breach, also referred to as *negligence*, is the failure to behave in a reasonably prudent manner. Ordinarily, the measure of this common prudence is the "reasonable (wo)man," a mythical average Joe, impersonated for trial purposes by the randomly selected members of the jury. When the defendant is a person with special skills and knowledge, like the therapists in *Tarasoff*, the law looks to a professional standard of care, defined by expert witnesses. There tends to be a great deal of perfect hindsight in the application of these standards by juries, but for the lawyer and psychotherapist considering an ethical dilemma, the concept can help to properly direct attention from the law back to psychology. The psychotherapist is not required to have a perfect solution, but only to deal with the problem in a way that conforms to the standards of the profession. A crisis is the worst time for a psychotherapist to stop acting like a psychotherapist.

The Duty to Warn and Protect

Psychotherapists certainly have a duty in tort law to behave professionally toward their patients. What made the *Tarasoff* case unusual was that the victim of the alleged malpractice was not the patient, but a stranger. Tatiana Tarasoff was murdered not by the psychotherapist, but by his patient, and the therapist's supposed failure to meet professional standards lay in the steps he took, or failed to take, to control his patient or warn a complete stranger.

The traditional rule in American law held that Peter generally had no duty to protect Mary from Paul's misdeeds—unless there existed a "special relationship" between either Peter and Paul or Peter and Mary that would create an expectation of or right to protection (American Law Institute, 1965, § 315). Such a relationship usually involves Peter's care of or control over Paul or Mary. For example, a parent has a duty to protect others from any harm that his child may cause, and a jailer has a duty to protect weaker inmates or civilians from the meaner ones. One could also take on a duty voluntarily, by promising to do something clearly necessary to the well-being of Paul or Mary.

In *Tarasoff*, the California Supreme Court applied these tenets of the common law for the first time to the therapist–client situation: "by entering into a doctor–patient relationship the therapist becomes sufficiently involved to assume some responsibility for the safety, not only of the patient himself, but also of any person whom the doctor knows to be threatened by the patient" (*Tarasoff*, 1976, p. 344). Given that special relationship, "once a psychotherapist does in fact determine, or under applicable professional standards should have determined, that a patient poses a serious danger of violence to others, he bears a duty to exercise reasonable care to protect the foreseeable victim of that danger" (p. 345). This duty, the court suggested rather broadly, could be fulfilled by committing the patient, or warning the victim, or taking other steps reasonable under the circumstances. Note that "warning" the victim or the authorities was not indispensable, but simply one way a professional could discharge the duty. Note also that the duty did not apply to the whole world—anyone who might eventually be hurt by the client—but only to "foreseeable" victims, that is, people that the psychotherapist could reasonably be expected to identify as being at real risk.

Tarasoff's reputation far exceeded its actual geographical reach. It was a decision of a California court and so created a binding legal rule only within that state. Courts in almost every state have endorsed the general legal principles regarding a duty to protect, but far fewer have explicitly extended these principles to cover the therapist–client relationship. Most courts that have specifically considered the question of the psychotherapist–client relationships have endorsed the *Tarasoff* analysis (*Bradley v. Ray*, 1995). Many of these decisions were issued by lower courts, however, and so do not represent the final word about their states' law (see Table 6.1). In many instances, the duty of professionals to third parties has been addressed in cases that do not involve psychotherapists.

Predictably, problems have arisen when courts attempt to apply the rule to specific situations. For example, what exactly is a "foreseeable victim"? How is this duty to protect to be carried out? Courts have also differed markedly on their definition of who has to be protected. Certainly courts have not fully grasped that the best way for a psychotherapist to protect third parties may often be to keep treating the client without any other measures that might interfere with treatment (Felthouse, 1989). Although most courts have required the protection of only reasonably identifiable victims (*Novak v. Rathnam*, 1987), some have gone so far as to expand the duty to all potential victims, regardless of how difficult it might be for a psychotherapist to know of their existence or identity (*Schuster v. Altenberg*, 1988).

In an attempt to eliminate some of this confusion, 23 states have passed laws regarding the duty to protect (see Table 6.2). These statutes generally do three things: first, they define when a duty will arise; second, they set out the ways in which a psychotherapist may discharge the duty, thereby relieving himself of liability for breach of that duty; and third, they provide immunity to therapists for breach of any client confidences disclosed in the discharge of the duty. For example, the California statute, passed in 1985, says a duty will arise only "where the patient has communicated a serious threat of physical violence against a reasonably identifiable victim or victims" (CAL. CIVIL CODE, 2000, § 43.92). The statute also says that the duty will be discharged by making "reasonable efforts" to notify the victims and law enforcement officials of the threat. Although the California statute does not provide immunity for the disclosure of confidential information (such a provision is made elsewhere in California law), most statutes do.

Such statutes do narrow the potential zone of liability. California's statute limits the duty to situations in which the patient has threatened

TABLE 6.1
Court Decisions Setting Out Basis and Extent of Duty to
Warn or Protect in States Without "Tarasoff" Statutes

State	Citation	Duty to Protect Under Some Circumstances	No Duty to Protect
AL	King v. Smith, 539 So.2d 262 (Ala. 1989)		X
AK	Chizmar v. Mackie, 896 P.2d 196 (Alaska 1995)	X	
CT	Frazer v. U.S., 674 A.2d 811 (Conn. 1996)	X	
DC	White v. U.S., 250 U.S. App. D.C. 435 (1986)	X	
GA	Bradley Center v. Wessner, 296 S.E.2d 693 (Ga. 1982)	X	
HI	Seibel v. City and County of Honolulu, 602 P.2d 532 (Haw. 1979)		X
IL	Siklas v. Ecker Center for Mental Health, Inc., 617 N.E.2d 507 (Ill. Ct. App. 1993)	X	
IA	Cole v. Taylor, 301 N.W.2d 766 (Iowa 1981)		X
KS	Boulanger v. Pol, 900 P.2d 823 (Kan. 1995)		X
ME	Joy v. Eastern Maine Medical Center, 529 A.2d 1364 (Me. 1987)	X	
MIS	Grisham v. John Q. Long V.F.W. Post, 519 So.2d 413 (Miss. 1988)	X	
MO	Scheibel v. Hillis, 531 S.W.2d 285 (Mo. 1976)	X	
NC	Davis v. North Carolina Dept. of Human Resources, 465 S.E.2d 2 (N.C. Ct. App. 1995)	X	
ND	NO CASE ON POINT		
NV	Doud v. Las Vegas Hilton Corp., 864 P.2d 796 (Nev. 1993)	X	
NM	Wilshinsky v. Medina, 775 P.2d 713 (N.M. 1989)	X	
NY	Schrempf v. State of New York, 496 N.Y.S.2d 973 (1985)	X	
OK	Wofford v. Eastern State Hospital, 795 P.2d 516 (Okla. 1990)	X	
OR	Cain v. Rijken, 700 P.2d 1061 (Or. 1985)	X	
PA	Dunkle v. Food Service East, Inc., 582 A.2d 1342 (Pa. Super. Ct. 1990)		X
RI	Rock v. State of Rhode Island, 681 A.2d 901 (R.I. 1996)		X
SC	Sharpe v. South Carolina Dept. of Mental Health, 354 S.E.2d 778 (S.C. Ct. App. 1987)		X
SD	Tipton v. Town of Tabor, 567 N.W.2d 351 (S.D. 1997)		X
TX	Van Horn v. Chambers, 970 S.W.2d 542 (Tex. 1998)		X
VT	Peck v. Counseling Service of Addison County, Inc. 499 A.2d 422 (Vt. 1985)	X	
WA	Peterson v. State of Washington, 671 P.2d 230 (Wash. 1983)	X	
WI	Schuster v. Altenberg, 424 N.W.2d 159 (Wis. 1988)	X	
WV	NO CASE ON POINT		
WY	NO CASE ON POINT		

"physical violence." Yet even these statutes leave questions: When is a potential victim "reasonably identifiable?" What constitutes "reasonable efforts" to prevent the harm? When is a threat serious enough to trigger an obligation to warn? In theory, what is reasonable is to be judged on the basis of what a properly trained psychotherapist exercising his normal professional judgment would think reasonable. Some insight comes from looking at similar cases, but so far no published case has applied the duty to protect in a situation in which the risk to others is HIV infection.

The *Tarasoff* problem is often discussed as a tension between the therapist's duty to protect others from his patient's violent tendencies and his duty to keep conversations with his patient confidential. Although this might be true from an ethical standpoint, there is, in fact, very little legal tension at all. It has been widely recognized by courts across the United States for decades that a client's right to confidentiality has many exceptions. Such exceptions generally allow for disclosure of information made in good faith to protect third persons or the general public from potential dangers posed by the client (*Simonsen v. Swenson*, 1920). Thus, in most cases outside the HIV realm, where a psychotherapist comes to a professionally reasonable and good faith opinion that a client is a threat to a third person, that client's right to confidentiality will not cover the therapist's disclosure of the danger. In cases involving individuals with HIV, however, a duty to warn third parties would run head-on into statutes, existing in virtually every state, that preserve the confidentiality of HIV-related information.

HIV Privacy Law

HIV confidentiality laws vary considerably among the states (Burris, 1993b; see Table 6.3). Psychotherapists who maintain records that contain HIV-related information should make a point of knowing what their state law requires of them, if anything. These statutes generally have broad language prohibiting release of information except in narrowly defined circumstances. Some of them deal with the issue of notification of third parties or health authorities concerning a threat posed by a client. These provisions, too, vary in their specificity in defining who can be warned and under what circumstances. The most narrowly tailored of these provisions allow notification only of people with whom the client is likely to have sex or share needles in the future, and then only after the physician has offered counseling to the client and warned the client that notification is going to take place. Normally, these laws require that the client's identity not be revealed (Cal. Health & Safety Code, 1999, § 121015; Conn. Gen. Stat., 1997, §19a-584; N.Y. Public Health Law, 1997, §2782(4)). Maryland's law is exceptional in actually requiring that the identity be revealed (Md. Health-Gen. Code Ann., 1997, §18-337). Some direct that the notification be conducted

TABLE 6.2
State Statutes Defining or Limiting Psychotherapists' Duty to Warn or Protect Third Parties

State and Statute	Basis and Extent of Duty			How Duty is Discharged					
	Duty Limited to Identifiable Victims	Patient Has Intent & Ability for Violence	Patient Makes Actual Threat of Violence	Notify Victim or Police	Notify Both Victim & Police	Attempt to Commit	Attempt Voluntary Hospitalization	Other Reasonable Steps	Immunity for Disclosure
AZ A.R.S. § 36-511	X	X	X		X	X	X	X	X
CA Civ. Code § 43.92	X		X		X	X	X	X	X[a]
CO C.R.S.A. § 13-21-117	X		X		X	X	X	X	X
DE 16 D.C. § 5402	X	X	X		X	X	X		X
FL F.S.A. § 455.671	X	X	X	X					X
ID I.C. § 6-1902	X	X	X		X				X
IN I.C. §34-4-12.4-3			X[b]	X		X		X	X
KY K.R.S. § 202A.400			X		X[c]	X[d]			X
LA L.S.A.-R.S. 9:2800.2	X	X	X		X	X			X
MD Cts. & Jud. Pro. § 5-609	X		X		X	X			X
MA M.G.L.A. ch. 123 § 36B	X	X	X	X		X	X	X	X
MI M.C.L.A. § 330.1946	X	X	X		X	X			X
MN M.S.A. § 148.975	X		X	X[e]					X
MT M.C.A. § 50-1-529	X		X		X				X
NE N.R.S. § 71-1, 206.30	X		X		X				X
NH R.S.A. § 330-A:22	X		X	X		X[f]			X
NJ N.J.S.A. § 2A:62A-16	X	X		X		X	X		X
OH R.C. § 5122.34									X

(continued)

TABLE 6.2
(continued)

State and Statute	Basis and extent of duty			How Duty is Discharged					
	Duty Limited to Identifiable Victims	Patient Has Intent & Ability for Violence	Patient Makes Actual Threat of Violence	Notify Victim or Police	Notify Both Victim & Police	Attempt to Commit	Attempt Voluntary Hospitalization	Other Reasonable Steps	Immunity for Disclosure
SD[g] S.D.C.L. § 36-33-31	X		X		X				X
TN T.C.A. § 33-10-302	X	X	X			X	X		X
UT U.C.A. § 78-14a-102	X		X	X[e]	X				X
VA Code § 54.1-2400.1	X	X	X	X	X	X		X	X
WA R.C.W.A. § 71.05.120	X		X		X				X[h]

[a]Immunity is provided for by separate statute (California Evid. Code § 1024).
[b]Liability can also arise when the patient stops short of making an explicit threat.
[c]Both victim and police notification is required if the victim is identifiable. Where the victim cannot be identified, the statute requires only police notification.
[d]Attempts to commit will only discharge duty if the victim is not identifiable.
[e]The statutes do not mention law enforcement and allow only for victim notification.
[f]Not only must the therapist attempt to have the patient committed, but the commitment also be obtained.
[g]Statute applies only to marriage and family therapists.
[h]Immunity is provided for by a separate statute. (Wash. St. § 71.05.390).

TABLE 6.3
Statutory Protection of HIV and AIDS Information

	AL	AK	AZ	AR	CA	CO	CT	DE	DC
Specific privacy protection for HIV/AIDS information			Y	Y	Y	Y	Y		Y
State law provides for spousal/partner notification									
Person with HIV infection required to reveal name of partner or spouse									
Health care provider or health department may contact persons at risk of exposure	Y			Y	Y	Y	Y		
Health care provider or health department required to contact persons at risk for exposure				Y					
Program permits disclosure of name of source to spouse/partner									
Permissible or mandatory disclosure to									
School official									
Health care provider	P		P		P	P	P	P	
Penal institution	M				M		P		
Insurance company							P		
Blood bank/organ donor			P	M	M			P	
Blood or organ recipient					P				
HMO/health care or mental health facilities			P		P		P		
Epidemiologists/researchers			P	P		P		P	
Subpoena or court order	Y		Y		Y		Y	Y	Y
Other		M	M	M	P	P	P	P	P
Penalties for impermissible disclosure									
Criminal	Y	Y	Y	Y	Y	Y		Y	Y
Civil			Y	Y	Y		Y	Y	

*A Y indicates states with HIV-specific privacy protection by statute. Such information may also be protected by sexually transmitted disease statutes, general health care privacy protections, or common law.
Note. From L.O. Gostin et al., Legislative Survey of State Confidentiality Laws, with Specific Emphasis on HIV and Immunization (Final Report presented to Centers for Disease Control and Prevention, Council of State and Territorial Epidemiologists, and the Carter Presidential Center, 1996). Adapted by permission.
P = permissible; M = mandatory.

(continued)

by a health department (ARIZ. REV. STAT. ANN., 1997, §36-664(K)). Other states have been less exacting, allowing disclosure to contacts or family members without specifying intermediate steps and even, in a few places, without reason to believe that the people notified are at risk (TEX. HEALTH & SAFETY ANN., 1997, §81.103). Georgia's statute, for example, allows disclosure not just to a spouse or sexual partner but to a client's child if the physician "reasonably believes" that the child is at risk of being infected (GA. CODE ANN., 1997, §24-9-47).

These notification rules apply almost universally to physicians only, despite concerns by other health care and mental health professionals about their own legal duties. A general confidentiality rule, however, actually

TABLE 6.3
(continued)

	FL	GA	HI	ID	IL	IN	IA	KS	KY
Specific privacy protection for HIV/AIDS information	Y	Y	Y		Y		Y	Y	
State law provides for spousal/partner notification									
Person with HIV infection required to reveal name of partner or spouse									
Health care provider or health department may contact persons at risk of exposure	Y	B	Y		Y	Y	Y	Y	Y
Health care provider or health department required to contact persons at risk for exposure									
Program permits disclosure of name of source to spouse/partner		Y							
Permissible or mandatory disclosure to									
School official	P				P				
Health care provider	P	P	P	P	P	P	P	P	P
Penal institution	P							P	P
Insurance company		P	P						
Blood bank/organ donor	P		P		P		P		
Blood or organ recipient									
HMO/health care or mental health facilities	P								P
Epidemiologists/researchers	P							P	P
Subpoena or court order	Y		Y		Y	Y	Y		Y
Other	P	P	P	P	P	P	P		P
Penalties for impermissible disclosure									
Criminal	Y	Y			Y		Y	Y	Y
Civil		Y	Y		Y		Y		Y

(continued)

clarifies their obligations as well. When the duty to warn third parties is a product of judge-made common law, a legislative enactment requiring non-disclosure of HIV-related information supersedes the judicial rule and therefore should protect social workers, nurses, psychologists, and others from being successfully sued for failure to warn. Where, however, the duty to warn is statutorily imposed, as it is now in at least 23 states, the tension between the duty to warn and duty to maintain confidentiality is at its strongest. The resulting legal question may come down to rather arcane issues of statutory interpretation, particularly whether the specific commands of the later HIV confidentiality law should be read to have repealed the more general requirements of the *Tarasoff* law in the HIV context.

Psychotherapists working in local, state, or federal agencies are normally subject to additional privacy law. The federal and many state constitutions are increasingly interpreted to protect the privacy of medical information, although in all but a few state constitutions, the right of privacy is

TABLE 6.3
(continued)

	LA	ME	MD	MA	MI	MN	MS	MO	MT
Specific privacy protection for HIV/AIDS information	Y	Y		Y	Y	Q		Y	Y
State law provides for spousal/partner notification									
Person with HIV infection required to reveal name of partner or spouse									
Health care provider or health department may contact persons at risk of exposure	Y		Y		Y	Y		Y	Y
Health care provider or health department required to contact persons at risk for exposure									
Program permits disclosure of name of source to spouse/partner					M				
Permissible or mandatory disclosure to									
School official						P		M	
Health care provider	P	P		P	P	P	P	P	P
Penal institution	P	P							
Insurance company		P							
Blood bank/organ donor	P	P					P		
Blood or organ recipient									
HMO/health care or mental health facilities	P								
Epidemiologists/researchers	P	P							P
Subpoena or court order	Y	Y			Y	P			
Other	P	P	P	P	P	P	P	P	P
Penalties for impermissible disclosure									
Criminal	Y	Y	Y		Y	Y			Y
Civil		Y	Y	Y	Y	Y		Y	Y

*A Y indicates states with HIV-specific privacy protection by statute. Such information may also be protected by sexually transmitted disease statutes, general health care privacy protections, or common law. *Note.* From L.O. Gostin et al., Legislative Survey of State Confidentiality Laws, with Specific Emphasis on HIV and Immunization (Final Report presented to Centers for Disease Control and Prevention, Council of State and Territorial Epidemiologists, and the Carter Presidential Center, 1996). Adapted by permission. P = permissible; M = mandatory.

(continued)

not explicitly stated (Chlapowski, 1991; Kreimer, 1991; Silverstein, 1989; *Whalen v. Roe*, 1977). Privacy protection has been found by courts to be particularly necessary for HIV-related information (*Doe v. Borough of Barrington*, 1990).

Assisted Suicide

Tort law, and the law of privacy, fall into the larger class of "civil" cases, those brought by private parties to recover money damages. Some of the case studies in this book raise issues in criminal law, the branch of law dealing with the government's enforcement of rules of conduct whose

TABLE 6.3
(continued)

	NE	NV	NH	NJ	NM	NY	NC	ND	OH
Specific privacy protection for HIV/AIDS information	Y		Y	Y	Y	Y	Y	Y	Y
State law provides for spousal/partner notification									
Person with HIV infection required to reveal name of partner or spouse							Y	F	
Health care provider or health department may contact persons at risk of exposure	Y	Y	Y			Y			Y
Health care provider or health department required to contact persons at risk for exposure						Y			
Program permits disclosure of name of source to spouse/partner									Y
Permissible or mandatory disclosure to									
School official		M				P	P		
Health care provider	P	P	P	P	P	P	P	P	P
Penal institution						P	P		
Insurance company					P	P			
Blood bank/organ donor						P	P		P	P
Blood or organ recipient									
HMO/health care or mental health facilities		M				P			P
Epidemiologists/researchers	P			P	P		P	P	
Subpoena or court order					Y		Y	Y	Y	Y
Other	P	P	P	P	P	P	P	P	P
Penalties for impermissible disclosure									
Criminal		Y				Y	Y	Y	
Civil		Y	Y	Y		Y		Y	Y

(continued)

violation is punished by fines or imprisonment. Most notable is the issue of assisting in a suicide. Nearly all states have some prohibition of helping another commit suicide (see Table 6.4). Some states prohibit the conduct by statute, others in court decisions defining the act to fall within the general category of homicide (*Compassion in Dying v. State of Washington*, 1996; Young, 1992). In 1997, the Supreme Court ruled that there was no "right to die" that conferred on a citizen the right to have assistance in committing suicide (*Washington v. Gluckberg*, 1997; *Vacco v. Quill*, 1997). In practical terms, the Court upheld the authority of states to make assisting suicide a crime. The decision answered some questions about end-of-life care but by no means all of them. For our purposes, there is still some uncertainty as to exactly what conduct would constitute "assisting a suicide."

Taking active part in a suicide—loading a gun or providing a fatal dose of medication—would almost surely count as assisting a suicide, but many things a psychotherapist could do in the course of providing client

TABLE 6.3
(continued)

	OK	OR	PA	RI	SC	SD	TN	TX	UT
Specific privacy protection for HIV/AIDS information	Y	Y	Y	Y		H	I	Y	Y
State law provides for spousal/partner notification									
Person with HIV infection required to reveal name of partner or spouse								Y	
Health care provider or health department may contact persons at risk for exposure	Y		Y	Y				Y	Y
Health care provider or health department required to contact persons at risk for exposure		Y				Y	J		
Program permits disclosure of name of source to spouse/partner									
Permissible or mandatory disclosure to									
School official	P				P	M			P
Health care provider	P	P	P	P	P			P	P
Penal institution									
Insurance company					P				
Blood bank/organ donor						P	P	P	P
Blood or organ recipient						P		P	
HMO/health care or mental health facilities					P			P	
Epidemiologists/researchers	P							P	P
Subpoena or court order	M	M	M	M			Y		
Other	P	P	P	P	P			P	P
Penalties for impermissible disclosure									
Criminal	Y				Y	Y		Y	Y
Civil	Y	Y	Y	Y				Y	Y

*A Y indicates states with HIV-specific privacy protection by statute. Such information may also be protected by sexually transmitted disease statutes, general health care privacy protections, or common law. *Note.* From L.O. Gostin et al., Legislative Survey of State Confidentiality Laws, with Specific Emphasis on HIV and Immunization (Final Report presented to Centers for Disease Control and Prevention, Council of State and Territorial Epidemiologists, and the Carter Presidential Center, 1996). Adapted by permission. P = permissible; M = mandatory.

care might be of practical assistance to a person considering suicide. Mental health professionals can play a valuable role in a client's decisions about dying. As described by a group of mental health professionals in a brief to the Supreme Court,

> Professionals can, for example, help patients to address issues such as pain, depression, dignity, tranquility, financial concerns, and the effectiveness or futility of available medical treatments. In addition, they can assist the patient to communicate with other health care providers, family members, social service providers, or others concerning the patient's needs, concerns and preferences, to help ensure that the patient receives necessary support and that the treatment provided comports with the patient's wishes. Finally, professionals can promote

and monitor appropriate involvement by significant others in a patient's end-of-life decisions, and they can counsel both patients and survivors in the inevitable process of grieving. (Washington State Psychological Association, 1997)

In theory, a wide range of acts could meet the statutory or common law definition of assisting in a suicide, from pulling the trigger for a person too weak to do it, to providing a gun and bullets or prescription drugs to a person who wants to kill himself or herself, to telling a person how to get the necessary means for suicide, to simply counseling a person who is thinking of suicide in a way that facilitates a decision to die. Many states' assisted suicide statutes have very broad definitions of assistance, allowing, at least in theory, for a wide range of prosecutions. For example, the California statute purports to punish anyone who "deliberately aids, advises, or encourages another to commit suicide" (CAL. PENAL CODE, 1997). General criminal laws are susceptible to a similarly broad interpretation. The North Dakota murder statute provides that anyone who "intentionally or knowingly causes the death of another human being" is guilty of murder (N.D. CENT. CODE, 1985). Under this statute and according to the state supreme court, murder does not require that a person shoot, hit, or throw an object at a person, but only that one engage in conduct that contributes to or results in the death of another person (*State v. Morrissey*, 1980).

In practice, courts have interpreted "assistance" narrowly, requiring some affirmative and direct conduct, such as providing the means for suicide, and not simply discussions about suicide (*Donaldson v. Van de Kamp*, 1992). Most of the rather small number of assisted suicide cases have dealt with defendants who do the actual killing, at the request of the victim or under a mutual suicide pact, and many actually focus on the question of where assisting suicide begins and murder ends, not on where the line is drawn between assisting suicide and complete innocence (*State v. Cobb*, 1981; *State v. Sexson*, 1994). Thus, in *People v. Matlock* (1959), the California Supreme Court held that a person who acceded to the victim's request to be strangled was guilty of murder rather than assisted suicide. The many cases against Dr. Jack Kevorkian, who has supplied clients with a variety of "suicide machines" and may, on occasion, have helped turn them on, fall squarely on this line between assisted suicide and murder (*People v. Kevorkian*, 1995). His ultimate conviction on murder charges came only after he publicized a videotape showing him personally administering a fatal dose (Belluck, 1999). Only a few cases have dealt with lesser forms of help, like filling a bathtub for a woman who wanted to drown herself (*State v. Bouse*, 1953). No cases have been brought against therapists or family members for providing emotional support to individuals who planned to take their own lives, which probably is a more accurate measure of what the law "is" than the broad language of statutes and court decisions. Moreover, commentators

TABLE 6.4
State Criminalization of Assisted Suicide

State	Court Decisions Impose Criminal Penalties for Assisting in Suicide	Homicide Includes Assisted Suicide	Statute Explicitly Prohibits Assisting in Suicide	Statute Authorizes Assisting a Suicide Under Certain Circumstances
AL		Ala. Code § 13A-6-1		
AK			Alaska Stat. § 11.41.1120	
AZ			Ariz. Rev. Stat. Ann. § 13-1103	
AR			Ark. Code Ann. § 5-10-104	
CA			Cal. Penal Code § 401	
CO			Colo. Rev. Stat. § 18-3-104(1)(B)	
CT			Conn. Gen. Stat. §§ 53A54A,-56	
DE			Del. Code. Ann. tit. 11, §§ 632, 645	
DC[a]			D.C. Code Ann. § 6-2428	
FL			Fla. Stat. Ann. § 782.08	
GA			Ga. Code Ann. § 16-5-5	
HI			Haw. Rev. Stat. § 707-702	
ID[a]			Idaho Code §39-152	
IL			Ill. Comp. Stat. 720 5/12-31	
IN			Ind. Code §§35-42-1-2, -2.5	
IA			Iowa Code §707A.2, 707A.3	
KS			Kan. Stat. Ann. § 21-3406	
KY			Ky. Rev. Stat. Ann. § 216.302	
LA				
ME			Me. Rev. Stat. Ann. tit. 17-A, §204	
MD				
MA	Comm. v. Mink, 123 Mass. 422 (Mass. 1877)			
MI			Mich. Comp. Laws § 752.1027	
MN			Minn. Stat. Ann. § 609.215	
MS			Miss. Code Ann. § 97-3-49	
MO			Mo. Rev. Stat. § 565.023 (1)(2)	
MT			Mont. Code Ann. § 45-5-105	
NE			Neb. Rev. Stat. § 28-307	

(continued)

TABLE 6.4
(continued)

State	Court Decisions Impose Criminal Penalties for Assisting in Suicide	Homicide Includes Assisted Suicide	Statute Explicitly Prohibits Assisting in Suicide	Statute Authorizes Assisting a Suicide Under Certain Circumstances
NV			Nev. Rev. Stat. § 449.670	
NH			N.H. Rev. Stat. Ann. § 630:4	
NJ			N.J. Stat. Ann. §2C:11-6	
NM			N.M. Stat. Ann. § 30-2-4	
NY			N.Y. Penal Law §§ 0.30, 120.35, 125.15(3), 125.25(1)(b)	
NC	State v. Willis, 121 S.E.2d 854 (1961)			
ND			N.D. Cent. Code §12.1-16-04	
OH	Blackburn v. State, 23 Ohio St. 146 (Ohio 1872)			
OK			Okla. Stat. Ann. tit. 21, §§ 813 et seq.	
OR				Or. Rev. Stat. §§ 127.800 et seq.
PA			18 Pa. Cons. Stat. Ann. § 2505	
PR			P.R. Laws Ann. tit. 33, § 4009	
RI			R.I. Gen. Laws §§ 11-60-1, 11-60-3.	
SC	State v. Jones, 86 S.C. 17, 67 S.E. 160 (1910)			
SD			S.D. Codified Laws §§ 22-16-37	
TN			Tenn. Code Ann. § 39-13-216	
TX			Tex. Penal Code Ann. §22.08	
UT				
VT				
VA				
WA			Wash. Rev. Code Ann. §9A.36.060	
WVa			W. Va. Code § 16-30-8(a)	
WI			Wis. Stat. Ann. § 940.12	
WY				

[a]Do not impose explicit criminal sanctions on assisted suicide, but nonetheless condemn assisted suicide in statutes allowing withdrawal of medical treatment.

have interpreted the Supreme Court's assisted suicide decisions as suggesting that assisted suicide laws could be found illegal if they created significant barriers to proper treatment of pain and emotional distress at the end of life (Burt, 1997).

Only one state has legalized assisted suicide. The Oregon Death With Dignity Act (1997) allows a terminally ill patient to request a fatal dose of medication from a physician. The request must be made orally at least twice and once in writing. The written request must be witnessed, and it cannot be filled until the patient has been advised of alternatives and evaluated by another physician to confirm the terminal diagnosis and the patient's competence to make the decision. Patients who are not competent must be referred for mental health counseling. Waiting periods and documentation are also specified.

LEGAL PROCESS AND LEGAL MEANING

Although the work of judges and lawyers and legislators might look academic and abstract, the outcome of a dispute about what the rules mean is that someone loses property, freedom, or even life. Likewise, the meaning given to the rules of statutes and court decisions is powerfully influenced by the social values and positions of the parties in a legal dispute and the process through which a disagreement becomes a lawsuit and then the subject of a judicial opinion. In this part of the chapter, I discuss how culture and legal process influence the application of the law and a psychotherapist's risk of being sued.

Uncertainty in Legal Interpretation

The legal system operates on the premise that rules have coherent, comprehensible meanings. As mental health providers are particularly well-qualified to attest, meaning in life is problematic. Most rules are interpreted similarly by most of the people much of the time, but even the apparently clearest of rules gets murky in some factual contexts, often because of the degree to which the interpretation of rules depends on unspoken, unrecognized social understandings about meaning and values (Kairys, 1998). Consider a nearly universal law, "thou shalt not kill." Many faiths subscribe to this law, but few take it literally. Although the rule would clearly prohibit murder as a sport in every culture, killing of all sorts is or has been at times considered morally justified, if not heroic. The rule is usually interpreted as species-specific, so hunting and butchering and fishing are excluded from the rule. It gets even harder when the rules are less straightforward: Consider

Tarasoff's rule that a psychotherapist has a duty to take reasonable steps to protect foreseeable victims from serious dangers posed by a client. As an abstract principle, it is rather clear, but after that . . . . In most but by no means all cases we will know what is meant by the words *psychotherapist* and *client*. In many cases, where there are threats of deliberate violence, defining *serious danger* would not be a big problem, but what about a dangerous driver or lover? We really get into trouble on core legal terms like *foreseeable* and *reasonable*, which ultimately have little specific meaning. In any case that comes to trial, they mean what a jury thinks they mean. Given that most cases filed do not go to trial, it is crucial to understand the other processes by which these terms are assigned meanings in particular contexts in the legal system.

The opinion-writing process is one way that meaning is assigned to disputed legal terms. A judicial opinion, like the one in *Tarasoff*, exemplifies this backward-looking approach, which results in the case law we use to talk about the rules. In judicial opinions, the facts are laid out plainly, doubts resolved, dilemmas dissected in comfortable hindsight. In their zeal to illuminate principles, first the lawyers in the litigation and then the judges have carefully selected and cleaned up the facts, defining the legal issues and throwing out anything "irrelevant" to the chosen conclusion. The case becomes a neat illustration of a self-evident principle. It ceases to resemble life.

This abstracted quality of the case needs to be borne in mind for at least a couple of good reasons. First, case decisions do not necessarily say what they seem to say. For example, most therapists probably believe that the psychologists in *Tarasoff* "lost," that is, that the court ruled that they had failed to properly protect Tatiana. In fact, the court said no such thing. The specific ruling was that the Tarasoffs could proceed with a lawsuit alleging a failure to protect through a warning, and they would be entitled to discovery and, depending on what evidence they developed, to a trial. They did not exercise this option, settling the case for an amount reported to be about $50,000 (Slovenko, 1988). Even in the late 1970s, that was a very low amount for a case involving a fatality, strongly suggesting that the Tarasoffs and their lawyers had doubts about their ability to prove that the therapist actually did anything wrong.

Thinking of law from a judge's perspective is also misleading because most legal interpretation happens in a completely opposite way. When one faces a legal dilemma, one is looking forward, not backward. By definition, a legal question with no obvious answer has never been faced in its exact form before or, to be more accurate, it has never been discussed in a judicial opinion before. (If it had been, there would be an obvious answer.) Client and lawyer are in the position of finding a reasonable interpretation of the rules, predicting, by analogy and a feel for jury and judge attitudes, what the law will be if one's acts lead to litigation. Good judgment and research can bring confidence, but uncertainty is unavoidable.

Legal Meaning and Social Context

Law is an arena for social dispute. That seems obvious in the case of the legislative and executive branches. One would not be surprised to see mental health providers lobbying politicians for a statute to limit *Tarasoff* liability, making arguments from principle and, if they are able, large campaign contributions. A well-organized effort might generate newspaper editorials and opinion pieces. At some level of sincerity and knowledge, legislators and constituents would debate the merits of making therapists responsible for controlling their dangerous clients, or of allowing assisted suicide, and so on. Courts also play a part in political debate. Judges and juries themselves are part of the public; they leave neither their opinions nor their values at the court house door, and what happens in courtrooms also can have an educative, or cathartic, or mobilizing effect on society. What *Tarasoff* has been for therapists, cases like *Roe v. Wade* (1973) or the prosecutions of Jack Kevorkian are to those fighting over "rights" to life or death. For better or for worse, a major court case will often assume a symbolic role far greater than its actual weight as a legal precedent. Being the defendant in a case like that entails being caught up in something larger than one's own acts and opinions. It also affects how the rules, however clear, will actually be applied.

The legal culture has its idiosyncrasies, but it is continuous with the rest of American social life. Judges and lawyers are better educated and more affluent than the average person. The typical lawyer is not out to fundamentally alter a society in which he or she is doing fairly well. It should be no surprise, then, that things like wealth, education, and connections are as helpful in the courtroom as they are on the street. Professional status, particularly in health care, earns deference from the court not simply as a matter of culture but as one of doctrine (Bersoff, 1992). It is perhaps in this light that the *Tarasoff* case strikes some as so extraordinary: not the notion that a person should take reasonable steps to prevent an obvious harm, but that a court should presume to demand such behavior of a professional and undertake to interrogate and punish him for the manner in which he exercised his discretion. Surely it also made a difference in the outcome of the case that the victim was an "innocent coed" and not, say, a prostitute with HIV (Aiken & Musheno, 1994; Galanter, 1974).

Ringing phrases like "We live in a system of laws not men," and "every man is equal before the law" suggest a great equality—unless you happen to be a woman. Or poor. Frequently, equality in the law takes the form immortalized by Anatole France in his observation about "the majestic egalitarianism of the law, which forbids rich and poor alike to sleep under bridges, to beg in the streets, and to steal bread" (*Macmillan Dictionary of Quotations*, 1989, p. 192). When the case concerns HIV, social attitudes about the disease and the behaviors that cause it are frequently far more important to a judge's decision than the words of the legal rules. In one study, for example, Musheno and colleagues found that negative imagery concerning HIV was a consistent feature in decisions denying legal claims of people with HIV (Musheno, Gregware, & Drass, 1991).

Law works to normalize and perpetuate existing social relations, including relations of power–weakness and wealth–poverty. Examples are legion. Until very recently, the institution of marriage was treated by the law as so "private" that ordinary rules against violence and rape were unavailable to married women (Taub & Schneider, 1998). Gay or lesbian sexual relations are branded as "sodomy" and thus criminal. Although law also sometimes allows the have-nots, outcasts, misfits, and progressives to successfully challenge the established order and to make substantial change, it is unwise to confuse the exception with the rule (Galanter, 1974; Rosenberg, 1991). Therapists who are sued go into court with some advantages—they have professional authority and the legal and financial resources of a liability insurance company. If the therapist is White and male, all the better. If the plaintiff has HIV, and the therapist has breached a "right" like privacy in order to "protect" innocent life, the picture gets even brighter for the defendant (Musheno et al., 1991).

Legal Procedure

It is by no means easy for a disagreement to become a lawsuit, and the barriers start well before any lawyers get involved. In the past 20 years, there has been extensive research on what has come to be called *disputing*, the process through which people recognize that they have been hurt by someone else's behavior and decide whether to take legal action.

The Disputing Phase

In the classic article in the field, Felstiner, Abel, and Sarat (1980–81) found that a legal dispute emerges in three steps: "naming," when an "unrecognized perceived injurious experience" gets recognized as such (e.g., the asbestos worker finding out he has lung cancer); "blaming," which "occurs when a person attributes an injury to the fault of another individual or social entity" and comes to believe that something might be done about it; and "claiming," "when someone with a grievance voices it to the person or entity believed to be responsible and asks for some remedy" (pp. 635–636).

A claim is transformed into a dispute when it is rejected by the allegedly responsible person.

Contrary to the myth of American litigiousness, empirical research suggests that people rarely take up the opportunity to sue (Weiler et al., 1991). Psychological factors, particularly attributions of responsibility, are of obvious significance (Coates & Penrod, 1980–1981). Research among people with HIV has detected a tendency toward self-blame in the face of mistreatment and an unwillingness to sue (Musheno, 1995; Weitz, 1989), explaining why the level of discrimination might be far higher than the level of discrimination litigation (Burris, 1996).

The literature on disputing suggests some of the barriers people have to go through to begin a lawsuit. First, they have to blame someone else for a bad event and feel efficacious enough to resist the mistreatment, neither of which is psychologically easy. The person must know about the law that might provide relief and feel both willing and able to seek access to the judicial system. For people whose usual relations with the state are as the object of criminal prosecution or bureaucratic supervision, the legal system may not appear to be either inviting or fair. Even those who trust the legal system, or feel it is worth their while to use it, have to be able to find a lawyer, which will depend on either their ability to pay or the likelihood that their grievance could turn into a sufficiently lucrative settlement or damages award. It is therefore no surprise that the Harvard Malpractice Study found that only one of every eight people who were injured by medical negligence ever filed a suit (Weiler et al., 1991). *Tarasoff* suits are themselves infrequent. A recent article reported that only 50 of the more than 40,000 members of the American Psychiatric Association are sued each year for breach of a duty to protect, of whom only 6 are found liable (Beck, 1990).

The Litigation Phase

For the small percentage of injured people who actually file a lawsuit, the legal system provides a long and often arduous process of pretrial fact-gathering, legal argument, trial, and appeal, throughout which lawyers maneuver for advantages in ongoing negotiations for a settlement. A suit begins with a document called the *complaint*, a terse recitation of the facts the plaintiff believes he or she is able to prove, and the legal claims arising from those facts. The complaint is not designed to present the plaintiff's complete case, but only to give the defendant notice of the main issues. Complaints are usually sketchy, in part for tactical reasons and in part because plaintiffs rarely have the full story when they sue. People often have a choice of more than one court system. *Tarasoff* was brought in California state court. A parallel system of federal courts primarily handles cases involving federal law but is available for state law cases (like *Tarasoff*) if the plaintiffs and the defendants are from different states and the amount claimed in damages is greater than $50,000.

Perhaps the most important, and usually the most protracted, stage of civil litigation is *discovery*, the process of collecting the facts through exchange of documents, written questions and answers, and depositions (out of court testimony by parties and witnesses). Modern civil litigation operates under the theory that there should be no dramatic courtroom surprises. All the evidence should be known before a jury is ever empaneled.

Defendants who believe they have been wrongly sued have an opportunity to avoid the rigors of discovery through what is usually called a *motion to dismiss*, or *demurrer*. This motion, made to the court soon after the case is filed, focuses on fatal legal defects in the plaintiff's case. The focus is on legal defects because, prior to discovery, there is very little factual evidence. Indeed, for purposes of deciding a motion to dismiss, a court assumes that all the sketchy facts presented in the plaintiff's complaint, as well as all inferences that can be reasonably drawn from those facts, are true. *Tarasoff* provides an excellent example. The famous story of therapists who carelessly failed to protect an obvious victim, Tatiana Tarasoff, from a clearly murderous client, Prosenjit Poddar, is taken from the plaintiff's unproven allegations. In response to the complaint, the defendants filed demurrers arguing that even if all the facts were just as the Tarasoffs claimed, the family had no claim because the defendants had no duty to protect her. Their version of the facts was never presented to a court, first because the trial judge dismissed the case and later because the defendants agreed to a settlement.

Poddar himself was prosecuted under the criminal branch of the law. Prosecutions are brought by the government. Prosecutors decide whom to charge, and with what offenses, their judgment subjected to only the most minimal check of a grand jury or judge, who reviews the evidence as described by the prosecutor. Most crimes are now defined by statutes, although "common law" crimes remain. The Model Penal Code (1995) a comprehensive sample law, has been widely adopted by the states and has brought some uniformity. Poddar pled not guilty by reason of insanity. The jury found him guilty of second-degree murder.

After a civil or criminal trial court has issued a final order—finished with the case—there may be an appeal to the appellate courts. The *Tarasoff* plaintiffs appealed the dismissal of their case to the intermediate appeals court, and, unsuccessful there, to the state's Supreme Court. The court heard the case argued twice before the justices wrote their final opinion on the duty to protect. Because the case concerned California law only, there was no basis for a final appeal to the U.S. Supreme Court. Shortly before issuing its first opinion in the *Tarasoff* case, the same California Supreme Court threw out Poddar's criminal conviction on the ground that the trial judge had given the jury incorrect instructions on the law (*People v. Poddar*,

1974). At his new trial, Poddar was convicted of the lesser crime of voluntary manslaughter and, after a stay in prison, was released on condition that he return to his native India where, as of 1983, he was said to be happily married (Slovenko, 1988). For a more extended explanation of the American court system and some of its basic concepts, see Burris (1993a) and Herman and Burris (1993).

ASSESSING LEGAL RISK

Being sued is a risk of doing business as a psychotherapist. The rational psychotherapist deals with this by taking out insurance, keeping good records, and avoiding careless or illegal behavior. Knowing, or learning, the applicable legal rules can help a therapist avoid obvious mistakes—like assisting in a suicide in the belief that the client has a legal right to that help. In most of the case studies covered in this book, there are key questions about the law that do not have a clear answer. In that case, incorporating the law into one's decision-making process may involve a risk assessment which, on the basis of this discussion, could take the form of the following list.

Recognize and Deal With One's Emotional Reaction to the Risk

When it comes to being sued, with its flavor of disgrace and ruin, few therapists are perfectly rational. In this respect, the fear of law is analogous to the fear of HIV. Any psychotherapist dealing with HIV has probably run into the problem of talking about the risk of transmission. People who are afraid of getting HIV from a waiter sneezing on the food are not crazy; indeed, if one defines sanity by the degree of deviation from the norm, they may be among the most normal, because they are engaged in the almost universal practice of gauging risk by qualitative factors like horror, familiarity, degree of control, and the ability to visualize the disaster (Schneiderman & Kaplan, 1992; Slovic, Fischhoff, & Lichtenstein, 1982; Tversky & Kahneman, 1982). These factors also influence health care providers' thinking about the law. Faced with the sort of legal–ethical dilemma described in this book, the psychotherapist can easily visualize the chain of events that leads from warning a client's sex partner to being humiliated on the witness stand by Johnnie Cochran. Fear of the power of law, rather than appreciation of the nuances and insights of law, is the dominant response. Accurately assessing legal risk, then, requires the same approach as defusing the fear of HIV. One must try to assess that risk at each link in the chain of feared events not in terms of its horror, but its likelihood, which depends on many tangible factors that are easily overlooked in a general panic.

The quantifiable risk is never a complete answer to fear of a risk. Even being told that the chances of being infected with HIV, or being sued, are one-in-a-million does not make some people more willing to run the risk. Having committed to a rational, systematic assessment of the likelihood of being sued, one must also confront one's qualitative concerns head-on. This is not a matter of writing off the fears as statistically "wrong," but of one's moral or social or professional responsibility to address the fear. This is familiar terrain for the psychotherapist, who at this stage of the legal risk analysis has the chance to think about his or her own reactions to powerlessness, to an alien system of thought, to financial or professional fears, and to weigh those reactions against his or her ethical values. At some point, minimizing one's legal risk, no matter how it may salve the fear of being sued, may be harmful to one's professional self-regard and standing, an unworthy motive for the ethical professional. The complete risk assessment involves considering the facts as well as the emotions and putting them in a perspective that restores some measure of choice to the psychotherapist.

Be Sure Your Acts Are Consistent With Professional Standards

Professionals who adopt the decision-making process introduced in this book have taken substantial measures toward avoiding legal liability. There are few, if any circumstances, in which it is wise to allow fears of being sued to divert one from the course dictated by professional ethics. Being sued is, after all, significantly different from losing a lawsuit. Acting professionally cannot guarantee that clients will not sue, but it significantly reduces the chances of their prevailing.

Identify Potential Plaintiffs

There will be no suit if no one sues. Who might want to? Why would they want to? Very often, a look at just these two questions is enough to reassure the psychotherapist that the chances of being sued are theoretical; at the very least, the process helps the psychotherapist identify important stakeholders in the dilemma and the need to address their concerns and, ideally, involves them in decision making.

Assess the Willingness and Ability of Potential Plaintiffs to Sue

Given the research on disputing, we have to start with the proposition that most people would prefer not to file a lawsuit or do not realize that they can. One may be able to make a reasonable guess about this simply from knowing the potential plaintiff's personality, education, or social status. Even if someone wants to sue, a legal risk assessment has to consider whether this would-be plaintiff could get a lawyer. Does the plaintiff have the money to pay up front? Does the plaintiff have legal claims, or claims to sympathy, that are strong enough to attract a lawyer on a contingency basis? Asking these questions helps focus not on the existence of a legal claim but on its strength. *Tarasoff's* Poddar could have sued psychotherapist Moore for breaching his privacy, provided that he could have found a lawyer, but the case would almost certainly have been dismissed in an instant.

CONCLUSION

At its practical best, the law offers a way to identify and apply rules and important values to confusing facts, to set responsibility and illuminate alternatives. Sometimes the process may yield something close to certainty, but law is a process, not a solution. Years ago, an eminent authority on the tort system put it plainly:

> in the great bulk of cases ... there is no method of ascertaining in advance whether conduct is negligent or non-negligent. At most, a method has been devised for testing conduct after it becomes known. The method is not difficult to state, but its satisfactory employment must rest upon the capacity of judges to know when it is applicable, and the capacity of juries to exercise a fair judgment on all the factors involved. (Green, 1928, p. 1046)

Given the irreducible uncertainty of law, particularly in the sort of troubling questions discussed in this book, almost all lawyers would advise the psychotherapist to be a psychotherapist—that is, to make decisions informed by law but always and fundamentally on the basis of intelligent and ethical application of the therapist's own professional knowledge and talent.

REFERENCES

Aiken, J., & Musheno, M. (1994). Why have-nots win in the HIV-litigation arena: Socio-legal dynamics of extreme cases. *Law and Policy, 16,* 267–297.

American Law Institute. (1965). *Restatement (second) of torts.* St. Paul, MN: Author.

Ariz. Rev. Stat. Ann. § 36-664(K) (1997).

Beck, J. C. (1990). Current status of the duty to protect. In J. C. Beck (Ed.), *Confidentiality versus the duty to protect: Foreseeable harm in the practice of psychiatry* (pp. 9–22). Washington, DC: American Psychiatric Press.

Belluck, P. (1999, March 27). Dr. Kevorkian is a murderer, the jury finds. *New York Times,* p. A1.

Bersoff, D. N. (1992). Judicial deference to nonlegal decisionmakers: Imposing simplistic solutions on problems of cognitive complexity in mental disability law. *Southern Methodist University Law Review, 46*, 329–372.

Bradley v. Ray, 904 S.W. 2d 302 (1995).

Burris, S. (1993a). A little law for non-lawyers. In S. Burris, H. L. Dalton, & J. L. Miller (Eds.), *AIDS law today* (pp. 3–17). New Haven, CT: Yale University Press.

Burris, S. (1993b). Testing, disclosure, and the right to privacy. In S. Burris, H. L. Dalton, & J. L. Miller (Eds.), *AIDS law today* (pp. 115–149). New Haven, CT: Yale University Press.

Burris, S. (1996). Dental discrimination against the HIV-infected: Empirical data, law and public policy. *Yale Journal of Regulation, 13*, 1–104.

Burt, R. A. (1997). The supreme court speaks: Not assisted suicide but a constitutional right to palliative care. *New England Journal of Medicine, 337*, 1234–1236.

CAL. CIVIL CODE, § 43.92 (West, 2000).

CAL. HEALTH & SAFETY CODE, §121015 (West, 1999).

CAL. PENAL CODE, § 401 (West 1997).

Chlapowski, F. S. (1991). The constitutional protection of informational privacy. *Boston University Law Review, 71*, 133–160.

Coates, D., & Penrod, S. (1980–81). Social psychology and the emergence of disputes. *Law and Society Review, 15*, 655–680.

Compassion in Dying v. State of Washington, 79 F.3d 790 (9th Cir. 1996) (*en banc*).

CONN. GEN. STAT., § 19a-584 (1997).

Doe v. Borough of Barrington, 729 F. Supp. 376 (D.N.J. 1990).

Donaldson v. Van de Kamp, 4 Cal.Rptr.2d 59 (Cal.App. 2 Dist. 1992).

Felstiner, W. L. F., Abel, R. L., & Sarat, A. (1980–81). The emergence and transformation of disputes: naming, blaming, claiming .... *Law & Society Review, 15*, 631–654.

Felthouse, A. R. (1989). The ever confusing jurisprudence of the psychotherapist's duty to protect. *Journal of Psychiatry and Law, 17*, 575–594.

GA. CODE ANN., § 24-9-47 (Harrison, 1997).

Galanter, M. (1974). Why the "haves" come out ahead: Speculations on the limits of legal change. *Law and Society Review, 9*, 95–160.

Givelber, D. J., Bowers, W. J., & Blitch, C. L. (1984). *Tarasoff*, myth and reality: An empirical study of private law in action. *Wisconsin Law Review, 1984*, 443–497.

Green, L. (1928). The negligence issue. *Yale Law Journal, 37*, 1029–1047.

Herman, D. H. J., & Burris, S. (1993). Torts: Private lawsuits about HIV. In S. Burris, H. L. Dalton, & J. L. Miller (Eds.), *AIDS law today* (pp. 334–366). New Haven, CT: Yale University Press.

Kairys, D. (1998). Introduction. In D. Kairys (Ed.), *The politics of law* (pp. 1–20). New York: Basic Books.

Kreimer, S. (1991). Sunlight, secrets and scarlet letters: The tension between privacy and disclosure in constitutional law. *University of Pennsylvania Law Review, 140*, 1–147.

Macmillan Dictionary of Quotations. (1989). New York: Macmillan.

Md. Health-Gen. Code Ann., §18-337 (1997).

Model Penal Code. (1995). Official draft and explanatory notes. Philadelphia: American Law Institute.

Musheno, M. C. (1995). Legal consciousness on the margins of society: Struggles against stigmatization in the AIDS crisis. *Identities, 2*, 102–122.

Musheno, M. C., Gregware, P. R., & Drass, K. A. (1991). Court management of AIDS disputes: A sociolegal analysis. *Law & Social Inquiry, 16*, 737–774.

N.D. Cent. Code, §§ 12.1-16-01 to 12.1-16-03 (1985).

Novak v. Rathnam, 505 N.E.2d. 773 (Ill. App. Ct. 1987).

N.Y. Public Health Law, § 2782(4) (1997).

Oregon Death With Dignity Act, Or. Rev. Stat. §§127.800 et seq. (1997).

Pa. Stat. tit. 63, §§ 1201 et seq., §§1901 et seq.

People v. Kevorkian, 517 N.W.2d 293 (Mich. App. 1994), *judgment vacated*, 527 N.W. 714 (Mich. 1994), *cert. denied*, 115 S.Ct. 1795 (1995).

People v. Matlock, 336 P.2d 505 (Cal. 1959).

People v. Poddar, 518 P.2d 342 (Cal. 1974).

Roe v. Wade, 410 U.S. 113 (1973).

Rosenberg, G. N. (1991). *The hollow hope*. Chicago: University of Chicago Press.

Schneiderman, L. J., & Kaplan, R. (1992). Fear of dying and HIV infection versus hepatitis B infection. *American Journal of Public Health, 82*, 584–586.

Schuster v. Altenberg, 424 N.W.2d 159 (Wis. 1988).

Silverstein, M. (1989). Privacy rights in state constitutions: Models for Illinois? *University of Illinois Law Review, 1989*, 215–296.

Simonsen v. Swenson, 177 N.W. 831 (Neb. 1920).

Slovenko, R. (1988). The therapist's duty to warn or protect third persons. *Journal of Psychiatry and Law, 16*, 139–209.

Slovic, P., Fischhoff, B., & Lichtenstein, S. (1982). Facts versus fears: Understanding perceived risk. In D. Kahneman, P. Slovic, & A. Tversky (Eds.), *Judgement under uncertainty: Heuristics and biases* (pp. 163–178). Cambridge, England: Cambridge University Press.

State v. Bouse, 264 P.2d 800 (Or. 1953).

State v. Cobb, 625 P.2d 1133 (Kan. 1981).

State v. Morrissey, 295 N.W.2d 307 (N.D. 1980).

State v. Sexson, 869 P.2d 301 (N.M. App. 1994).

Tarasoff v. Board of Regents of the University of California, 551 P.2d 334 (Cal. 1976).

Taub, N., & Schneider, E. M. (1998). Women's subordination and the role of law. In D. Kairys (Ed.), *The politics of law* (pp. 328–357). New York: Basic Books.

Tex. Health & Safety Ann. §81.103 (1997).

Tversky, A., & Kahneman, D. (1982). Availability: A heuristic for judging frequency and probability. In D. Kahneman, P. Slovic, & A. Tversky (Eds.), *Judgement under uncertainty: Heuristics and biases* (pp. 163–178). Cambridge, England: Cambridge University Press.

Vacco v. Quill, 521 U.S. 793 (1997).

Washington State Psychological Association, the American Counseling Association, the Association for Gay, Lesbian and Bisexual Issues in Counseling, and a Coalition of Mental Health Professionals. (1997). Brief as amici curiae in support of respondent. *Washington v. Glucksberg,* 521 U.S. 702 (1997).

Washington v. Glucksberg, 521 U.S. 702 (1997).

Weiler, P. C., Hiatt, H. H., Newhouse, J. P., Johnson, W. G., Brennan, T. A., & Leape, L. (1991). *A measure of malpractice: Medical injury, malpractice litigation, and patient compensation.* Cambridge, MA: Harvard University Press.

Weitz, R. (1989). Uncertainty and the lives of persons with AIDS. *Journal of Health and Social Behavior, 30,* 270–281.

Whalen v. Roe, 429 U.S. 589 (1977).

Young, H. H. (1992). Assisted suicide and physician liability. *The Review of Litigation, 11,* 623–656.

II

CASE EXAMPLES
USING A SYSTEMATIC
DECISION-MAKING MODEL
WITH HIV/AIDS CLIENTS

7

A DECISION MODEL FOR ETHICAL DILEMMAS IN HIV-RELATED PSYCHOTHERAPY AND ITS APPLICATION IN THE CASE OF JERRY

BOB BARRET, KAREN STROHM KITCHENER, AND SCOTT BURRIS

The previous six chapters provide the context in which ethical issues in HIV-related psychotherapy arise. Understanding the complexity of sorting through the dynamics of personal responses to clients and to ethical, legal, cultural, and end-of-life aspects of this work is really only the first step toward effective clinical practice. Knowing when an obligation to others overrides confidentiality or determining the benefit of becoming more personally involved with a client requires a systematic model that minimizes decisions contaminated by countertransference issues that could pose a danger to clients and others (Barret, 1996). This chapter introduces the reader to a systematic decision-making model and then applies that model to a case that involves an HIV-positive client who is having anonymous, unprotected sexual encounters.

A MODEL FOR MAKING ETHICAL DECISIONS

The model of ethical decision making applied to cases in this section of the book calls for (a) carefully reviewing personal reactions; (b) determining facts; (c) making a preliminary plan; (d) analyzing the preliminary plan in terms of a professional code of ethics as well as foundational ethical principles; (e) examining the legal consequences of the preliminary plan; (f) identifying and assessing options to refine the preliminary plan by balancing clinical, ethical, and legal considerations; (g) choosing a course of action; and (h) implementing the course of action and evaluating the outcomes. Also included are consultation and documentation. Consultation should occur whenever the clinician is uncertain and may involve conversations with legal and ethical experts, reviews of the literature, and meetings with co-workers and supervisors. Information obtained from each consultation should be clearly documented. Proper documentation means also that the decision-making process will appear in written case notes or client charts so that each step of the practitioner's thinking and the analytical process is evident. Documentation protects the practitioner from potential legal difficulties and also serves as an additional point of reflection, a checking out to determine that all options and steps have been taken. Before applying this model to a specific situation, we describe each step and discuss the implications of that step for the practitioner.

Pause and Identify Your Personal Responses to the Case

Before taking action, it is important to pause and sort through what often is a complex set of personal and professional reactions to the client. This step asks the clinician to look closely at the feelings he or she has

---

EXHIBIT 7.1
A Model for Making Ethical Decisions: Application

1. Pause and identify your personal responses to the case.
2. Review the facts of the case.
3. Conceptualize an initial plan based on clinical issues.
4. Consult the ethics code and assess the ethical issues based on the five foundational principles:
   - autonomy
   - beneficence
   - do no harm
   - fidelity
   - justice.
5. Identify the legal issues.
6. Identify and assess the options.
7. Choose a course of action and share it with your client.
8. Implement the course of action: monitor and discuss outcomes.

Note. Consultation should take place whenever you have any doubts or questions about the legal or ethical issues or your own ability to be objective. Consultation with co-workers, colleagues, supervisors, professional ethics committees, and attorneys should be an integral part throughout the process. Each step of the decision-making process must be carefully documented.

while sitting with the client. The clinician also is challenged to identify the ways personal beliefs and values about the client and the situation may affect treatment. For example, responses to a client who has been abandoned by all family members might differ from those toward a client who has significant family and social support. Furthermore, anger at a client who continues to practice unsafe sex may interfere with treatment. Being aware of feelings and values and the ways they may affect treatment or even one's ability to be understanding and empathic demands careful reflection. Anticipating ways to manage one's own issues while providing services to the client is essential. Both positive and negative countertransference can render the treatment ineffective and may discourage the client from seeking further help.

Review the Facts of the Case

In this step the clinician focuses on what facts are actually known rather than what appears to have taken place. It is essential to separate facts from assumptions and to place established facts against the backdrop of HIV disease as well as other specific circumstances facing the client. For example, being aware of side effects of medication or symptoms of dementia places facts in perspective. Moreover, it may be useful to compare one's knowledge of basic HIV disease transmission and progression against that of the client's. Suicidal urges early in disease progression may be handled quite differently from those evident during end-stage AIDS. Although the facts may look similar, disease symptoms and progression may change what the clinician decides to do. Similarly, it is important to consider other important defining client characteristics. For example, what is the client's racial or ethnic background? Does he or she have strong religious views that may affect treatment? Each of these influence the clinician's definition of his or her role with the client, understanding about what it means to benefit or harm the client, and final course of action.

Conceptualize an Initial Plan Based on Clinical Issues

At this point most practitioners will have at least a sketch of what they want to do. It is important to keep the focus on what is in the client's best interest instead of jumping ahead to considerations about what ethical boards, lawyers, or judges would say. Too often, concerns about suits and censure cloud clinical judgment. This step zeros in on planning from a clinical perspective in light of this client's psychological makeup and prognosis. It focuses on one major question: If the clinician's sole concern is the clinical treatment of the client, what would be the preferred course of action?

Consult the Ethics Code and Assess the Ethical Issues

Chapter 3 provides a useful guide to determining and balancing the ethical issues as they pertain to ethical standards, the five aspirational portions of the APA Ethics Code (APA, 1992), and the five foundational principles (autonomy, beneficence, do no harm, fidelity, and justice). Examining one's initial plan in light of ethical standards and the five principles is an essential step. Where the Ethics Code requires (or prohibits) particular action, no further analysis may be needed. If the Ethics Code does not require particular action, the aspirational sections (Preamble and General Principles) should be consulted to determine what specific values are active in a specific instance. If no further requirement is determined, the five foundational principles can clarify ethical decisions. When considering the five principles, the clinician should be aware of his or her own values and countertransference issues, as well as what is known about the client and the client's values and beliefs. What this means is that there is a certain subjectivity that influences the balance between the principles. Ethical decision making is complex because moral principles often conflict in ways that are not easily resolved, and not all personal values are necessarily moral ones. The guidelines below may be helpful:

- The facts of a case or particular situation may influence which moral principles are most relevant or important.
- Overriding a moral principle should be done only for good moral reasons.
- Do no harm takes precedence over beneficence. Most ethicists suggest that all other things being equal, not harming others is generally a stronger ethical obligation than benefiting them. Another approach is to do the least amount of avoidable harm.
- Try to create the greatest balance of value over disvalue. In other words, accentuate the positive.

Before moving forward, it is important for the clinician to consider his or her organization's policies related to the case. Some institutions have very clear HIV-related policies, whereas others have never considered the types of situations clinicians may encounter. Becoming familiar with how one's workplace policies may play a role in the plan is a step that is best undertaken sooner rather than later.

At this point, the clinician writes down the options that have become clear. Developing a matrix of the advantages and disadvantages of each option helps in ranking the options. Listing the ethical benefits and drawbacks to the client, and others, and the possible impact of each option on the therapeutic relationship and psychological treatment is a professionally sound way of sorting out the information that has been generated.

Identify the Legal Issues

The legal issues involved with each option must be considered. This can be done by becoming familiar with the literature, consulting with colleagues and co-workers, or perhaps speaking with an attorney familiar with HIV-related treatment issues. In this step, the practitioner acts both to protect himself or herself and to consider possible legal consequences for the client. Be aware that sometimes there may be conflict between what is legal, ethical, and psychologically therapeutic. For this reason, determining the legal issues for each option is helpful.

Identify and Assess the Options

A tentative plan should emerge from the process of going through the preceding steps. The clinician's next step is to refine the plan so that it: (a) requires the therapist to consider the positive and negative consequences of his or her initial response to the case; (b) advances clinical interests as much as possible; (c) permits the therapist to operate within the guidelines of his or her professional code of ethics and agency policies; (d) minimizes harm to the client and relevant others; (e) maximizes all other foundational principles to the extent possible; and (f) allows the therapist to operate within the law. The tentative plan must "fit" with current treatment goals and strategies. It is essential to determine how the plan will affect the therapeutic relationship and possible ways that it could change treatment goals or strategies as well as the client's probable response. If more than one strategy seems compelling, further consultation may help resolve the impasse.

In the end, the revised plan should take into account the personal responses isolated in the initial step, the facts of the case, ethical codes and principles, whatever legal directives that have appeared, and the employing agency's or association's policies and procedures. Those who work in a clinic or other setting must consider institutional policies. Again, we remind readers that sometimes the most ethical response may conflict with the law and institutional policies.

Choose a Course of Action and Share It With Your Client

Having determined what to do, the clinician informs the client about what is going to happen, including the supporting rationale for the decision. This may precipitate a crisis, so having an effective plan for managing unanticipated events can be essential. Any concerns about the client's decision-making ability or reasoning should be discussed openly. The clinician should explain clearly and precisely how the chosen course of action facilitates the client's treatment plan and try not to react defensively to the client's potential anger and confusion. The overriding directive is to empower the client by making him or her an ally in the treatment plan.

Implement the Course of Action: Monitor and Discuss Outcomes

The plan is evaluated both as it is being implemented and after the crisis has passed. Determining how the client used the intervention to become more responsible or to improve coping skills is one method of evaluation. Assessing the impact on the client–therapist relationship and future psychotherapy is another method. Isolating what has been learned provides information that will be useful to the clinician with other clients. Moreover, watching the way the clinician's actions influence the client's safety (and the safety of others) over time also serves as a point of evaluation. The client's overt and often subtle reflections on the clinician's plan may generate feelings that should be faced both in and out of the psychotherapy relationship. Being sensitive to the ways in which the client's life becomes more complex as a result of what happened is especially important. It is critical to keep the focus balanced between the positive and negative influence of the clinician's action. Each step should be documented in the client's file.

At first glance, following these steps may appear cumbersome and time consuming, and it is true that some clinical situations do not allow sufficient time to walk through each step at a leisurely pace. However, routine use of this model will lead to greater efficiency. Role-playing situations that are likely to occur will also develop proficiency in this process. Even reading about case application of the model can lead to greater proficiency.

The next section demonstrates how the model can be applied in therapy with an actual client. The narrative is presented from the perspective of the clinician, Bob Barret, one of the few in his community doing HIV-related psychotherapy, with consultation from an ethics expert, Karen S. Kitchener, and a legal expert, Scott Burris.

APPLICATION OF THE MODEL: THE CASE OF JERRY

Case Presentation (by Bob Barret)

Jerry, age 29, resident of North Carolina, gay, and HIV-positive, seeks counseling to deal with depression and anxiety. He has been in a relationship with another man for several months. Jerry fears that his relationship is ending and that he will be asked to leave the apartment that they have been sharing. Jerry's fears stem from his partner's repeated assertions that he does not think that he can deal with Jerry's HIV status and the many arguments that they have been having.

Jerry is worried about living alone. He has always had a relationship since he came out 6 years ago. Although he is trying to manage his sense of loss and panic over the potential deterioration of his relationship and his health, he has not been able to verbalize his feelings to his partner; generally, his response is "Fine, I'll get out whenever you say!" followed by a trip to a bookstore and finding someone with whom to have sex. After prodding, Jerry admits that he has anal intercourse with these men and that he does not use a condom.

Jerry begins the session by talking about his sexual encounter of the previous night. Although he feels guilty about not telling his partner about his anonymous encounters, he expresses little concern about engaging in unsafe sex. He states that sex helps him forget all of his troubles for a while. He says he does not believe that he will ever have another relationship if his partner kicks him out. "No one will want to touch me if they know I have HIV," he says. "That's the way I got HIV, and anyone stupid enough to have sex with me deserves just what they get!" He then begins to talk about illness, deterioration, and the possibility of facing death alone.

Pause and Identify Your Personal Responses to the Case

Pausing enables me to sort through my initial negative reaction to what Jerry has just said. I feel anger about his attitude and behavior. His final statement, "Anyone stupid enough to have sex with me deserves just what they get!" is particularly troublesome. I struggle to find an empathic response that might help us understand his internal experience of his behavior in the hope that he may see the danger of his actions. Having unprotected sex places him at risk reinfection, which could lead to further declines in his health. Furthermore, my concern for the health of others also prevents me from being more empathic. Although I believe that each of us is responsible for our own health, the callousness of his remark does little to enhance my willingness to be empathic toward him.

Attempting to mask this reaction is likely to be difficult and may distract me from other important aspects of providing treatment to him. My distrust might contaminate my ability to be supportive in other areas of his life. I also feel a sense of obligation to my community to do what I can to stop the spread of HIV disease. Jerry's behavior clearly violates that value. Simultaneously, I believe that it is important for him to be in therapy and that one way to change this behavior can be through increased self-understanding. Confronting him too harshly early on may drive him away, and that would mean that he continues the risky behavior without anyone monitoring him; not responding genuinely may give him the idea that I approve of what he is doing.

As he continues to talk about his situation, I am distracted by my own confusion, and I sort through various ways to lead him back to what he said so I might understand it more fully. My initial decision is to ask him to tell me more about these episodes and to try to suspend my judgment. What I learn is that he goes to a nearby park infrequently and may initiate unprotected anal intercourse with people he meets there. Rarely does he see these individuals again, and his intent is just to have fun.

My strongest impulse is to tell someone. I don't like this reaction and see it as an attempt to reduce my sense of personal responsibility. As I sort through those feelings I recognize there is no one to tell. There are no authorities, nor are other experts readily available to me. I wrestle with my own sense of helplessness and disapproval of Jerry and his behavior. I try to settle myself by reviewing the facts of the case.

Review the Facts of the Case

The facts of the situation are quite clear. Jerry has HIV disease, and his use of condoms in his primary relationship indicates that he can act responsibly about his HIV infection. His sexual behavior with others may place them at risk, but even that is not altogether certain; many researchers speak of "sufficient" exposure to HIV infection being necessary to seroconvert. Still, unprotected anal intercourse is the most risky behavior for transmitting HIV. The men he has unsafe sex with are not easily identifiable, and his intent is not to harm them but to release his own anxiety. Furthermore, in my state there is no law that forbids this behavior, and knowledge about HIV disease and its transmission is widespread. All of these "facts" really are only self-reports; it could be that he is not having sex with anyone. I need more information before I can decide what is factual and what might be his testing of our relationship. From earlier questions I know that he is oriented to time and place and that he does not present with symptoms of dementia. He also knows the risk he is taking. His psychological history does not reveal ongoing problems that might be a factor in this situation.

Conceptualize an Initial Plan Based on Clinical Issues

I believe that Jerry has an adjustment disorder with mixed emotional features. Although a more specific diagnosis is likely to be apparent later in treatment, on the whole he seems to be reacting somewhat normally to life with HIV. As he attempts to integrate his view of himself as a person with HIV disease, he experiences much anger and frustration, and he feels significant shame as a result of the stigma that is attached to HIV. Not being one who analyzes his emotions to any great extent, Jerry is simply acting out internal emotional responses. Psychotherapy will help him more properly identify what is happening so he can make more responsible plans for himself and others.

My temporary plan is to review the seriousness of his behavior with him and to ask him to sign a safe sex contract with me. I will emphasize that this will protect him from getting reinfected and protect others from risk of HIV. My basic strategy is to buy myself enough time to sort through the more complex aspects of this situation. I know I will continue to worry that his poor impulse control may result in "slips" from our contract. I also worry that if he is arrested and tells the arresting officers that I knew what he was doing, my reputation and that of other clinicians could suffer. My plan is to get Jerry to agree to maintain his safe sex contract and to regularly check with him about his experience as he tries to be more responsible. I will talk with him about the risks to himself as well as others and encourage him to discuss his behavior with his physician. I will explain the dilemma he and I are both in and my personal struggle to accept him when he is placing others at risk.

Consult the Ethics Code and Assess the Ethical Issues (by Karen Strohm Kitchener)

This case raises several treatment issues but a single difficult ethical issue: how to deal with the fact that although Jerry is HIV-positive, he continues to have anonymous, unsafe sex with other men. In other words, Dr. Barret must balance a responsibility to Jerry, which implies keeping the information about his sexual practices confidential, with a responsibility to society, which suggests protecting those with whom Jerry is having unsafe sex.

The ethical dilemma raised by this case is the one most commonly written about by those addressing the ethical issues raised by HIV-related practice. As discussed in chapter 2, it is frequently dealt with in terms of whether the *Tarasoff* ruling would apply (*Tarasoff v. Board of Regents of the University of California*, 1976); in other words, whether there is a legal duty to warn a third party about a client's HIV status. In this case because Jerry is having unsafe sex with partners who do not know of his HIV status, Dr. Barret should ask whether he has an ethical duty to warn Jerry's partners and, if so, how he might go about doing so in an ethical manner.

It is quite possible that different practitioners will analyze this case and come to different courses of action. There may be no single course of action that would be honored as "right" by legal and ethical experts. What is important is determining any requirements of the Ethics Code (APA, 1992) and developing a line of reasoning that ensures that behavior is ethical.

According to Standard 5.02, psychologists have a primary obligation to respect the confidentiality of those with whom they work. This suggests that Dr. Barret has a primary responsibility to protect Jerry's confidence. On the other hand, Standard 5.05 indicates that psychologists disclose confidential information without the consent of the individual only as mandated by law, or where permitted by law for a valid purpose, such as "(1) to provide needed professional services to the patient or the individual or organizational client, (2) to obtain appropriate professional consultations, (3) to protect the patient or client or others from harm, or (4) to obtain payment for services, in which instance disclosure is limited to the minimum that is necessary to achieve the purpose" (Standard 5.05). Although this standard is frequently understood to require psychologists to break confidentiality when a client's actions pose a threat to a third party, in fact that is not the case (Canter, Bennett, Jones, & Nagy, 1994). The standard gives psychologists permission to break confidentiality only in cases where it is required or permitted by law. In other words, it does not address the ethical question of whether or when a psychologist should break confidentiality to protect a third party from harm.

The aspirational principles from the Ethics Code (APA, 1992) confirm the original dilemma of responsibility to the individual and to society. On one hand, Principle E: Concern for Others' Welfare admonishes psychologists to contribute to those with whom they interact professionally; on the other hand, Principle F: Social Responsibility requires that they be concerned about the community and the society in which they live. In other words, these principles would suggest that the psychologist has a responsibility to both the client and to society. Principle E adds, however, that "When conflicts occur among psychologists' obligations or concerns, they attempt to resolve these conflicts and to perform their roles in a responsible fashion that avoids or minimizes harm." This statement suggests that Dr. Barret must ask, How can I respond in this situation in a way that does the least amount of avoidable harm?

Furthermore, Standard 5.03, Minimizing Intrusions on Privacy, suggests that if confidentiality is to be broken it should be done in a way that minimizes intrusions on privacy. Thus, these standards suggest that if Dr. Barret decides to break confidentiality he should ask how he can do so in the least intrusive way and in a way that discloses only information that is germane to the purpose for which the communication is made.

Three other standards offer some guidance in this case. First, Standard 1.14, Avoiding Harm, suggests that psychologists act in a way to "avoid harming their patients or clients . . . , and to minimize harm where it is foreseeable and unavoidable." HIV-positive individuals and those in high-risk groups often have good reasons to fear being identified; thus, breaches of confidentiality may have serious negative consequences for the infected individual. As a result, when psychologists are working with individuals who are HIV-positive, they should foresee the possibility that clients may at some point engage in unsafe sexual activity. If they believe that they have an ethical responsibility to break confidentiality under these circumstances, clients should be informed at the outset of treatment that this may occur.

In general, the APA Ethics Code suggests that Dr. Barret ought to identify a course of action with Jerry that minimizes harm, and if Dr. Barret decides to break confidentiality, he should do so in a way that minimizes intrusion on Jerry's privacy. The foundational principles introduced in chapter 3 offer further guidance in cases like Jerry's. First, the responsibility to maintain confidentiality rests on two fundamental ethical assumptions: respect for autonomy and fidelity. The principles of beneficence and do no harm also can inform decisions in this case, and the principle of justice should remind Dr. Barret that Jerry must be treated fairly.

Autonomy

Maintaining confidentiality respects the individual's rights to make decisions about with whom and where private information is shared. Thus, breaking confidentiality could be seen as a violation of the individual's autonomy. On the other hand, as noted in chapter 3, autonomy does not mean that people have absolute freedom to do what they wish. Although individuals have a right to decide how to act and think, they do not have the right to engage in activities that threaten the rights of others to engage in similar activities. In this case because of the infectious nature of HIV, engaging in unsafe sexual activities with uninformed partners may be seen as a threat to others' ability to make autonomous choices as well as a threat to their lives. As a result, other ethical principles may trump Jerry's autonomous wish to remain silent about his HIV status with uninformed partners.

Fidelity

Although the principle of autonomy does not provide an adequate rationale for keeping information about Jerry's HIV status confidential, the principle of fidelity offers a different perspective. As noted in chapter 3, therapists establish an implicit or explicit contract with clients before initiating therapy. This contract includes the promise to maintain confidentiality. Thus, breaking confidentiality involves breaking a promise. Melton (1988) has argued that those who have been infected with the HIV virus have not had a particularly strong relationship with the mental health community, and making a habit of breaking promises could exacerbate the problem because fear of exposure would lead to mistrust. If those who are in high-risk groups or who are HIV-positive do not seek mental health services because of such a fear, psychologists would have less opportunity to intervene with educative efforts. As Beauchamp and Childress (1989) pointed out, it is not yet clear "which rule of confidentiality would save the most lives in the long run in these circumstances: One that permits or perhaps requires

notification of spouses or lovers or one that guarantees strict confidentiality"
(p. 340).

Do No Harm

Because of the stigma associated with being HIV-positive, breaking confidentiality may have negative consequences for Jerry himself and destroy his faith in both the therapist and other potential helpers, thereby violating the principle of do no harm. For example, disclosure could put him in danger of being arrested for illegal sexual activity in some states, or the humiliation may lead him to consider suicide. Dr. Barret must assess the potential negative consequences of disclosure on Jerry before deciding on a course of action.

Beneficence

Beneficence, which involves protecting others from harm as well as doing good, is also important in this case. HIV is an infectious disease that may be terminal. A strong ethical argument can be made for intervening in a way that protects Jerry's partners from the harm that would result from contracting the disease. In addition, Jerry is placing himself at risk of opportunistic infections when he engages in unprotected sexual activity. On the other hand, Jerry has come seeking psychotherapy. As he comes to understand himself and his behavior, there is the possibility that he may resolve the underlying psychological distress that is leading him to act out and decide to act more responsibly in his sexual encounters. Although breaking confidentiality may help others and protect him from further infection and arrest in the short run, there is also the possibility that such an action would result in Jerry rejecting all psychological assistance and acting out in other irresponsible and socially dangerous ways.

Justice

The principle of justice is usually associated with deciding how psychological services should be distributed fairly. In this case, the principle is a reminder that Jerry deserves to be treated fairly and should not be discriminated against because of his HIV status or his sexual orientation.

Identifying a way to balance these principles is not easy. The principles of autonomy, fidelity, beneficence, and do no harm suggest there are good ethical reasons both to maintain and break confidentiality. The question that Dr. Barret must answer is this: Can I design a course of action that protects Jerry from the harm that would occur if I broke confidentiality, that maintains trust, and that may protect Jerry's partners from infection? Certainly, this ought to be the first priority. As Melton (1988) suggested, "the question is how to protect third parties from serious harm, with minimal intrusion on the privacy of the client" (p. 944). This is a particularly important consideration in this case; Jerry's current partner already knows of his HIV status, and Dr. Barret does not know the identity of those with whom he is engaging in one-night stands. Although some states may require Dr. Barret to inform the public health department or the police, a better course of action might be to engage Jerry in therapy in a way that helps him deal with his fears of losing his partner and living alone. If he does so, Jerry might not feel the need to engage in unsafe sex with other men. If the therapist can do so, then he may have found a way to proceed that upholds the responsibility to benefit both Jerry and society and does the least amount of avoidable harm.

In summary, cases like Jerry's sometimes lead practitioners to think in terms of dichotomies—to break confidentiality or not to break confidentiality. This case suggests the need for greater sophistication. First, it underlines the importance of informed consent, including informing clients of the limits of confidentiality. Second, it suggests that psychologists must consider the harms that might occur if confidentiality were broken and those that might occur if it were not. Last, it suggests that psychologists must ask themselves whether there are ways to intervene with clients like Jerry that are responsive both to their social responsibility and to their responsibility to avoid harming such clients.

Identify the Legal Issues (by Scott Burris)

Goethe's motto "Without haste, but also without rest" is an apt one for cases like this. Jerry is not a bomb about to go off in a crowded room. He is not a loaded gun pointed at the head of an anonymous sex partner. This is not an emergency. Dr. Barret has time to gather facts, deliberate, and document. If he does these things with reasonable dispatch, he will have done 95% of what he can do to comply with the letter and spirit of the law and avoid being sued. Only if he does these things does it make much sense to talk about the law.

Jerry's case presents the first of a number of "duty to warn" scenarios that appear in this book, and so it is worth stating at the outset that the psychotherapist's duty to warn or otherwise protect third parties from a danger posed by a patient is very, very limited. The duty is still seen by courts as an exception to the broad, general principle that no one should depend on the kindness of strangers for protection. The starting point of any legal analysis will be the proposition that we do not have to intervene when we see danger brewing for another, if we have not caused the danger or done something to make it worse (American Law Institute, 1965, §§315–324). Fifteen years into the HIV epidemic, there has yet to be a judicial opinion anywhere in the United States ruling that a psychotherapist is responsible to warn sexual or needle-sharing contacts of a patient with HIV, and I for one do not expect that there ever will be.

In one way, then, Jerry's case raises a very important ethical issue for me as an attorney. My obligation is to Dr. Barret's welfare. Dr. Barret does not just want to minimize his legal risk at all costs. He wants to make a decision about Jerry that is informed by legal analysis and a good estimate of the legal risk for both Jerry and himself. Unfortunately, health care providers, including psychotherapists, often take a dim view of the legal system, which can look hostile, alien, and threatening to one's professional reputation and livelihood. I know enough psychology to recognize that people often judge risks more by the awfulness of the potential outcome than by the actual likelihood of the outcome occurring. Health professionals also often perceive the law to be far more mechanical and determinantal than it actually is, failing to see the extent to which rules can be interpreted differently by different lawyers and judges. So here's my concern: If I just tell Dr. Barret not to worry and skip the details, I am myself acting paternalistically and depriving him of information that might help him in his dilemma. Yet if I tell him about the many legal rules that might apply and how a court might interpret them in this case, I might obscure my basic message that his risk is low or make him feel that he has no choice but to do exactly what I recommend.

Reflecting on my own role, I see that I do not want to use my special knowledge of the law to take a decision away from my client. The burden of what to do about Jerry has to remain on Dr. Barret. I'll try to use the legal consult to reduce his legal anxiety and broaden his analysis of the situation. Consistent with his concerns, I'll talk about both the risks he faces and the possible legal implications of his actions for Jerry.

Protecting Jerry's Partners: Confidentiality and the Duty to Protect

Like most psychotherapists, Dr. Barret is aware of the *Tarasoff* rule, that a psychotherapist has an obligation to take reasonable steps to prevent a patient from harming others under at least some circumstances. He is also aware that most states have cases or statutes that protect the confidentiality of therapeutic confidences generally or that specifically protect the privacy of HIV-related information shared with a health care provider (see chapter 6, Tables 6.2 and 6.3). There is an obvious tension here, with the psychotherapist apparently liable for trouble whichever course he takes. Because these rules are part of state law, rather than the law of the federal government, they vary from place to place. Looking at the several North Carolina laws and cases that apply to this situation helps narrow the issues in Jerry's case and eliminate much of the apparent tension.

The law has a variety of interpretive rules that are useful when legal obligations seem to be in conflict. For *Tarasoff* situations involving HIV, the most important are the rules that favor the specific over the general rule and the legislative over the judicial one. Depending on the state, the psychotherapist's duty to protect may be the product of a court decision or of a statute passed by the legislature. If the legislature has also passed a statute dealing specifically with the release of HIV-related information, that statute will often determine what the psychotherapist's obligation is, because a statute trumps a court-made rule, and a statute setting out the behavior required in a specific situation trumps a statute setting out a more general rule of conduct. At least two cases across the country have held that a strict HIV confidentiality law overrode any duty a health care provider might have to warn a patient's spouse of his HIV (*N.O.L. v. District of Columbia*, 1996; *Santa Rosa Health Care Corp. v. Garcia*, 1998).

Our first question, therefore, is not whether Dr. Barret has a *Tarasoff*-like duty to warn, but whether he is even allowed to release the information under the state's HIV confidentiality law, which forbids the release of HIV information except in certain defined circumstances. The one exception that might apply here allows a release when it "is necessary to protect public health and is made as provided by the Commission in its rules regarding control measures for communicable diseases and conditions" (N.C. Gen. Stat., 1997, §§130A-143(4)). The Commission for Health Services is the state health department's policy-making body, and its rules set out a variety of very specific obligations for people with HIV and their physicians to avoid risks to sex partners. These rules do not mention psychotherapists, nor do they deal with the right or obligations of people (other than physicians and a few other professionals) to report dangerous behavior to the health department (N.C. Admin. Code, 1997). Strictly speaking, then, the Commission's rules do not set out a means by which a *psychotherapist* can report a patient like Jerry, so the exception in the confidentiality law does not apply, and Dr. Barret cannot rely on it to excuse him from his obligation to keep Jerry's information private. Compliance with this sort of statute would be a defense against *Tarasoff* liability in any state.

If we nonetheless assume that the law does not totally forbid disclosure to protect Jerry's sex partners, we have to face the question of whether it *requires* some reasonable steps to protect them. Courts in North Carolina have taken a very narrow view of the obligation of a psychotherapist to control a dangerous patient or otherwise to protect third parties from the patient's dangerous behavior. North Carolina courts have restricted the duty to the situation of a patient who has already been involuntarily committed and then is negligently released or allowed to escape. The duty is based on the psychotherapist's actual knowledge of a threat and the ability, in light of the commitment, to control the patient (*Currie v. U.S.*, 1987; *Davis v. North Carolina Department of Human Resources*, 1995; *King v. Durham County Mental Health*, 1994). They have not found an obligation to commit someone in the first place; nor does Jerry seem to meet the criteria for involuntary commitment in North Carolina, which require that the patient be mentally ill (N.C. Gen. Stat., 1997, §§122C-3(21), 122C-261, 122C-263). Even if a court were to find that a psychotherapist may sometimes have a duty to take some action in this sort of outpatient setting, I think it unlikely that such a duty would be found to arise under the circumstances here. The usual *Tarasoff*-type victim has no idea of the risk the patient poses, or can do little to avoid it. This is not the case with Jerry's anonymous partners, who must know of HIV and who can insist on safe sex. The pervasive and well-known nature of the HIV risk would also make it difficult for any of these partners to make a case against Jerry or Dr. Barret: They would have to both prove that Jerry (and not some other partner) was the source of their infection and convince a judge and jury that they were not as or more responsible than Jerry for exposing themselves to the risk.

What if Dr. Barret decides he wants to take some action? On paper, the HIV confidentiality law limits his options to, at most, notifying the health department, and even that might be illegal, but in practice I doubt Jerry could successfully sue Dr. Barret for taking any of the several protective steps open to him. The law is more than just rules. Often, particularly in litigation, you can better understand what happens as a clash of stories— real human dilemmas enacted on a Perry Mason stage. If Dr. Barret feels he has to warn the health department, or the police, or the men in the park, that sex with Jerry could be fatal, he is going to look like a hero to a whole lot of jurors and judges, many of whom will overestimate the risks of transmission and underestimate the value of safe sex. Jerry's claim of privacy will likely fall on deaf ears against Dr. Barret's plea of saving lives. The rules on HIV notification, which are full of specific duties for physicians and people with HIV to tell partners and avoid risk, could be taken as evidence of the legislature and health authorities' intention to allow health care providers to intervene in cases like this. A court might rule that the omission of psychotherapists from the legal language was simply an oversight.

The good news for Dr. Barret is that his legal risk is very low. North Carolina law does not create a duty to protect Jerry's sex partners; even if it did, the HIV confidentiality law limits Dr. Barret's response to, at most, warning the health department. And even if he had that duty and failed to fulfill it, none of Jerry's sex partners could successfully sue. Thus Dr. Barret is free, from a legal point of view, to make his own best professional judgment about what to do. That's also the bad news: There is no clear legal command that takes the responsibility for this decision off his shoulders.

The Stakes for Jerry

Dr. Barret is not in serious legal danger, but if he chooses to bring in the health authorities there may be more or less serious consequences for

Jerry. The Commission for Health Services' rules require people with HIV to avoid sexual or other behavior that poses a risk of transmission to others. The rules explicitly require them to inform prospective partners of their HIV infection (N.C. Admin. Code tit. 15A, 19A.0202, Aug. 1997). Local health authorities have the power to confine Jerry or order him to change his behavior (N.C. Gen. Stat., 1997, §§130A-145). This is quite typical across the county. Intervention, even in the form of a warning, from the health department might help get Jerry's attention. Ideally, health department interventions are nonpunitive and are carried out with a sophisticated understanding of the psychosocial complexities of HIV and risky sex. (The experiences of local health departments with compulsory HIV control measures are discussed in Bayer & Fairchild-Carino, 1993; one health department's protocol is presented in Gellert, Page, Weismuller, & Ehling, 1993.) Nevertheless, Dr. Barret would probably want to get some information on the attitudes and practices of local health officials before going to them for assistance.

We also have to deal with the homophobia still embodied in North Carolina law. The state is one of 16 that still has a statute forbidding sodomy or "the crime against nature," which its courts interpret to include consensual homosexual activity between adults (*North Carolina v. Jarrell*, 1975). Jerry could be punished just for having sex. His HIV status could expose him to additional criminal prosecution for anything from assault to attempted murder. The prevalence of both homophobia and AIDS phobia in the community might make it hard for Jerry to get a fair trial and expose him to substantial vilification and a long jail term even for behavior that was not actually very dangerous (Dalton, 1993). Such prosecutions are rare, but the possibility justifies Dr. Barret's caution in taking Jerry's situation to the police or the public health authorities.

My Conclusions

The law doesn't clearly tell Dr. Barret what to do, but neither will it conclusively preclude any of the responsible options Dr. Barret has identified. Despite the tension between them, Dr. Barret does not have to choose between privacy and protection; his real task is to come up with a defensible resolution to the problem. Ethics, and the judgments of professional peers, are primary measures of the legal reasonableness of his actions. How he makes and implements the decision will also affect the perception of the outcome: moving with all deliberate speed, gathering information and assistance, and documenting the process are all associated with both the substance and appearance of reasonableness. If he is judged at all, he will be judged largely for his ability to defend his choices as harmonizing responsibility for third parties and respect for privacy. My best advice is to develop a treatment plan for Jerry, in consultation with other psychologists, with such documentation as necessary to demonstrate that he has dealt with the dilemma in a professionally acceptable manner.

Identify and Assess the Options (by Bob Barret)

As I reflect on Dr. Kitchener's comments my confidence rises. I am trying to find a balance between my obligation to Jerry and the responsibility I feel for my community as well as for Jerry's potential sex partners. My biggest worry continues to be that if I do report Jerry, he will mistrust all mental health practitioners and continue with his unsafe behavior. If I can keep him in treatment, I have a better chance to help him change his irresponsible behavior. I do not want to harm Jerry in any way, but at the same time I do not want to be a silent observer while he is engaged in behavior that is potentially harmful to others. Finding the balance between minimizing harm and minimizing intrusion continues to be my goal. The foundational principles of autonomy (keeping my promise), beneficence (as he understands himself better he will become more responsible), and justice (can I find a way to help him without reporting him to authorities while being reasonably confident that he is not doing harm to others?) guide me as I assess my plan. Keeping him in psychological treatment offers the best hope for a desirable outcome. I want to create a place for Jerry to examine his behavior without his having to censor what he tells me. The best way for me to help him is to maintain confidentiality and hope he trusts me enough to tell me the truth. Dr. Kitchener's advice reassures me, and I begin to reflect on Mr. Burris's assessment of my legal situation.

Although I worry slightly about being sued, my main concern is with my professional responsibility. I do not want to be called before a court, but neither do I want to create public mistrust about my profession. The law may say that my duty to warn others does not apply in these circumstances, but I feel a moral obligation to protect others from harm if I can. Because the North Carolina Health Department's rules about disclosure in HIV-related cases are limited to physicians, my risk of being charged might be greater if I did break confidentiality, especially because the courts of my state have not generally held psychotherapists responsible for protecting the public welfare. Mr. Burris points out that breaking confidentiality may create a greater legal risk for me than honoring the privacy of our communications. I pay close attention to his encouragement to consult with other psychologists and to document each step I take fully.

My anxiety has been reduced after the two consultations. After carefully documenting what each of the experts said to me, I move to formulate my plan. Although this situation has created more activity for me than I find with most of my clients, I like being on the cutting edge of our profession.

I am attracted to the demand for creative approaches and to the exercise of considering alternative points of view. In some small way I have the sense that I am contributing to creating the standard of care in an area that is so new.

There are several actions that I can take. I reject contacting the local health department because they are not likely to do anything other than interviewing Jerry. Likewise, local law enforcement is not going to take any action. Consultation, encouraged by both Dr. Kitchener and Mr. Burris, seems like an appropriate step. Jerry had previously signed a release so I could speak with his physician, so I know I can have that conversation without breaking confidentiality. At the same time I want to emphasize my grave concern to Jerry about what he is doing. My plan is to insist that he sign a safe sex contract with me and to check with him in our weekly sessions to see if he is honoring that agreement. I worry that this plan is only as good as Jerry's promise to honor it, but at least I am on solid ethical and legal grounds. In the next session I decide to go over the details about HIV transmission and safe sex practices, carefully checking to see that Jerry understands these facts and then ask him to sign a contract that states the risky behaviors and includes the steps he will take to avoid placing others at risk. I also want to review the risk that Jerry is taking in terms of his own health. Speaking about the risk of unsafe sex when his immune system has already been compromised might help him maintain these new behaviors. I also want to let Jerry know that I am going to advise his physician about my treatment plan and ask that he discuss the contract on his next visit there. I get in touch with another psychologist in my community and review the plan (keeping Jerry's identity concealed) and document that step as well.

What continues to trouble me is that Jerry may not be capable of adhering strictly to our contract and that others may become infected. I do not like knowing that he (and others) are adding to the numbers of the HIV-infected population, and I wonder if there is anything I can do that would placate my need to respond to the community's vulnerability. My role as a social activist had been cast long before I met Jerry, so thinking about what I might do was not exactly a new task for me. When I saw my first "Jerry" I struggled with finding peace with myself as I continued to provide him treatment. Although his behavior did become more responsible, I was not sure when or how often he "slipped." So, I began to identify other options I could pursue that would help me feel better about what I was doing. First, I approached the local health department and asked them to post information about risky behavior and safe sex in adult bookstores and other areas of sexual activity. I also got in touch with a local reporter who covered HIV issues. She agreed to write a story that featured the risks that many were taking as they engaged in unprotected intercourse. One part of her story featured sex between men in public places. This story created lots of controversy but helped me feel like I had lived up to my obligation to my community. A warning had been issued and that was about the best I could do given the inability to identify those whom my client was placing at risk. As I recall that action I remind myself to check back with the health department to see if those signs are still in place.

Choose a Course of Action and Share It With Your Client

The next time that Jerry comes in I tell him about my concern about his behavior, emphasizing that he is placing himself at risk of illness. We talk about the implications of his spreading HIV to others as well as the impact of this behavior on his relationship. Reluctantly, he agrees to sign an ongoing safe sex contract and to explore his behavior more fully with me. His interest in being more responsible seems sincere, and our relationship feels more secure. I also speak with him about my plan to talk with his physician and the need for public heath warnings to those who have anonymous sex. At first Jerry resists letting me talk with his physician. However, I remind him that effective medical treatment demands as much information as possible and that if his medical team and I work together he will manage his illness more effectively. He tells me that he will discuss this situation with his doctor and that he will ask the doctor to call me for further consultation. He signs a release before he leaves. Later in the week his doctor calls and we talk about his behavior. We agree that each of us will bring up his sexual activity each time we see him and that I will inform the physician if Jerry appears to be placing others at risk. Once again I document this consultation in Jerry's file.

Implement the Course of Action: Monitor and Discuss Outcomes

Over the next several months, Jerry demonstrates that he can be responsible sexually. His relationship ultimately fails, and with the assistance of psychotherapy Jerry explores his emotional response to HIV. He comes to see that part of the motivation for participation in unsafe sex has been his anger. He is angry about being infected, angry about the stigma that accompanies HIV, angry that his family has been absent from his life. His sadness and fear about his limited future fuel the anger. Once he begins to understand why he is angry he starts thinking about his future in a new way. Soon thereafter he decides to move to a larger city, one that would have a visible HIV-infected population and one that might offer new opportunities. Before he leaves I review the file and document everything that has transpired. I also refer him to an HIV-wise psychologist there and reinforce the importance of maintaining his commitment to safe sex in his new community. For a few months after he left I got occasional notes from him. It was obvious that he was happier and that the decision to move had been a good one for him.

I discuss this situation with colleagues from time to time and scan the literature for information that would validate the course of action that I selected. Often I felt very alone and unsettled by the lack of absolute guidance. After years of HIV work I have learned that each patient is different and, although the facts may look similar, there is no standard procedure to follow in each instance. That is part of the challenging nature of this work and one reason my interest in it continues. As my HIV-related work has become more "routine" I no longer have to spend as much time in analyzing situations like this one. Still, the law changes, the standard of care becomes clearer, and I know I need to stay current through professional reading and receiving additional training. Developing a means to incorporate it into awareness will create a guide that will help movement through difficult situations like this one.

REFERENCES

American Law Institute. (1965). *Restatement (second) of torts.* St. Paul, MN: Author.

American Psychological Association. (1992). Ethical principles of psychologists and code of conduct. *American Psychologist, 47,* 1597–1611.

Barret, R. L. (1996). Countertransference issues in HIV-related psychotherapy. In M. Winiarski (Ed.), *HIV mental health into the 21st century* (pp. 39–51). New York: New York University Press.

Bayer, R., & Fairchild-Carino, A. (1993). AIDS and the limits of control: Public health orders, quarantine, and recalcitrant behavior. *American Journal of Public Health, 83,* 1471–1476.

Beauchamp, T. L., & Childress, J. F. (1989). *Principles of biomedical ethics.* Oxford, England: Oxford University Press.

Canter, M. B., Bennett, B. E., Jones, S. E., & Nagy, T. F. (1994). *Ethics for psychologists: A commentary on the APA Ethics Code.* Washington, DC: American Psychological Association.

Currie v. U.S., 836 F.2d 209 (4th Cir. 1987).

Dalton, H. (1993). Criminal law. In S. Burris, H. Dalton, J. Miller, & The Yale AIDS Law Project (Eds.), *AIDS law today: A new guide for the public* (pp. 242–262). New Haven, CT: Yale University Press.

Davis v. North Carolina Department of Human Resources, 121 N.C. App. 105, 465 S.E.2d 2 (N.C. Ct. App. 1995).

Gellert, G., Page, B., Weismuller, P., & Ehling, L. R. (1993). Managing the noncompliant HIV-infected individual: Experiences from a local health department. *AIDS & Public Policy Journal, 8,* 20–26.

King v. Durham County Mental Health, 113 N. C. App. 341, 439 S.E.2d 771 (N.C. Ct. App. 1994).

Melton, G. B. (1988). Ethical and legal issues in AIDS-related practice. *American Psychologist, 48*, 941–947.

Melton, G. B., and Jue. (1988). TO COME.

N. C. ADMIN. CODE tit. 15A, r. 19A.0202 (Aug, 1997).

N. C. GEN. STAT. §§ 122C-3(21), 122C-261, 122C-263 (1997).

N. C. GEN. STAT. § 130A-143(4) (1997).

N.O.L. v. District of Columbia, 674 A.2d 498 (D.C. 1996).

North Carolina v. Jarrell, 24 N.C. App. 610, 211 S.E.2d 837 (N.C. Ct. App. 1975).

Santa Rosa Health Care Corp. v. Garcia, 41 Tex. Sup. Ct. J. 535 (Tex. 1998).

Tarasoff v. Board of Regents of the University of California, 551 P.2d 334 (Cal. 1976).

8

THE SECRETIVE HIV-POSITIVE SPOUSE: THE CASE OF RUBEN

SALLY JUE, KAREN STROHM KITCHENER, AND SCOTT BURRIS

ORIENTATION TO THE MAJOR ETHICAL ISSUES HIGHLIGHTED IN THE CASE

One of the most complex situations that mental health providers face involves working with a married man who is secretly having sex with other men. This chapter describes the dilemma created for the therapist when a client learns that he is HIV-positive and tries to keep this fact a secret from his wife. This case occurred in California.

CASE PRESENTATION (BY SALLY JUE)

Ruben initiated therapy because his male partner, Jim, recently tested positive for HIV, and Ruben is anxious about his own health. Ruben has had a sexual relationship with Jim for 6 months. Prior to his relationship with Jim, Ruben had occasional sex with other men. However, he considers his relationship with Jim "different" and more important. Ruben does not consider himself gay because he is "masculino" and because when he does have sex with other men, he is the "active" or penetrating partner.

Ruben is also a married man who lives with his wife, Elena, and their 2 children, ages 1 and 3. Ruben married Elena when he was 20 years old. They both immigrated to the United States from Mexico 5 years later. Both have been legal residents for 7 years but are not yet U.S. citizens. For the past 6 months, Ruben has struggled with his feelings for Jim and Elena. He clearly cares for Elena, loves his children, and enjoys being a father. Ruben speaks openly about the stress of keeping his relationship with Jim a secret, but he also states that it is common in his culture for men to have other partners as long as they are discrete and fulfill their familial obligations.

In the first three sessions, I spent most of my time providing information about HIV and safer sex and dealing with Ruben's fear and indecision about having an HIV test. Without offering any explanation, Ruben cut off all sexual contact with Elena and all contact with Jim since finding out about Jim's HIV status. He stated that he would remain celibate because he is now too afraid to have any kind of sex with anyone. After the third session, Ruben was tested at a confidential test site. At the following session, he told me that he tested positive. He is afraid to tell Elena and has continued to avoid sexual contact with her. She has begun asking if he is feeling tired or unwell. Ruben states that he just cannot tell her and becomes very emotional as he imagines her hurt feelings and the shame he would bring to himself and his family. He also fears that if Elena finds out the truth, she would find ways to keep the children from him and tell his parents, who would be deeply disappointed.

PAUSE AND IDENTIFY YOUR PERSONAL RESPONSES TO THE CASE

Pausing enables me to sort through my ambivalent feelings about Ruben and his situation. I can easily empathize with his fears of bringing shame and disappointment to himself and his family, and his fear of possibly losing contact with his children is valid—I have certainly seen this happen in other similar cases. However, I also feel Ruben is largely responsible for his current dilemma because he practiced unsafe sex with Jim, previous partners, and Elena. To avoid all sexual contact with his wife and offer no explanation, although protective, seems emotionally hurtful. These factors, plus the possibility that his children could also be HIV-positive although they are currently healthy, interfere with my ability to be more empathic.

My first impulse is to tell Ruben he must let his wife know that he is HIV-positive and that because there is a strong possibility that she and the children might be infected, they must get tested. This is important because early intervention leads to better health outcomes. Although Ruben, not his family, is my client, I cannot help being concerned about their health and feeling anxious about what my liability for their welfare might be.

Here is the dilemma: Strongly confronting Ruben about my belief that he should tell Elena may drive him away and destroy the trust that we have built. I feel it is important for Ruben to stay in therapy because it can offer a safe, nonjudgmental place to weather this crisis. However, not raising the possible health consequences to his family of his behaviors feels like negligence on my part and could give Ruben the impression that I approve of his silence.

I am also somewhat confused by how Ruben's definitions of marital fidelity and being gay differ from my own. This leads me to ask whether they are truly different cultural values and norms or merely Ruben's denial of his sexual orientation and rationalizations for his multiple relationships. In pursuing this train of thought, I now wonder if there might be other cultural factors I need to be aware of that could be helpful to me in continuing my work with Ruben. I make a note to call a colleague who has worked with gay Latino men and Latino families.

REVIEW THE FACTS OF THE CASE

I realize that I am nearly as immobilized by my feelings as Ruben is by his fears. To try to move forward, I review the facts of the case.

Jim and Ruben are HIV-positive, and Ruben had unprotected intercourse with Elena, Jim, and previous partners. Ruben then cut off all contact with Jim and all sexual contact with Elena, offering her no explanation. Because of his self-imposed celibacy, Ruben currently presents no danger to others. Ruben's severing of his sexual relations with Elena suggests concern for her welfare and a desire to protect her from harm. However, there is a clear possibility that he could have infected her during the years he had unprotected sex with other men, and she could have inadvertently passed HIV onto their children during pregnancy or delivery.

My Latina colleague confirmed Ruben's views on homosexuality and marital fidelity as common Latino cultural norms. She also told me that because of cultural gender role norms, it was unlikely that Elena would openly confront Ruben on the change in his behavior. However, cultural gender roles regarding a Latino man's responsibilities to his family might be used as a positive motivator for Ruben, especially because it is clear that he cares deeply for his wife and children.

Ruben is oriented to time and place, rarely drinks alcohol, and has no drug or psychiatric history. He does not display any symptoms of dementia. He has clearly stated that suicide is not an option because he would never abandon his family.

CONCEPTUALIZE AN INITIAL PLAN
BASED ON CLINICAL ISSUES

My initial diagnosis for Ruben is that he has an adjustment disorder with mixed emotional features. Ruben's reaction to his HIV status and his assessment of its possible impact on his familial relationships appear within normal range. The latter particularly overwhelms him. Whether he discloses his HIV status or not, his relationship with Elena is irreversibly altered, and he knows this. At the moment, avoidance is the safest and easiest response for him. Ongoing treatment can assist him in sorting through his feelings and examining more responsible options and their possible consequences to himself and his family.

My initial plan is to find out what he thinks the impact of his HIV status is on himself and his immediate family. During this discussion, if Ruben does not raise the issue himself, I will bring up Elena's and the children's possible infection and need to have an HIV test. I will also emphasize the importance for Ruben, and possibly his family, to be regularly monitored by an HIV-knowledgeable physician, because early intervention leads to better health outcomes. However, in California a physician can, over the objections of the patient, breach confidentiality to inform known partners that they have been exposed to HIV. Although I am tempted by the prospect of getting myself off the hook about how to get Elena tested without alienating Ruben, I cannot, in good faith, encourage him to seek HIV medical care without letting him know about this law.

I will use Ruben's commitment to his cultural gender role as protector and provider for his family and his caring and concern for Elena and his children to try and motivate him to be honest with her. Although I still empathize with his dilemma, I can point out how withholding his HIV status from Elena contradicts his stated beliefs and feelings. I feel that he has some time to make a decision, however, because his celibacy prevents her from further risk of infection. I can also provide HIV referrals and more HIV information, do some reality testing of his fears, and help him explore various options for handling his situation.

I am reasonably comfortable with my initial plan, but I wonder how much of a responsibility I have for his family's well-being. Does Elena's need to find out about her HIV status supersede Ruben's right to confidentiality?

CONSULT THE ETHICS CODE AND ASSESS THE
ETHICAL ISSUES (BY KAREN STROHM KITCHENER)

As I think about how to respond to Ms. Jue, both the similarities and differences between this case and Jerry's (see chapter 7) case strike me. Both cases involve individuals who are HIV-positive and who refuse to inform their partner or partners of their HIV status. Consequently, both involve balancing the responsibility to keep information that client's share about their HIV status confidential and a responsibility to society, which would suggest that the therapist, in this case Ms. Jue, has some responsibility to protect the client's partner. The similarities stop there, however; the issues raised by Ruben are more complex. The therapist has taken Ruben at his word that he has stopped all sexual contact with his wife. If this is true and she is not already infected, then the danger of infecting her is not imminent. On the other hand, Ruben has had occasional sex with other men prior to his relationship with Jim; thus, he may have been infected for a very long time, and Elena and their children may already be infected. Moreover, Ruben could be fearful of admitting occasional slips in his resolve not to engage in sexual activity with his wife and thus continue to engage in potentially dangerous behavior with her if she is not infected. The case is further complicated by the cultural differences between Ms. Jue and Ruben.

Because there are so many similarities between the cases, I will summarize for Ms. Jue the main points from Jerry's case, first in terms of the American Psychological Association (APA, 1992) Ethics Code and then in terms of foundational ethical principles. I will then point out the differences.

APA Ethics Code

In terms of the APA Ethics Code, Ms. Jue should consider Standard 5.05, which gives psychologists permission to break confidentiality only when doing so is required or permitted by law even when a client's actions pose a danger to a third party. In addition, Standard 5.02 should remind her that she has a primary obligation to respect confidentiality. This is why it is important that she consult with a lawyer to learn about the laws in her state. The other standards that are important in Ruben's case include Standards 1.14, Avoiding Harm; 4.02, Informed Consent to Therapy; 5.01, Discussing the Limits of Confidentiality; and 5.03, Minimizing Intrusions on Privacy. These standards require that Ms. Jue consider how to avoid harming Ruben to the extent that it is possible and to minimize any harm when it is "foreseeable and unavoidable."

The standards on informed consent and a discussion of the limits of confidentiality should lead Ms. Jue to review her informed consent procedure to evaluate what she told Ruben about the limits of confidentiality. Because therapists who work with HIV-positive clients frequently face decisions about breaking confidentiality when clients are endangering others, Ms. Jue may have included a statement about the limits of confidentiality in her consent procedure. If she has, she may want to remind Ruben of this agreement and engage him in a discussion of whether his failure to inform

Elena of his HIV status does endanger her. This may help Ruben understand Ms. Jue's dilemma about breaking confidentiality and may help him begin to understand how his silence may threaten the welfare of both his wife and his children. Furthermore, the standards on confidentiality suggest that if Ms. Jue decides that she must break confidentiality, she should do so in a way that minimizes intrusions on Ruben's privacy. For example, she may need to disclose his HIV status in order to protect Elena; however, she does not need to disclose how Ruben contracted HIV or that he was in a relationship with a man.

The APA Ethics Code addresses cultural differences between therapists and clients in Standard 1.08, Human Differences, and 1.09, Respecting Others, and in Aspirational Principle D: Respect for People's Rights and Dignity. Principle D generally suggests that psychologists should respect cultural differences and eliminate the effects of biases and unfair discrimination on their work. Standard 1.08 is more specific. It requires psychologists who work with clients whose ethnicity, race, or sexual orientation differs from their own to get the necessary training, experience, or consultation to ensure that they perform competently. Standard 1.09 requires that psychologists respect the rights of clients to hold values and opinions different from their own. In this case, Ms. Jue has already taken action that is consistent with both standards by consulting with a Latina colleague about Latino beliefs and values, and she appears to be taking into consideration Ruben's value system as she conceptualizes her initial plan. Although there is no explicit standard that would tell her how much consultation is required, she needs to obtain enough to provide competent services to her client. Standards 1.08 and 1.09 and Principle D should remind her to continue to check in with her Latina colleague or others about Ruben's culture as she plans her treatment to ensure that it is culturally sensitive. For example, her Latina colleague might point out that Ruben may be tempted to engage in sexual activity with his wife just to prove that he is still a man.

Two other aspirational principles from the code are relevant to Ruben's case as they were in Jerry's case. They are Principle E: Concern for Others' Welfare and Principle F: Social Responsibility. These principles suggest that psychologists should aspire to benefit those with whom they are working and to benefit society. They also suggest that Ms. Jue should balance her obligations in a way that minimizes harm.

Foundational Ethical Principles

As the APA Ethics Code suggests, Ms. Jue must find a balance between her responsibility to help and not harm Ruben and her responsibility to Ruben's wife Elena and their children. As in chapter 7, the question to be addressed is this: How much responsibility does a therapist have for a client's partner? The identity of Ruben's partner is known, so if Ms. Jue begins to doubt that Ruben is remaining celibate she needs to consider whether she should break confidentiality to inform Elena about Ruben's HIV status if he refuses to do so. Furthermore, she is struggling with how she can maintain a trusting relationship with Ruben because she believes that he needs support and information to help him deal with his current crisis.

Although keeping confidentiality is based to some extent on the principle that autonomous people have the right to decide with whom they share their secrets, autonomy does not mean that individuals have the right to endanger other people. In this case, according to Ms. Jue's assessment, Ruben is not continuing to endanger Elena by engaging in sexual activity with her. However, by failing to let her know that she may be HIV-positive he is keeping her from the benefit of early treatment, and he may be contributing to the long-term harm of both her and their children. If Elena is HIV-positive, delaying treatment may mean that treatment is less successful. Ultimately, if Ruben and Elena get full-blown AIDS, their children may be left without parents. Furthermore, if Ruben has been infected with the HIV virus for many years and his children are infected, delaying treatment for them may also affect their long-term health.

An additional autonomy issue makes this case different from others. Elena apparently has no reason to believe that she is at risk of infection when engaging in sexual activity with her husband. Furthermore, cultural norms may exacerbate the assumption that she should trust him. In other words, Elena cannot make an autonomous decision about protecting herself even though her health may be at risk.

However, Ms. Jue's obligation to maintain confidentiality is also supported by the principle of fidelity, which requires promise keeping, truthfulness, and loyalty. The question is this: What has Ms. Jue promised Ruben in terms of confidentiality? If she has promised that she will keep confidentiality under all circumstances, she is in a very difficult situation. It is more likely, however, that she informed him when he entered therapy that there might be occasions when confidentiality would be broken. The principle of fidelity would also lead her to ask what she can do to maintain Ruben's trust as well as help Elena.

Her plan to engage Ruben in a discussion of the impact of his HIV status on himself and his family is probably a good one from both the perspectives of autonomy and fidelity. It allows her both to remain loyal to Ruben and to maintain his trust. These discussions as well as educational information about the nature of the HIV virus and treatment possibilities may allow Ruben to understand the implications of his disease for his wife and his children. As noted earlier, as a part of this discussion she may want to remind him of their original confidentiality agreement assuming it involved the caveat that she might break confidentiality if she considered him to be dangerous to someone else. As she suggested, using Ruben's commitment to his family may motivate him to disclose his HIV status to his wife. Such a discussion may also help to promote his autonomy in that he can take charge of planning how to deal with his HIV disease and its impact on his family. By reminding him of his original contract regarding confidentiality, he will be more fully aware of the dilemma that Ms. Jue is facing.

The principle of beneficence requires that psychologists act in ways that promote the welfare of those with whom they have a professional relationship and remove harm when it is possible and foreseeable. Because Ruben is her client, Ms. Jue has a stronger responsibility to help him than she has to Elena and the children. However, compassion alone has to leave her concerned about his wife and their children. Because it is likely Elena will find out about Ruben's illness at some point in time, part of helping Ruben may involve problem solving about how and when he can inform her and what he wants to tell her about how he contracted the disease. It may also involve having Elena come to therapy with him, so that Ms. Jue can help him inform her. Doing so would both help Ruben deal with an imminent problem in his life and would give Elena the information she needs in order to get tested. Beneficence also requires that she intervene with Ruben in ways that are culturally appropriate, as it appears that Ms. Jue is doing.

As in the case of Jerry, the principle of nonmaleficence would suggest that Ms. Jue needs to balance the good for Elena and the children that might come from breaking confidentiality with the harm that might occur to Ruben if she did so. Because of cultural issues, the stigma of being HIV-positive might be even stronger for Ruben than it was for Jerry. Furthermore, disclosure of his HIV status without his permission might irrevocably damage their therapeutic relationship.

Last, the principle of justice would require that Ms. Jue consider whether she is treating Ruben fairly. Researchers (Crawford, Humfleet, Ribordy, Ho, & Vickers, 1991) have suggested that many psychologists are biased negatively toward gay men, and Ms. Jue should ask whether some of her anger toward Ruben reflects homophobia, particularly because Ruben's homosexual activity may have infected an apparently heterosexual woman. She also should reevaluate whether she has enough knowledge of the Latino community to understand the issue from Ruben's perspective. If not, she would need to get further consultation or refer Ruben to someone who has more background working with Latinos (as suggested by Standard 1.08 of the APA Ethics Code).

Balancing the Ethics Code and Foundational Ethical Principles

At this point, Ms. Jue's treatment plan seems to balance her ethical responsibilities in a defensible way. By working with Ruben within his cultural framework to disclose his HIV status to Elena, she is respecting his autonomy and remaining faithful to their relationship.

By continuing to help him deal with his HIV status and identify ways to disclose his HIV status to his wife, she is benefiting Ruben and potentially benefiting Elena and their children. By consulting with a Latina colleague, she is trying to ensure that her treatment is fair and culturally sensitive. As Ms. Jue observes, Ruben has decided to become celibate so Elena is not immediately at risk for further infection.

If, however, Ruben decides to resume having intercourse with Elena or if he has occasional "slips" in his resolve and continues to refuse to inform her of his HIV status, the situation would change. Beauchamp and Childress (1989) have argued that as the risk of harm to a third party increases, so does the responsibility to intervene. This is particularly true when the potential harm is severe, as it would be if Elena was not HIV-positive and became so by participating in sexual activity with Ruben. Furthermore, Ruben is violating Elena's right to make an autonomous decision about risking her own health, and by keeping silent about his HIV status, he is violating his responsibility to be trustworthy and to deal with his own family with care. Under these circumstances, breaking confidentiality might be justified because the harm that might come to Ruben by breaking confidentiality, although regrettable, would not be as severe as the harm that might occur to Elena if she contracted HIV. The fact that she might become pregnant and unknowingly pass the HIV infection to an unborn child would add weight to the decision to breach confidentiality. Before doing so, however, Ms. Jue ought to inform Ruben of her intentions and give him the opportunity to tell his wife himself, thereby allowing him to exercise some autonomy in the method and time of informing her. In addition, she should check with a lawyer to identify if the law would preclude breaching confidentiality. If so, then she would need to consider that informing Elena would probably violate Standard 5.05 of the Ethics Code.

Needless to say, this is a kind of ethical case in which no decision feels perfectly correct, and no matter what Ms. Jue decides, she will probably feel some moral regret that a "perfect" solution cannot be found. She seems to be on a good track, however, walking a middle ground between either ignoring her concern for Elena or overreacting to it. As Ruben learns more about his disease and the implications for his family, his own moral responsibility may be awakened, and Ms. Jue can help him find a way to act as a responsible Latino man should to care for his family. Whatever the decision, Ms. Jue should remember that she needs to treat Ruben with care and compassion and that even "correct" decisions that are implemented without them can lead to poor moral outcomes.

IDENTIFY THE LEGAL ISSUES (BY SCOTT BURRIS)

The issues involved in the case of Ruben could be said to involve a psychotherapist's legal obligation to protect a third party from a threat of harm arising from a patient's behavior. As in Jerry's case, the law does not provide an unambiguous answer that solves Ms. Jue's dilemma. The law on the books in California, where Ms. Jue practices, creates at most a very limited duty to act, but unlike Jerry's case, we have here a specific, known victim—Elena—who would make a very sympathetic plaintiff were she to sue Ms. Jue for allowing her to become infected with HIV. For this as much as any other reason, I will advise Ms. Jue that she must take some action if Ruben comes to pose a threat of transmission to his wife.

Ms. Jue has done a good job of collecting the facts, but there are some important things that we do not know. We do not know whether Elena is already infected and, although I admire Ms. Jue's care in learning about and considering cultural norms in the situation, we cannot rule out the possibility that it was Elena who acquired HIV outside the marriage and infected Ruben. Because we do not yet know who is infected and who is at risk, the legal analysis has to address the possibilities that bear most directly on Ms. Jue: that Elena is not infected and so would be in danger should Ruben's celibacy lapse, and that she is already infected but has no reason to know it and so is perhaps missing necessary medical care.

Liability If Elena Is Subsequently Infected

Thus far, the case of Ruben does not involve a duty to warn or protect from future harm. As long as Ms. Jue believes Ruben will stick to his resolution, Elena is not at risk. Ms. Jue should critically examine Ruben's statements, psychological status, and what she knows of his behavior to be sure that his intention to be celibate is real and within his capacity to maintain, and she should document her analysis. She should also carefully monitor the situation for signs that Ruben's resolve may be weakening. Provided she does this, she would be in a good position to defend her conduct in the event of litigation.

Although we do not (yet) have a tangible threat of harm to address, the situation could change. Should Ms. Jue come to believe that Ruben has slipped or is about to slip, we have what is lacking in Jerry's case: an identified victim. Ms. Jue knows about Elena and the risk she faces, and she can readily get in contact with her. If the case develops this way, we will have the same questions that arose in Jerry's case, but under a different state's legal rules: Must Ms. Jue intervene by warning or controlling Ruben and, conversely, to what extent is she allowed by the law to take measures that entail revealing confidential information about Ruben?

Clients often come to me with a sense of legal interpretation as deduction: They think my job is to read a set of statutes and cases and derive from them an answer as to what the law "is" on any given point. Sometimes I can, if the question is simple enough and a law or court decision addresses it in no uncertain terms. In hard cases—in other words, in most of the cases that anyone would bother to ask me about—there is no such clear answer. Legal interpretation in these cases is a matter of prediction: The lawyer makes an educated guess about how the matter would get to court, who the litigants would be, and how judges and juries would react to the exact combination of legal rules and facts that the case would present. In making this prediction, the lawyer draws not only on what he or she knows about the legal system and the rules, but also on his or her experience of power, race, gender, status, and all the other social factors that influence legal interpretation and fact-finding.

Ruben's case makes for a difficult prediction job. A number of statutes, cases, and even the state constitution are relevant, but none unambiguously addresses this situation. Ruben's outsider status—as a bisexual or gay man, as a person with HIV, as an immigrant, even as an adulterer—makes this a very potent situation from a social point of view. I can make a reasonably reliable prediction, but I want Ms. Jue to understand, and be able to question, my reasoning process.

California has several provisions that provide privacy protection to medical information (Doughty, 1994). An HIV confidentiality law prohibits the negligent or deliberate release of the results of an HIV test (Cal. Health & Safety Code, 1998). Judges, however, have narrowly interpreted this law to forbid only the disclosure of an actual blood test result, from a medical record, by a person with access to that record (*Urbaniak v. Newton*, 1991). Because Ms. Jue learned of Ruben's status from Ruben himself and has no blood test result in her records, this statute does not seem to apply to her disclosure of Ruben's status to Elena or anyone else.

Physicians are authorized under the law to notify their HIV patients' sex or needle partners that they have been exposed to HIV and may be infected. The law forbids the physician from naming the patient, although in cases like Elena and Ruben's the identity will often be obvious. Moreover, the physician cannot make this disclosure before discussing the situation with the patient and giving the patient the opportunity to act. According to a strict interpretation of statutes, the legislature's decision to explicitly authorize physician notification of exposed partners should be read as entailing a decision not to authorize other health care and mental health professionals to do so. This statute does nevertheless provide some guidance, insofar as it spells out the procedures the legislature thought appropriate when it considered physician notification of people like Elena; if Ms. Jue does decide she has to notify Elena, she would be well-advised to follow the statutory requirements as closely as is feasible.

Constitutions in the United States normally protect citizens' rights against government misdeeds. California is unusual in having a provision of its state constitution that has been interpreted by courts to protect the privacy of medical records held by private citizens, including records of psychotherapy (*Urbaniak v. Newton*, 1991). The constitutional right of privacy is not, however, an absolute guarantee of nondisclosure: "an infringement of that right may be constitutionally permitted when the need for disclosure outweighs his interest in privacy" (*Cutter v. Brownbridge*, 1986, p. 844). I expect that a court would regard protecting Elena as a sufficiently strong reason for breaching Ruben's privacy.

California also has a statute that protects the privacy of medical records generally (Confidentiality of Medical Information Act, 1982). Like many state HIV laws, this one is structured to broadly prohibit release of information "regarding a patient's medical history, mental or physical condition, or treatment" to anyone (§56.05), except in a set of clearly delineated exceptional circumstances, none of which apply here (§56.10). Ms. Jue's information about Ruben comes from the records of her care for Ruben and so is protected by the medical records privacy law.

Two of the three privacy provisions probably do not forbid release, but the medical records law apparently does. It applies to medical records like Ruben's and purports to define the entire range of allowable disclosure. It makes no exception for warning someone like Elena or calling in the health department or the police. I am reasonably confident that Ms. Jue could rely on this law as a justification for not warning Elena, or otherwise protecting her in a way that involved release of Ruben's HIV status, but I cannot rule out a court, sympathizing with Elena's position, finding a loophole.

Must Ms. Jue find some way to protect Elena? California is, of course, the birthplace of the *Tarasoff* ruling (*Tarasoff v. Board of Regents of the University of California*, 1976), yet my interpretation of the medical records privacy law not only requires Ms. Jue to keep silent but would seem to bar the warning required in the *Tarasoff* case itself. As often happens, two bodies of law applying to the same conduct seem to require different behavior.

Here is how I work through this. The *Tarasoff* decision came down in 1976. At that point, the law was clear: A psychotherapist who was aware of a patient's threat of harm to a third party would be required to warn or otherwise protect that person from the threat, even if the protection entailed a breach of confidentiality. In 1981, the legislature passed its sweeping Confidentiality of Medical Information Act. The law seemed to prohibit the sort of release made in *Tarasoff* and, as a law passed by the legislature, it trumped the *Tarasoff* court decision. Now the law seemed to oblige the psychotherapist to take reasonable steps to protect the third party, but only to the extent it was possible to do so without revealing information protected by the statute. Finally, in 1985, the legislature passed another law that purported to limit the psychotherapist's duty to warn or protect to instances of "violent behavior" (Cal. Civ. Code, 2000, § 43.92). No such limitation would have been required if the legislature thought it had eliminated the duty to warn altogether by passing the privacy law. Moreover, the 1985 statute does not seem to preclude a duty to protect third parties from nonviolent threats a patient might pose (like HIV transmission). Trying to harmonize these various provisions as they might apply in Ms. Jue's case, I conclude that (a) Ms. Jue probably has a duty to take reasonable steps to protect Elena from being infected with HIV by Ruben, but (b) she may not satisfy this duty by disclosing Ruben's HIV status, because the release is not necessary to protect Elena against physical violence.

My research finds no case law directly addressing the intersection of privacy, the duty to warn, and HIV, but one recent case does support my interpretation by implication. *Reisner v. University of California* (1995) was a suit by the sex partner of the doctor's patient. The doctor knew that a transfusion had infected the patient but never told her. She later had sex with the plaintiff and infected him before she was diagnosed with AIDS and learned of the transfusion infection. The court affirmed the idea that a professional has a duty to protect third parties to whom a patient might spread HIV, but it did not have to deal with the confidentiality problem because, as the court noted, the plaintiff would have been protected by the physician revealing the diagnosis to the patient.

Right now, Ms. Jue seems to be fulfilling her duty to Elena by working through the problem with Ruben. If this fails, and Ms. Jue fears the resumption of unprotected sex with Elena, what can she do? Well, she could notify Elena against my legal opinion, in which case I expect she would be wrong on the law but not likely to be sued by Ruben or to lose if he did sue. It is worth mentioning here that "willful, unauthorized communication of information received in professional confidence" is "unprofessional conduct" for a California psychologist (Cal. Bus. & Prof. Code, 2000, §2960(h)). Acting against my legal advice could hurt her were she to be charged with unprofessional conduct by the state Board of Psychology, because it would support the claim that her decision was "willful" rather than merely incorrect.

Another option would be to inform the health authorities, who probably have some experience working through such cases (Gellert, Page,

Weismuller, & Ehling, 1993). This, too, would contravene my strict reading of the law on the books, but it comports with the law of a judge or juror's common sense, and Ruben would again have a very hard time convincing anyone in the legal system that he had been wronged and deserved compensation. Whatever the law, if the moment comes when Ms. Jue believes she is all that stands between Elena and infection by Ruben, Ms. Jue has to act and, unless her judgment or execution are wildly unreasonable, she will not, I think, end up paying damages to Ruben.

Liability for Delaying Elena's Medical Care

What about a legal duty to ensure that Elena gets timely diagnosis and treatment? A lawyer could argue this claim, but it stretches the obligation to a third party well past the point a court would probably be willing to go. Ms. Jue did not create the harm, nor has she made it worse. Obviously she should work to get Ruben to deal with Elena's risk and document her efforts, but the health care issue alone would not, I think, justify a breach of confidentiality under California or any other state's law.

This file should be kept open. Ms. Jue's initial plan sounds like a good one, but if Ruben changes his behavior or talk, it should be revised.

IDENTIFY AND ASSESS THE OPTIONS (BY SALLY JUE)

I was relieved to find that my initial plan adheres to the Ethics Code and upholds the foundational ethical principles. As long as Ruben remains celibate, I have some time to try to convince him to tell Elena about his HIV status and to help him find a way to do so that minimizes harm to them both. By discussing how Ruben's HIV status affects himself and his family, I can remain true to the principles of autonomy, fidelity, and nonmaleficence. By continuing to seek cultural consultation from my Latina colleague, I can uphold the principles of beneficence and justice. However, should Ruben give any indication that he is incapable of maintaining his celibacy or that he has had unprotected sex with Elena, I need to seriously consider breaching confidentiality and informing her of his HIV status if he still chooses not to do so himself.

Having a better understanding of federal and state laws and relevant case decisions is helpful in understanding the law, but it is also frustrating because, according to Mr. Burris, a strict reading of the laws would seem to support maintaining Ruben's confidentiality, even if he does have unprotected sex with Elena. For me, a strict reading of the law may violate what I perceive to be the ethical and compassionate course of action. However, it was reassuring to hear that if I believe that I am "all that stands between

Elena and infection by Ruben," and I document the events, clinical assessments, and ethical decision-making process that would lead me to breach confidentiality, my legal risk would be relatively low. As for problems with the licensing board or ethics committee, if I continue to consult with others to provide quality clinical care for Ruben, I hope to minimize the possibility of him filing a complaint.

Although my initial plan is ethically and legally defensible in its original form, I have decided to refine and strengthen it after reviewing Dr. Kitchener's and Mr. Burris's input.

In addition to engaging Ruben in discussion about the impact of his HIV status on himself and his family, I will also review the limits of the confidentiality statement Ruben signed upon entering treatment with me and discuss with him whether his failure to inform Elena of his HIV status endangers her and threatens the welfare of his family. This discussion maximizes the principles of autonomy and fidelity by maintaining my loyalty to Ruben and his trust. Because Elena has no reason to believe that she could suffer potential harm from having unprotected sex with him, I will appeal to Ruben's protective instincts to help resolve this dilemma. Because I also feel some responsibility to minimize harm to Ruben's family, I need to be clear with him about the limits of confidentiality. I will tell Ruben that if he tells me he has had unprotected sex with Elena, or if my clinical assessment indicates he is not being honest about having unprotected sex with her, or that he is incapable of maintaining his celibacy with her, I would have to inform Elena of his HIV status unless he decides to tell her himself.

For now, I have no reason to doubt Ruben's ability and motivation to remain celibate. His concern and care for his family appear genuine, and his history has demonstrated ongoing responsible behavior such as a stable work record and monthly support payments to his parents in Mexico for nearly 5 years. Entering treatment shows his capacity to seek help in resolving his problem constructively. I also have no reason to believe Ruben has been dishonest with me or with himself. He has openly discussed painful conflicts in his struggle toward resolution. However, I do have doubts about how long he can maintain his celibacy with Elena. Another addition to my original plan would be to continually assess and carefully monitor and document Ruben's ability and commitment to remaining celibate with Elena and any indications that demonstrate otherwise. Although I tend to be optimistic, it does not hurt to be prepared for the worst.

Given Ruben's feelings for Jim and their 6-month relationship prior to his HIV test results, I feel it prudent to check in with Ruben about the status of that relationship as well. Ruben may decide to reestablish contact with Jim and could also resume sexual relations with him. I hope that he and Jim decide to practice safer sex so that they do not reinfect each other—another area for me to explore.

I will also continue to seek cultural consultation with my Latina colleague to ensure that my work with Ruben remains culturally sensitive. She can assist me with separating cultural factors from more personal countertransference issues. Her input has helped alleviate my anxiety about identifying and managing my cultural differences with Ruben.

CHOOSE A COURSE OF ACTION AND
SHARE IT WITH YOUR CLIENT

During Ruben's next visit, as we explore how he is coping with his HIV status, I review the limits of the confidentiality statement he signed when he began treatment with me and how it applies to his case. He tells me that he still does not want Elena to know and that this discussion gives him added incentive to remain celibate with her. When, at the suggestion of my Latina colleague, I ask how long he thinks he, as a healthy man with normal desires, can hold out, Ruben admits he has been seeing Jim again. He states that he not only missed Jim but that it was comforting to talk to someone else who is HIV-positive. Ruben continues to refuse going to an agency for any kind of assistance or information, saying it felt safer and more confidential getting any information he wanted through Jim. Jim would also help him find a doctor. Jim has also insisted on safer sex, and Ruben feels his desires are being met with Jim.

Ruben tells me he hopes that he can still trust me to keep his "secrets" from Elena. Again, I remind him this is not an issue unless he gives me reason to believe he has or would have unprotected sex with her. I make it clear that breaching his confidentiality is not a decision I would want to make, nor would I do so without first consulting him and thinking through the issues carefully. I reiterate that I also need to be able to trust him to be honest with me.

IMPLEMENT THE COURSE OF ACTION:
MONITOR AND DISCUSS OUTCOMES

Two weeks later, Ruben reports that Elena has become "more seductive" and has hinted at wanting another child. When he refuses to have sex with her, she expresses hurt feelings and asks him if he still loves her. Ruben feels very guilty and has a harder time resisting having sex with her. He says there is no way that he will use a condom or avoid vaginal intercourse because she is his wife and such behavior changes would make her suspicious. He also states that he has read that not every incidence of intercourse leads to HIV infection, so he believes that a lapse or two to make her happy would be all right.

I remind Ruben that he may have already infected Elena and his children. Because he and Jim practice low-risk sex to prevent reinfection, he would need to do the same to prevent infecting or reinfecting Elena. If she does become pregnant, he would also run the risk of infecting his unborn child. Again, I suggest we explore some options for informing her of his HIV status without revealing how he became infected. At this point, Ruben becomes upset and says he would never get Elena pregnant and that she and the children are probably fine because they are as healthy as ever. When I remind him that he too, appears completely healthy and is experiencing no physical problems, he becomes silent and refuses to discuss the issue further.

At the end of the session, I let Ruben know that I have experienced him as a responsible, caring person and a good father and husband and that it is sometimes very difficult to do the right thing for others when such action could come at great cost to oneself. I suggest that it is impractical to remain celibate indefinitely, that his current behavior distresses Elena, and that he at least think about how to tell her of his HIV status. Ruben acknowledges that he has not thought about the long-term consequences of his plan. Although he agrees to think more about this, he is clearly unhappy and still very ambivalent about disclosing his HIV status to Elena.

I am having some doubts now about Ruben's ability to remain celibate with Elena. He is clearly struggling with this and is starting to rationalize that Elena might "get lucky" and not become infected by one or two lapses. This new rationalization introduces the possibility that he may have unprotected sex with Elena and that his refusal to discuss the possibility that she may already be HIV-positive shows an inability or reluctance to consider the potential consequences of such behavior to his wife and children. This is worrisome to me because I now have to consider breaching Ruben's confidentiality. I am only partially consoled by Dr. Kitchener's opinion that under these circumstances "breaking confidentiality would probably be justified because the harm that might come to Ruben, although regrettable, would not be as severe as the harm that might occur to Elena if she contracted HIV," possibly became pregnant, and unknowingly passed the infection to an unborn child.

I feel so frustrated. In the past, I had managed to convince my clients to tell their spouses or partners and to refrain from high-risk sex while struggling with their decision, or there has not been an identifiable victim. Sometimes I become angry with Ruben for putting all of us in this position, but when I put myself in his place, I am not sure I would be doing any better. This helps me to regain my empathy for Ruben and to separate his less likable behaviors from my positive feelings for him as a person.

Before Ruben's next visit, I feel I need to reassess the circumstances under which I would breach his confidentiality and how I might have to inform Elena of his HIV status. Ruben still has not sought medical care. If he does not have a physician by his next visit, I will not be able to convince him to allow me to enlist a physician's assistance in this matter. That would have been the easier route because, in California, a physician has a clearly stated right to breach confidentiality in cases such as Ruben's. I have no reason to believe Jim would tell Elena. I suspect Ruben would be even more resistant to Jim telling Elena, because that might lead to disclosure of Ruben's sexual relationship with him. At this point, much to my frustration, it appears that (to paraphrase Mr. Burris's expression) I might be the only person standing between Elena being infected by Ruben.

Breaching Ruben's confidentiality would be a clear violation of the APA's Ethics Code, Standard 5.05, which allows me to break confidentiality only when doing so is required or permitted by law when a client's action poses a danger to a third party. In this case, according to Mr. Burris's consultation, the law does not permit me to disclose Ruben's HIV status to Elena. Although I have adhered to the Ethics Code standards on informed consent to therapy, discussing the limits of confidentiality, human differences, and respect for people's rights and dignity, these standards would not appear to take precedence over Standard 5.05. On the other hand, Principle E: Concern for Others' Welfare and Principle F: Social Responsibility, suggest that I need to take into consideration the harm to Elena and the children if I do not break Ruben's confidentiality because I have some responsibility to minimize harm to them. Perhaps I will have a clearer idea of how to proceed if I reanalyze the situation based on the foundational ethical principles.

To preserve as much of Ruben's autonomy as possible and (I hope) minimize any damage to our relationship, I feel that I need to let Ruben know of my intent before I inform Elena and seek his input on how best to do this to minimize the fallout to them both. If Ruben has no suggestions, I will give him the following options: I can call Elena and ask her to meet with me with or without Ruben; Ruben can ask her to come to a session, and I will tell her during the session; or I can call her while Ruben is with me to ask her to come in. I will make it clear to Ruben that I will only tell her his HIV status; answer any HIV-related questions that she might have; and if she desires, give her referrals for testing or counseling. This plan honors Ruben's client relationship with me, minimizes intrusion of his privacy and thus reduces harm to him, and maximizes beneficence for Elena by giving her all of the information that she needs to protect herself. This plan also preserves some autonomy for both Ruben and Elena.

My greatest fear is that Ruben will tell Elena not to talk to me and that she will do as he asks. Should that occur, I do not know what I would do. Mr. Burris's consult suggests that involving the authorities would contradict a strict reading of the law but not the law of a judge or jurors' common sense should Ruben decide to sue me for damages. I am not at all comfortable calling the public health department. To do so seems to be the most intrusive and traumatic for Ruben, Elena, and myself and would violate fidelity by destroying Ruben's trust in me and possibly all other mental health professionals, as well as violate the other ethical principles. Calling the authorities also strikes me as a flagrant violation of the Ethics Code.

Before finalizing my contingency plan, I call Dr. Kitchener because circumstances have changed since her initial consultation. She asks me what information I got from the lawyer. Based on that information, she points out that if anyone filed a complaint against me, an ethics committee or licensing board might find me in violation of the APA Ethics Code if I break Ruben's confidentiality. She agrees that if I decide to breach Ruben's confidentiality, it would be best to tell Ruben before I call Elena. Although it may not be ethically required, it is more defensible because it gives him some control on how I would inform her and gives me the opportunity to salvage our relationship as much as possible. She suggests that I remind him of the consent form he signed, that I let him know I believe he is endangering Elena and possibly his children, and that it is my responsibility to inform Elena, and then ask him whether he would like to be part of the conversation. Dr. Kitchener also suggests that informing the authorities would be a last resort, but that if necessary, I could try to use it as leverage to get Ruben to allow me to talk to Elena.

To honor the ethical principle of justice, I also check in with my Latina colleague. I want to be sure that, as a heterosexual woman, I am not overidentifying with Elena. I also ask her input on how best to implement my contingency plan. She asks if I would make the same decision if Elena happened to be Ruben's gay male partner, spoke no English, and knew nothing about HIV. Seeing I would make the same decision helps me determine my countertransference has not interfered with my ability to be fair. She also suggests I continue to respect and appeal to Ruben's cultural values and role as the protector and provider for his family and to reassure Elena of his care and concern for her.

Although I am feeling more secure with my contingency plan, I experience some apprehension in possibly having to implement it with Ruben, because it violates California law. Although my plan also clearly violates the Ethics Code standard on disclosures, I have upheld other standards set forth in the code and feel that the code's aspirational principles support my decision to minimize harm to Elena and the children. On a personal level, however, I am not sure my relationship with Ruben will survive this dilemma, and this thought makes me sad.

At Ruben's next session, he tells me that Jim has been his primary source of emotional support so he does not want to give up that relationship. With Jim, Ruben feels that he can be himself and has no secrets, and for now there is no pressure from Jim to give more than what he is currently able.

Ruben also states that things are better at home. When I ask what made things better, he becomes somewhat evasive. After some probing, he reluctantly admits he had unprotected sex twice with Elena. He tells me that he could not help it, that they both felt better, that she was happier, and that there was less tension at home. He hopes they "got lucky," meaning she was not infected.

I then ask Ruben if he plans to tell Elena about his HIV status. To my dismay he becomes tense and shakes his head. Although I am relieved I had taken the time to think through my contingency plan, I still feel terrible about having to share it with Ruben. I take a deep breath and remind Ruben of the consent form he had signed and our recent discussion about it. I let him know that by having unsafe sex with Elena, I believe he is endangering her and also the children, because if he and Elena become ill, their ability to care and provide for their children will change. I add that if he does not tell her, I would feel the need to inform her of his HIV status, even if it means breaching his confidentiality, because of the potential harm to Elena and possible unborn child and the negative long-term consequences for himself. I tell Ruben that I have given this matter a great deal of thought and that although I prefer not to do this, I feel he leaves me no choice unless he is willing to disclose his HIV status to his wife.

At this point, Ruben becomes upset and angry. He says I obviously care more about Elena than him and that he should have known "you women would stick together." I empathize with Ruben's anger and the difficult position he is in and reiterate that I am doing what I feel is best for the entire family in the long run. I point out that Ruben's celibacy has already distressed Elena, that she may already be HIV-positive, and that delaying medical treatment leads to poorer health outcomes.

I ask Ruben if he has found a doctor yet. He says he has not looked for one because he feels healthy and he does not want a doctor to tell Elena either. This tells me that I will not be able to work with a physician on this issue and that I really will have to deal with it myself.

Ruben reiterates that he cannot bring himself to tell Elena because of the shame involved and the fear of losing his family. When I suggest that delaying disclosure while continuing unprotected sexual relations with Elena could also lead to losing his family, Ruben refuses to explore this topic further and says he just cannot make the disclosure himself.

I tell Ruben he then leaves me no choice. I will need to talk to Elena, but because of our relationship, I will only tell Elena his HIV status, what she needs to do to lower her risk during sexual relations with him, and any HIV information and referrals she may want. I make it clear to Ruben that I want to minimize any further distress as much as possible and that any other information he has revealed to me would remain confidential. I go over some options for informing Elena: Ruben can bring her to his next session, he can be in the room when I call her to see if she will come in to see me, or I can do a home visit with or without him while the children are at school. I then ask Ruben which approach is more comfortable for him, because I would like him to have some control over the situation and hope that it might help salvage our relationship.

Ruben is now more agitated and upset. I sense he is feeling cornered and more desperate. He says that he will tell Elena not to talk to me. I ask him to reconsider because if he prevents me from reaching Elena and continues to have unprotected sex without telling her his HIV status, he would force me to report him to the public health department. I feel terrible saying this and doubt I could even do this, but I am hoping it will compel Ruben to pursue a less drastic alternative. I then tell Ruben that I would really hate to do this because it would be the most intrusive and traumatic course of action for all of us. I ask him not to put us in this position and remind him that the choice is his.

Ruben accuses me of not caring about him and betraying his trust. He says that he is only trying to protect Elena's feelings and keep his family together and that my telling her would destroy everything and is not the act of someone who cares about him or his family. I again express empathy with Ruben's feelings by acknowledging that doing what is best for the family in the long run could be very painful in the short term and that because I do care, I am having this discussion with him rather than acting without informing him. I appeal again to Ruben's cultural gender role as protector and provider for his family by asking him if he has considered how he would feel knowing he could have protected his wife and family but did not. I reassure him that if he works with me on this, I would do whatever I could to assist him and Elena through this crisis.

Although Ruben looks as if he is on the verge of tears, at least he has not walked out. I gently tell him that I know he is in a terrible dilemma in which there is no easy way out, but that it would be easier for both of us if we do this together. Ruben asks how this might affect the family's ability to remain in the United States if they were to visit relatives in Mexico or if he and Elena applied for citizenship. I tell him I do not have answers to these questions but that I have a colleague who is an immigration lawyer who has worked with several individuals with HIV. I could call him and find out or give his number to Ruben for a free telephone consultation. Because Ruben was tested at an anonymous site and has not yet sought medical care, there is no record of his HIV status. Elena would be equally protected if she too gets tested at an anonymous site. This is a relief to him, and he asks me to call my colleague to obtain more information.

My willingness to address this issue seems to reassure Ruben that despite our disagreement over his dilemma with Elena, I am still willing to help him. He tells me that he is still angry and upset with me, that he does not want to tell Elena, but that he really does not want me to involve the authorities. He says he feels that I am forcing him to do something he does not want to do, that he has no choice. I tell him that in a way, he is right, but that I would like to give him as much choice as possible given the limits of confidentiality. We review our options again. He does not think that he can go back to being celibate with Elena without her raising more questions. I am relieved that he is honest about this despite his anger with me and knowing such a statement strengthens my need to inform Elena. He tells me that although he would prefer that I not force the issue, he would rather be here while I call Elena to make sure that I do not tell her anything beyond his HIV status. It is clear that Ruben's trust has been shaken. I agree that this is a good idea and ask if Elena is home now. Ruben says she probably is. I tell him that I will ask her to come in and talk to me and that Ruben can attend if he wants to. Ruben says that he will come with her, and he repeats that he wants to make sure I only tell her what we agreed to discuss—his HIV status, HIV information, and testing.

I call Elena and introduce myself as Ruben's counselor. I let her know that Ruben is with me and that we would like her to come in as soon as possible to discuss something important. She asks if Ruben is all right. I tell her that he is handling things as well as can be expected. She is concerned, and we agree that the three of us will meet first thing tomorrow morning. Before Ruben leaves, I ask him if he wants to talk about how he will handle Elena's concerns before then. He tells me not to worry about it and says he cannot deal with any more discussion until tomorrow.

I am exhausted when Ruben leaves. I wonder if he and Elena will show up tomorrow. It is clear that he is very ambivalent about disclosing his HIV status, and his forced consent stems more from his fear of me involving the authorities, something I still do not feel good about bringing up. I am relieved that he did not walk out, that he continued to honestly express himself during the session, and that he was receptive to finding out how all of this might affect his citizenship application in the future and his ability to visit relatives in Mexico.

In addition to documenting our discussion and Ruben's reactions, I also add that he gave no indication of being suicidal or self-destructive. His love for his family and his commitment to being a good provider and father remain strong, so it is unlikely he would do anything further to jeopardize that role. Just to be sure, I check in with my Latina colleague about today's session. She reaffirms that Ruben's commitment to his family and role has remained strong and consistent and that he is unlikely to become suicidal overnight. His interest in becoming an American citizen also demonstrates a long-term goal for himself and his family. She suggests that Elena would probably not be openly angry with Ruben but would be more likely to internalize her feelings. I also document leaving a message for my immigration lawyer colleague to give me a call.

When Ruben and Elena arrive for their appointment, both are looking stressed, and none of us look like we got much sleep. Elena immediately asks what is wrong and looks worried. Ruben refuses to look at either of us. Uncomfortable as it is, I begin by telling her that what I am about to say will be difficult for all of us, but that Ruben and I asked her to come out of concern for her and their children's well-being. As I look at Ruben, it is clear in his refusal to look at us or say anything that he still will not tell Elena himself. I continue by informing her that Ruben is HIV-positive and ask her if she knows what this means. Elena is clearly worried about Ruben's health so I answer her questions about HIV and current treatments and reassure her that with early intervention, there is no reason that Ruben cannot live a long and relatively healthy life. I then ask her if she knows how HIV is transmitted. A look of horror crosses her face as she realizes the implications for herself. Ruben, by now, is very uncomfortable and has moved away from Elena. She asks him what this means. He cannot answer her, so I let her know that if she has had unprotected intercourse with him, it is important she and her children be tested to determine her own HIV status. She begins to cry and asks Ruben how this could have happened. When he tells her he does not know, I do not challenge his statement. Instead, I reemphasize the importance of finding out her own status, for herself and her family, because early intervention leads to better health outcomes. I offer to give them whatever referrals and support they need.

For the moment, Ruben is relieved because Elena has not become angry with him or questioned him further about how he became infected. Because she is focused on her own feelings and is clearly upset, he becomes the family protector again. He comforts her and offers to go with her for testing. We make an appointment for her at an anonymous test site and they agree to return together next week. I let them know they can call me if they need anything.

After Ruben and Elena leave, I am completely drained, although things turned out better than I expected. Difficult as it has been, I feel that although I have violated a strict reading of the law and some Ethics Code standards, I did the right thing and that my decision and its implementation are defensible on a clinical and ethical basis.

At some point, however, I know Ruben will become angry again, regardless of Elena's test results, and I have some fears about my potential liability because I technically violated California law. I wonder if there is anything I can do to lower my risk, so I make a note to call Mr. Burris for another consultation. From my personal perspective and the perspective of foundational ethical principles, I feel I made the right decision and implemented it in an ethically and clinically sound manner. However, I am uncertain about how the licensing board and the APA Ethics Committee might respond to my actions should Ruben file a complaint with them, so I also make a note to call Dr. Kitchener to ask her advice on this matter.

Karen Strohm Kitchener's Ethical Debriefing Consultation

Ms. Jue has clearly had to deal with one of the most complex ethical cases that therapists may have to face. It has called for not just a single ethical decision, but a series of them.

As I mentioned to her in our telephone conversation, there are generally two ways that complaints like this might come before the Ethics Committee. The first would involve the client making a complaint, which is probably unlikely in this case. Ruben has already told his therapist that the shame involved with his infection is too great to share with his wife. It seems unlikely that he would share the information in a public venue to bring a charge against his therapist. Another therapist would probably not be in a position to bring a case against Ms. Jue unless he or she had access to Ruben's case file. Unless Ruben sought treatment from another therapist, this would probably not occur. Even if it did, the therapist would have to have Ruben's permission to break confidentiality and file a case. A *sua sponte* complaint might be brought against her by the Ethics Committee if the complaint became public, as it might if a lawsuit were filed. If any of those scenarios occurred, she might be found in violation of the APA Ethics Code. No one, of course, can speak for the Ethics Committee and predict exactly how the members would view the situation. I have not served on the Ethics Committee since the 1992 revision of the Ethics Code, so I have not adjudicated a case involving Standard 5.05. However, it seems to me that to find her guilty of violating Standard 5.05, the committee would need to determine whether Ms. Jue's actions violated California law. Apparently, the legal advice she received is that this question is not as clear-cut as it initially may seem. If the committee did determine that she violated Standard 5.05, it might take into consideration her careful reasoning, her careful documentation of her reasoning, and her consultation with others about this difficult issue.

Ultimately, the basic issue revolves around the importance of confidentiality in the therapeutic relationship. The APA has decided it is primary unless the law requires or permits that it be broken. In my mind, a question remains about whether a greater good would be done by breaking confidentiality in cases such as Ruben's and, therefore, protecting his wife, or breaking it and violating his trust and, perhaps, decreasing the chances that other people who are HIV-positive would seek psychotherapy. I wish that I could say something more reassuring to Ms. Jue; however, this case underlines how difficult some ethical decisions can be even when trying to follow the Ethics Code and make good ethical decisions.

Scott Burris's Legal Debriefing Consultation

I still rate Ms. Jue's legal risk as low. Malpractice litigation is a process that as often begins with an injury to a relationship as to a person, and I think it is too soon to tell whether Ruben really feels that Ms. Jue did him a wrong. His situation was untenable, and although risky, his only chance of reestablishing a harmonious family situation lay through disclosure. He may come to see this, even if he loses his family. He may feel, or come to feel, that Ms. Jue was closer to his own desires than he was when she forced the issue.

This is, admittedly, the optimistic view. However, even if he loses his family and blames Ms. Jue—and is willing to go public with a suit—his legal case against her is weak. Her disclosure was discreet, private, and made with care and consideration for Ruben's feelings. Ms. Jue has a very good argument: It was done with Ruben's consent, insofar as he helped arrange the meeting and attended, without protest, while the disclosure was made. Although Ms. Jue's procedure might strike other psychotherapists as coercive, I am not at all convinced that a court of law would see it that way. Ultimately, a court and a jury would see a man claiming he was damaged because his psychotherapist told his wife that he was putting her life at risk.

Ms. Jue's conduct of the case illustrates the central legal theme of this book. In a crisis, she continued to act as a trained mental health professional. She endeavored to ascertain and apply clinical standards and ethical rules. She consulted with colleagues and documented her judgments and activities. She made professionally reasonable decisions under difficult circumstances. She acted with reasonable deliberation and did not allow her sense of moral urgency to become incautious, counterproductive haste. Whether the outcome is good or bad, and no matter what happens to her in court or before her licensing board, she will know that she made the best decisions she could.

Sally Jue's Final Comments

Violating one of the Ethics Codes and a California law do not sit well with me, but I still strongly feel that I made the right decision and could adequately defend my actions should they find their way to an ethics committee or licensing board. Mr. Burris's debriefing also alleviates my anxiety about legal liability. Both consultations remind me again of the importance of making and documenting deliberate, carefully reasoned decisions and the benefits of consultation. I cannot imagine having to struggle with this case on my own. For now, it appears that my best course of action is to remain vigilant about my personal feelings and the potential ongoing clinical, ethical, and legal issues and to continue to seek consultation as needed.

Difficult as it has been, I feel that I have learned much from this experience that will benefit my work with other clients. Nevertheless, I experience regret about causing Ruben and his family so much pain and only hope that, selfish as it sounds, they will allow me to continue to be part of their struggles.

REFERENCES

American Psychological Association. (1992). Ethical principles of psychologists and code of conduct. *American Psychologist, 47,* 1597–1611.

Beauchamp, T. L., & Childress, J. F. (1989). *Principles of biomedical ethics.* Oxford, England: Oxford University Press.

Cal. Bus. & Prof. Code, §2960(h) (2000).

Cal. Civ. Code, §43.92 (2000).

Cal. Health & Safety Code, §§120980, 121015 (1998).

Confidentiality of Medical Information Act, Cal. Civil Code §56-56.37 (1982 & Supp. 1998).

Crawford, I., Humfleet, G., Ribordy, S. C., Ho, F. C., & Vickers, V. L. (1991). Stigmatization of AIDS patients by mental health professionals. *Professional Psychology: Research and Practice, 22,* 357–361.

Cutter v. Brownbridge, 183 Cal.App.3d 836 (Cal. Ct. App. 1986).

Doughty, R. (1994). The confidentiality of HIV-related information: Responding to the resurgence of aggressive public health interventions in the AIDS epidemic. *California Law Review, 82,* 111–184.

Gellert, G., Page, B., Weismuller, P., & Ehling, L. R. (1993). Managing the noncompliant HIV-infected individual: Experiences from a local health department. *AIDS & Public Policy Journal, 8,* 20–26.

Reisner v. University of California, 31 Cal.App.4th 1195, 37 Cal.Rptr.2d 518 (Cal. Ct. App. 1995).

Tarasoff v. Board of Regents of the University of California, 551 P.2d 334 (Cal. 1976).

Urbaniak v. Newton, 277 Cal. Rptr. 354 (Cal. Ct. App. 1991).

9

THE HIV-POSITIVE SEX WORKER: THE CASE OF RHONDA

VIVIAN B. BROWN, KAREN STROHM KITCHENER,
AND SCOTT BURRIS

ORIENTATION TO THE MAJOR ETHICAL ISSUES HIGHLIGHTED IN THE CASE

A challenging ethical situation facing psychotherapists involves resolving the issues surrounding the duty to protect when those at risk are both clearly identified and not clearly identified. In some communities laws have been passed that make it a crime for individuals who know they have HIV to have unprotected sex. In others, the responsibility of the clinician to inform at-risk third parties is unclear. Some of the conflict may be the internal struggle between the clinician's belief that keeping the client in treatment will lead to behavior change and the awareness that in the interim someone might become infected. The case of Rhonda illustrates this dynamic.

CASE PRESENTATION (BY VIVIAN B. BROWN)

Rhonda, age 20, uses heroin, crack cocaine, and speedball. As the substance abuse specialist in a community health center in Georgia, I have been working with Rhonda for the past 8 months. She presented for both HIV and substance abuse treatment immediately after finding out that she was HIV-positive. Her initial reaction to this news was anxiety and panic.

During recent months, Rhonda has participated in a Narcotics Anonymous group for women who are HIV-infected, but her commitment to her sobriety has been shaky. She continues to work as a prostitute so she can provide money to her mother, who has custody of her two children. She appears to have pushed the issue of her HIV status to the bottom of her worry list. She uses her time with me to talk about her loneliness and her disappointment over losing her children. Her children were tested, and they are negative.

Rhonda wants to be a better mother to her children and continues to hope that she will be able to save money and stay clean so she can take the time to get a "real" job and then petition the court for custody. In the meantime, she visits her kids at least once a week, taking gifts with her when she does. She confided that during her childhood her mother ignored her and beat her often. She wants to be a better mother than that for her kids.

Rhonda has a partner, David, who pimps for her. She once tried to get him to use a condom, and he beat her up so badly that she had two broken ribs and a head injury. He said that condoms are for "tricks" and that he is no trick. Since then, she has been afraid to bring up the issue of condoms, and she has not told David about her HIV status. David apparently refuses to be tested for HIV.

Rhonda believes that the way back to a more secure life is possible only with David's help, and David insists that she continue with her sex work. I encourage her to always insist that her sex partners use condoms, and when she has the results have been mixed. On two occasions when she asked her partners to use condoms, she was beaten and not able to work for several days. As a result, Rhonda has grown more cautious about asserting her needs, and she frequently experiences bouts of despair during which she loses hope of ever being able to have her children.

Recently, Rhonda missed several appointments, and I think she has started using again. My supervisor is putting pressure on me to intervene because she may be infecting others.

PAUSE AND IDENTIFY YOUR PERSONAL RESPONSES TO THE CASE

When I am honest with myself, I know I am wavering in my commitment to work with her. I want to help her and know that she needs lots of support, but I am not at all comfortable with the knowledge that she may be infecting others with HIV.

As I pause to reflect on the case, I can feel my anxiety and my desire to get away from the dilemmas. I struggle to find a balance between all the risks involved. Having unprotected sex places Rhonda at risk of opportunistic infections that could lead to her deteriorating health and death; having unprotected sex with David, her partner and pimp, places him at risk of infection. My concern for David, however, is diminished somewhat by the fact that he is a batterer and that he is unwilling to be tested for HIV. It is hard to be empathetic toward David when he takes no responsibility for his own health or Rhonda's and when he places her at greater risk of harm. If she tells David about her HIV status, he might physically harm or kill her. If she insists on using condoms with her sex partners, they might physically harm her. In addition, it appears that she may have started using drugs again, and this also raises the risk of her being reinfected or of contracting opportunistic infections through needle sharing. She may also run from treatment.

I believe it is important for her to remain in treatment. However, I feel my anxieties and my supervisor's pressure may lead to my driving her away from treatment. I need to get hold of my anxieties about "doing no harm," in order to help Rhonda with her anxieties. I wrestle with my own sense of helplessness and hopelessness. I try to settle myself by reviewing the facts of the case.

REVIEW THE FACTS OF THE CASE

These are the facts: Rhonda has HIV disease but continues to engage in sex work, often without the use of condoms. Her partner and pimp David refuses to use condoms, refuses to be tested for HIV, and batters her. Her sexual behavior with others may place them at risk, but even that is not altogether certain. Certainly her intent is not to harm any of her partners but to keep herself from physical harm, to attempt to make money for her children, and to continue a relationship with her primary partner. Furthermore, knowledge about HIV disease and its transmission is widespread. It is possible that David also has HIV disease and has infected Rhonda.

I need more information about a number of issues, including Rhonda's decision-making ability. Her low self-esteem, her status as a victim and survivor of violence, and her head injury at the hands of David raise the issues of cognitive impairment and impaired decision-making ability. I also do not know for sure whether Rhonda has relapsed and is using drugs again. She has missed appointments, but this may be for other reasons including the fact that she may sense my discomfort with her and her behaviors. On the positive side, Rhonda has shown the motivation and ability to remain drug-free during recent months by participating in Narcotics Anonymous, even though her commitment has been shaky. Moreover, she has been working with me for 8 months, and we have had a fairly good relationship.

CONCEPTUALIZE AN INITIAL PLAN
BASED ON CLINICAL ISSUES

In her initial assessment, Rhonda was seen as exhibiting problems with substance abuse and anxiety. She entered treatment immediately after learning her HIV status, and she needed immediate crisis intervention to deal with her anxiety and panic and to help her begin to integrate her view of herself as a person living with HIV. She experiences considerable anxiety and fear about not living to see her children grow up, frustration and shame about losing the children, and depression and helplessness about her relationship. She has experienced a history of physical and sexual abuse beginning in early childhood, and she continues the pattern of abusive relationships into her young adulthood. Her substance abuse began when she was a teenager and involved with an older man who was an injection drug user and pimp. Her HIV status was the precipitating event that led to her wanting to give up drugs, but she has many pressures on her to continue her drug use and sex work.

Psychotherapy can help her more clearly identify what is happening in her life and what risks she needs to respond to so she can make more responsible plans for herself and her children. My initial plan is to review the seriousness of her situation with her and to ask her to make a commitment to continue treatment with me while we work together to come up with a plan to reduce all the risks to her and others. I will talk with her about the risks to herself as well as others and explore with her whether she might want to go into a residential drug treatment program for women living with HIV. I will discuss with her the dilemma she and I are both in and my personal struggle to work with her as we move through reducing all the risks. I also will consult with an ethics expert on these dilemmas.

CONSULT THE ETHICS CODE AND ASSESS THE
ETHICAL ISSUES (BY KAREN STROHM KITCHENER)

To some extent the ethical issues involved in Rhonda's case are similar to those involved in the case of Jerry discussed in chapter 7 and the case of Ruben in chapter 8. The client is HIV-positive and is having unsafe sex with several partners. What makes this case particularly difficult is that Dr. Brown knows the identity of one of the client's partners (David).

Consequently, she must weigh the responsibility to protect him from possible HIV infection. In addition, the client herself may be in real danger both from opportunistic infections and battering. She believes she is particularly vulnerable if she informs her partner of her HIV status. It is no wonder Dr. Brown is feeling helpless and hopeless.

Because many of the ethical issues are similar to those discussed in the cases of Jerry and Ruben, they are summarized here; the reader is referred to those cases for a more complete discussion. Issues that are unique to this case are discussed more fully here. As with the case of Jerry, the legal analysis will clarify whether there is a legal duty to warn and whether there is a legal mandate or permission to inform anyone. Dr. Brown should also be guided by ethical considerations.

APA Ethics Code

In the American Psychological Association (APA, 1992) Ethics Code, the standard that is most relevant is 5.05. It gives psychologists permission to break client confidentiality only to protect others from harm where it is required or permitted by law, but it does not obligate them to do so. In other words, if Dr. Brown gets legal advice that in her state the law forbids breaking confidentiality in AIDS-related cases, then it would also be unethical for her to do so according to the Ethics Code. Two of the code's aspirational principles, Principle E: Concern for Others' Welfare and Principle F: Social Responsibility, suggest that psychologists like Dr. Brown have responsibilities both to their clients and society. One section of Principle E is particularly relevant in Rhonda's case because it suggests that when "conflicts occur among psychologists' obligations or concerns, they attempt to resolve these conflicts and to perform their roles in a responsible fashion that avoids or minimizes harm." This statement is underscored by Standard 1.14, Avoiding Harm, which requires that psychologists avoid harming their clients or minimize harm when it is not completely avoidable. The fundamental question Dr. Brown must answer is this: Which course of action will create the least amount of avoidable harm?

Other standards mentioned in the case of Jerry are also relevant here. Standards 5.02, Maintaining Confidentiality, and 5.03, Minimizing Intrusions on Privacy, both suggest that any breaches of confidentiality, if they occur, should be done in ways that disclose the least amount of information possible and do so in the least intrusive way. Standard 5.02 should also remind Dr. Brown that maintaining confidentiality is a primary obligation of psychologists. In addition, Standard 5.01, Discussing the Limits of Confidentiality, requires that clients be informed early in the relationship if there are occasions when the psychologist will consider breaking confidentiality. This is especially true if therapists believe that they have some responsibility to protect others from their client's potentially dangerous actions or to protect clients from self-inflicted harm.

Foundational Ethical Principles

The foundational principles of fidelity and autonomy are particularly relevant to this case because both provide the basis for the rule of confidentiality. Confidentiality is based on the assumption that autonomous people have the right to make decisions about those with whom they share private information. In Rhonda's case this would include information about her HIV status. Respect for autonomy means that Rhonda has a right to keep her thoughts private; however, she does not have the right to engage in activities that threaten the rights or lives of others. Other things being equal, this would include both David and her sex customers. In this case, however, David and her sex customers are presumably adults who are also engaging in high-risk behaviors. They are aware that Rhonda is on the street and should be aware that such activity may lead to the transmission of HIV or other sexually transmitted diseases. Nevertheless, they refuse to use condoms when they engage in intercourse. Thus, they are making choices to engage in sexual behavior that they should know puts them at risk. Furthermore, David has refused to be tested for the disease.

As noted in chapter 3, autonomous decisions must be intentional, they must be based on adequate understanding, and they cannot result from coercion (Beauchamp & Childress, 1989). Because of the power differential between Rhonda and David and the threat she feels to her life, her decision about whether to tell him about her HIV infection may not be fully autonomous. This does not completely excuse Rhonda for her failure to tell him, but it does suggest that Dr. Brown's responsibility to warn David may not be as strong as it would be if David were not a threat to her and were not engaging in high-risk behaviors himself.

Moreover, Dr. Brown has questions about Rhonda's general competence because of her head injury and the possibility that she is again abusing drugs. If either or both are true, it would suggest that Rhonda's competence is limited; thus, there may be more of a justification for Dr. Brown to intervene in Rhonda's life, even hospitalizing her against her will if she believes Rhonda is a threat to herself.

The foundational principles of fidelity should also remind Dr. Brown that a breach of confidentiality involves breaking a promise and violates the trust that is essential both for therapeutic relationships and for the common bonds that allow people to engage in social interactions. As described in the case of Jerry, there may be a variety of other harmful consequences that occur as a result of breaking Rhonda's confidence. This seems to be particularly salient in this case because Dr. Brown is aware that Rhonda may "run from treatment."

The principles of beneficence and do no harm are also relevant. Because HIV is an infectious disease that could be fatal if untreated, there seems to be a prima facie argument in most cases for choosing a course of action that protects others from contracting the disease. However, because Rhonda is a client, Dr. Brown has a special obligation (fidelity) to promote her welfare (beneficence) and avoid harming her. She must consider whether she can protect Rhonda's sexual partners without harming Rhonda and if not, how she can do the least harm possible, especially because there is good reason to believe that Rhonda's life may be in danger if she reveals the information to David. Dr. Brown should consider how to confront Rhonda's cycle of self-destruction and despair. If she can intervene effectively with Rhonda, she may cease acting in a way that puts herself or others at risk. This seems to be what Dr. Brown is suggesting when she says they will work together to come up with a plan that reduces the risks to Rhonda and to others.

The foundational principle of justice would suggest that Dr. Brown consider whether she is dealing fairly with both Rhonda and others in Rhonda's life. She needs to impartially evaluate whether her anger that David is Rhonda's pimp and has battered her is biasing her ethical decision making. Although there may be ethically relevant issues regarding David's behavior that decrease her responsibility to protect him, she must carefully evaluate whether her feelings about David are leading her to treat him unfairly. Similarly, she should ask whether her own ambivalence about Rhonda's behavior is interfering with her ability to provide fair treatment. For example, can she still feel care and compassion for Rhonda and her life?

Balancing the Ethics Code and Foundational Ethical Principles

What then should a psychologist do to avoid or minimize harm, as the APA Ethics Code suggests? Here, considering the risk assessment factors introduced in chapter 3 may prove useful. Beauchamp and Childress (1989) suggested that in making decisions like this both the magnitude of harm and the probability of harm must be considered. In the case of Rhonda and David, the magnitude of harm and probability of harm need to be considered for both the options of informing David about Rhonda's HIV status and not informing him. First, Dr. Brown must evaluate the magnitude of harm and probability of harm for David if Rhonda continues to engage in unsafe sex with him. If David contracts HIV from Rhonda, the magnitude of harm could be great. On the other hand, the probability of harm is not completely clear because sexual intercourse with someone who is HIV-infected does not necessarily lead to the partner's infection (Lamb, Clark, Drumheller,

Frizzel, & Surrey, 1989; Martin, in press). In addition, David might already be infected.

Dr. Brown must also consider the magnitude and probability of harm to Rhonda if she informs David of her HIV status. From what Dr. Brown reports, both are probably very high because there is evidence that David has violently abused her in the past. Last, Dr. Brown must consider the extent to which David bears some responsibility for his own danger: He is knowingly engaging in high-risk behaviors without protecting himself, he is using Rhonda by keeping her on the street, he is exploiting the power differential in their relationship, and his actions threaten her well-being.

Another issue that Dr. Brown must consider is this: Rhonda is also engaging in sex work and is also exposing her sexual partners to HIV. Assessment of the magnitude and probability of harm are also relevant in evaluating Dr. Brown's responsibility to act in a way that might be protective of these partners. However, in this case Dr. Brown's options are limited because she does not know Rhonda's sex customers. She could inform the police about Rhonda's HIV infection and her prostitution, but this would involve a gross violation of her privacy, would disregard her autonomy, and would violate the principles of fidelity and doing no harm. Furthermore, it may have a chilling effect on Dr. Brown's ability to work with future clients like Rhonda if the word gets out that Dr. Brown turned her in. In the long run, society may benefit more if Dr. Brown continues to maintain confidentiality, continues to encourage her to use condoms, and helps her change her lifestyle. Last, Dr. Brown should remember that the Ethics Code only allows her to break confidentiality if it is permitted or mandated by law.

In summary, balancing responsibilities to clients with responsibilities to others whom the client may be placing at risk poses some of the most difficult ethical decisions that confront Dr. Brown and other therapists working with HIV-positive clients. In making such decisions, Dr. Brown clearly needs legal counsel. In addition, she must ask how she can avoid harm or minimize it when it is unavoidable. On the other hand, it may not be possible "to come up with a plan to reduce all the risks to Rhonda and others," as Dr. Brown hopes. She should consider ways to balance a responsibility to exercise reasonable care for Rhonda's sexual partners with the responsibility to protect her client's privacy and her life. A variety of options might be considered, from education to hospitalization.

The first step might be to reestablish trust with Rhonda; if she disappears, Dr. Brown cannot help her or protect others. Next, Dr. Brown should assess her competence. If she is competent she might work with Rhonda to educate her about HIV and help her consider alternative options like entering a residential treatment program for women living with HIV. Although Rhonda has not been interested in dealing with her HIV status in therapy, Dr. Brown has an ethical responsibility to confront Rhonda's behavior. For example, she may point out that if Rhonda becomes increasingly ill, David will find out about her illness and will probably be angry that she had not told him earlier, and she will be unable to help support her children.

Dr. Brown also must deal honestly with Rhonda about her own discomfort with her sexual activity and encourage her to practice safer sex if she is going to continue prostitution. If it is a crime for Rhonda to engage in unprotected sexual activity while she is HIV-positive, she should inform her of that. If she fails to do so, she is undermining their relationship as well as the principle of fidelity. If Rhonda is not competent to make reasonable decisions and her behavior poses a threat to herself or others, Dr. Brown may need to consider involuntarily hospitalizing her.

If none of these options works and Dr. Brown believes she must break confidentiality and the law mandates or permits her to do so, she should break it in the least intrusive way and in a way that discloses the least amount of information about Rhonda. For example, she may use the public health department's partner notification system so that David is informed that he might be HIV-positive but not informed of Rhonda's identity. If Dr. Brown chooses this option, she should talk with Rhonda about it ahead of time, reminding her of their initial consent agreement and giving her the opportunity to change her behavior and to tell David herself. This step allows her some autonomy over how and when the information about her HIV status is disclosed. It will also allow her to consider how she might protect herself from David's probable violence and may help convince her to consider options other than prostitution.

This case is like many others dealing with the duty to protect. No perfect moral solution may be found that protects the client and society without harming either. In these cases, the best a psychologist may do is minimize harm to the extent that it is possible, as the APA Ethics Code suggests.

IDENTIFY THE LEGAL ISSUES (BY SCOTT BURRIS)

Rhonda presents Dr. Brown with a set of serious ethical issues. I am glad that Dr. Brown has contacted me, because I think some legal information will be useful to her in handling the case. I think her risk of being sued, let alone found liable, is virtually nil, for cultural as much as legal reasons. Because I can see that Dr. Brown is very concerned with Rhonda's welfare, I also want to talk to her about Rhonda's legal risks in this situation.

Those Involved in the Case Are Very Unlikely to Sue and Very Unlikely to Win If They Do

In theory, a lawsuit could come from three directions: Rhonda could sue Dr. Brown for disclosing her HIV status to someone else, such as David or the police; David could sue Dr. Brown, alleging that her failure to disclose Rhonda's infection (or otherwise control her sexual behavior) caused him to get HIV; and one or more of Rhonda's sex clients could sue for reasons similar to David's. I do not think it too likely that Rhonda, David, or any of Rhonda's sex customers will be willing or able to pursue a lawsuit. The fact is that most people who have a legitimate reason to sue do not do so (Kritzer, Bogart, & Vidmar, 1991), and none of our plaintiffs have much of a legal case. Moreover, it takes a certain amount of drive and organization to find a lawyer, not to mention faith in the legal system and a willingness to invest current energy in the possibility of a payoff some time down the road. David and Rhonda sound like they have other, more pressing problems, and Rhonda's customers may be too embarrassed or feel too guilty to get involved in litigation (even assuming they ever knew Rhonda's name or who her therapist was and what her therapist knew about Rhonda's condition). Even if one of these people wanted to sue, I think he would have a hard time finding a lawyer willing to invest in the case. Whatever the law, a tort case depends to an enormous degree upon the underlying human story, and every one of our possible plaintiffs could be made to look awfully bad to a jury.

Georgia Law Favors Dr. Brown Whether or Not She Discloses

This case is subject to the law of Georgia, which, like most states, has a statute protecting "AIDS confidential information" (Ga. Code Ann., 1997, §24-9-47). This law would not allow Dr. Brown to disclose information directly to sex partners, but it does provide at least two ways that she could work with others to intervene. The statute generally allows cooperating health care providers to disclose information to other health care providers and their staff as necessary to provide care or otherwise carry out their routine business. The law allows a hospital or physician to disclose HIV information and contacts who may be at risk to health authorities, who are required to find and assist partners at risk. Physicians are also explicitly authorized to disclose a patient's infection to a spouse or sex partner. Dr. Brown is not a physician, so these laws do not authorize her to act, but she could consult with Rhonda's physician, acquaint him with issues of Rhonda's behavior and the risks she poses, and ask him to contact David and the health authorities.

Dr. Brown, or her superiors at the health clinic, are not required to report cases of HIV disease to the health department. The confidentiality law allows disclosure for reporting purposes, and a court would probably accept the argument that alerting the health department to the risks of Rhonda's conduct falls within this exception. It would then be up to the health department to take action (Ga. Code Ann., 1997, §31-2-1). As with Jerry's case, the psychotherapist would be well-advised to find out how, and how well, the local authorities handle cases like these before pursuing this avenue.

Dr. Brown may act to protect Rhonda's partners, but does the law require her to do so? The Georgia courts recognize that a health care provider may sometimes have a duty to protect a third party at risk of harm from a patient (*Bradley Center v. Wessner*, 1982). The duty has been limited, however, to situations in which the professional can "exercise control over the freedom of a mental patient, or claim the legal authority to confine or restrain the patient against his will" (*Keppler v. Brunson*, 1992). Unless Rhonda is at this point committable and Dr. Brown can actually get hold of her and confine her—neither of which seems true—Dr. Brown would have no duty to act under Georgia law. This is all academic, however, because the legislature has acted to preclude *Tarasoff*-type lawsuits in the HIV context (*Tarasoff v. Board of Regents of the University of California*, 1976). The HIV confidentiality law includes a blanket immunity from civil suit that expressly eliminates any duty to disclose and bars anyone from suing a health care provider for disclosing or failing to disclose any information protected under the statute (Ga. Code Ann., 1997, §24-9-47(j)).

Rhonda Faces Serious Legal Jeopardy If the Authorities Are Called In

Dr. Brown is not at legal risk, but Rhonda could be. Any involvement of police can substantially raise the stakes for Rhonda. In an ideal world, there would be a safe place for her to work through her current crisis. In our world, the best we can offer may be jail (Dalton, 1993). In many states, statutes specifically make it a crime to engage in sexual conduct that could spread HIV. In some states, a person with HIV who engages in prostitution commits a felony involving substantial jail time. This is the case in Georgia, which has a law that makes sex or needle sharing without disclosing one's infection a felony punishable by up to 10 years in prison. Prostitutes can be convicted under this statute even if no sex takes place, meaning that the normal arrest for prostitution (solicitation) goes from being essentially a nuisance offense to a major felony (Decker, 1987; Ga. Code Ann., 1997, §16-5-60). A local district attorney might also try to charge Rhonda with an even more serious crime, such as attempted murder. (Rhonda may eventually be found out even if Dr. Brown does not call in the police. Georgia has an administrative rule requiring the mandatory testing of anyone convicted of prostitution; Ga. Comp. R. & Regs., 1997, r.90-5-48-.05.)

Can the Law Protect Rhonda?

Dr. Brown is trying to get Rhonda into a safer place, starting with a residential drug treatment program. Like many women caught in an abusive relationship, she may have trouble getting away from her abuser. Georgia has laws that can be used to protect Rhonda from abuse. In addition to the various criminal penalties for violent behavior, Rhonda can get a court order protecting her from David, which could be tailored to her situation and needs to, for example, direct David to cease any contact with her or to vacate their common apartment (Ga. Code Ann., 1997, §19-13-4). Dr. Brown may wish to explore the resources available in the legal system to help Rhonda make a clean break with David.

Conclusion

Legal analysis, whether by judges, practicing lawyers, or academics, tends to mirror popular attitudes. There are exceptions, but Rhonda's case is not likely to be one. She and David, and, to a lesser extent, her sex customers, are perceived as among the "guiltier" people with HIV, caught, so it might be said, in the trap of their own vicious behavior. Attitudes like these strongly affect perceptions of the nature of harm in this situation and the legal responsibility for it. Dr. Brown is likely to look pretty good by comparison, as long as she follows a professionally responsible course that she can sincerely justify to herself and her colleagues.

Paradoxically, the hostile social attitudes that help insulate Dr. Brown from a lawsuit also make her job even harder. She is trying to see Rhonda, and even David, as people of worth struggling with enormously difficult histories and present-day circumstances. The law that will indulge every presumption in Dr. Brown's favor will, if it gets its hands on Rhonda, probably treat her mercilessly. In any sort of criminal trial, she would be painted as the Typhoid Mary of AIDS and be sentenced to a jail term so long she would never get out again. Finding a way to get Rhonda back on her track of responsibility and sobriety, without destroying her, will not be easy.

IDENTIFY AND ASSESS THE OPTIONS (BY VIVIAN B. BROWN)

After documenting the consultations I just received, I reassess my initial plans to determine the best way I can balance these responsibilities. I feel that my plans are consistent with ethical guidelines. The question I am struggling with is which course of action will lead to the least amount of avoidable harm.

Maintaining confidentiality respects Rhonda's right to make decisions for and about herself, including decisions associated with whom her private information is shared. However, this also means that I need to be clear about her ability to make rational decisions because of any possible cognitive impairment, the influence of drugs, or depression and anxiety.

Breaking confidentiality may have serious negative consequences for Rhonda, thereby violating the principle of do no harm. Although David may be at risk of transmission of HIV, Rhonda seems to be at greater risk from the potential for David's physical abuse.

A breach of confidentiality also violates the trust that Rhonda seems to have for me and our therapeutic relationship. If she leaves treatment because of my breaking a promise, she may be in danger of arrest for her illegal activities, of not getting treatment for her medical and her psychological needs, and of physical abuse. If Rhonda stays in treatment with me, she may reduce her risks and the risks of others.

There are several actions that I can take to balance these ethical issues with legal requirements. I have checked Georgia laws, and it is clear that if Rhonda is convicted of prostitution and tested positive for HIV in connection with that conviction (and is informed of the test results), the Penal Code elevates any subsequent prostitution conviction from a misdemeanor to a felony. I will need to inform Rhonda of this. This could have a serious effect on her and her children.

HIV infection in the absence of AIDS is not a reportable condition in Georgia. I could discuss the issues with Rhonda's physician at the health center, and he could disclose Rhonda's HIV status to David or the health authorities. However, this action would more likely lead to increased danger of harm to Rhonda from David. I could enlist her physician to join me in encouraging her to enter a residential treatment program.

With regard to harm toward David and her other sex partners, I remind myself that male-to-female transmission is estimated to be eight times more likely than female-to-male transmission. Again, David's likelihood of infection seems to be less than Rhonda's risk of being battered. Although there is a probability of harm to her other sex partners, it may be that the probability of harm to Rhonda is equally great because of the possibility of reinfection. I need to educate her about these issues.

I also will need to arrange a neuropsychological assessment for Rhonda to help determine if she has been cognitively impaired by the battering and whether she is able to make reasonable decisions.

Last, I want to get her into a safer place, namely a residential drug treatment program, and to discuss obtaining a restraining order. I need to help Rhonda see that if she becomes increasingly or visibly ill, David will find out about her illness, and she will be in increased danger. Although a retraining order is possible, and I will raise this with Rhonda, it is also possible that David will ignore it and be more likely to harm her physically.

I believe that the best course of action is to continue to engage Rhonda in therapy and to assist her in finding a safer place where she can deal with her fears regarding her illness, her desire to reduce or eliminate her drug abuse, and her desire to be with her children without fears of physical abuse from David and her other sex partners and without fear of arrest. I believe this course of action upholds my responsibility to both Rhonda and society with the least amount of avoidable harm.

There is one other area I want to address: the pressure I feel from my supervisor, the director of the health center. It seems clear to me now (after my consultations) that he is more concerned with Rhonda's sexual partners than with Rhonda's well-being. I feel somewhat frustrated with his lack of understanding for the complexity of the issues. I decide to schedule an appointment with him to discuss the consultations, my decision making, and my plan.

CHOOSE A COURSE OF ACTION AND SHARE IT WITH YOUR CLIENT

The next time I see Rhonda I begin sharing my concerns with her. I tell her about my concerns about her behavior—that she is constantly putting herself at increased risk. We discuss the risk of infections to her, the risk of being arrested because of her sex work, the implications of her being convicted for her and her children, the risk of spreading HIV to others, and the risk of her being physically harmed by David and her customers. Rhonda expresses her feelings of gratitude toward me for caring about her. She says she knows I am trying to help but that she cannot see any way out of her current situation. I share my thoughts and plans about the assessment and the possibility of her entering a residential treatment program. She listens and says that she will think about it. I ask her to also think about whether we both should meet with her physician to see what he thinks. We set up our next appointment in 2 days. I feel more secure that she will return to see me, but I know she will have a tough time thinking about her options.

IMPLEMENT THE COURSE OF ACTION: MONITOR AND DISCUSS OUTCOMES

I contact a neuropsychologist to schedule an assessment, explaining that the client has not accepted the need for an appointment yet. However, I want to be able to tell her that one is available, if she wants it.

In the next session, Rhonda reports that she is willing to explore the options I discussed. However, she fears that David will not allow her to go into drug treatment and that he may not allow her to stop work. I begin discussing the issues of obtaining a court order protecting her against David. Her fear increases, and she misses our next appointment.

I am aware that Rhonda is facing a number of significant losses—loss of her partner, loss of her children, loss of her drugs, loss of her work, loss of her image of herself as a "healthy" woman, and loss of her health. I feel the tensions and the shifting of balance between positive and negative influences of my actions as well as the balance between my responsibility to exercise reasonable care for Rhonda's sexual partners with the responsibility to protect her privacy and her life.

In her next session Rhonda shares with me that she was given a great deal of information about HIV before and after her testing and that her anxiety became so elevated that she increased her drug usage. I tell Rhonda all my concerns about her behaviors and how she is placing herself at risk in many ways. I also discuss with her that when she is taking drugs, or when she is very anxious, or if David has caused damage to her ability to think clearly, she may not make the best decisions for herself. I restate why it might be a good idea that she get a neuropsychological assessment. She consents, and in her presence I call the neuropsychologist to schedule the appointment.

When the report comes back on the neuropsychological assessment, it is clear that there is evidence of mild traumatic brain injury. I discuss this with the neuropsychologist, and we discuss whether Rhonda is competent enough to make reasonable decisions and whether a period of hospitalization would be beneficial. Both of us conclude that it would be better if Rhonda decides to enter a residential treatment program on her own.

I document these steps and decisions carefully. In my next appointment with Rhonda I discuss with her how hard it must be for her to face all the losses and changes we have been exploring. Rhonda again shares her despair and feelings of hopelessness. I decide to set up an additional appointment with her to provide extra support and possibly to share the information regarding the neuropsychological assessment. I feel quite tense about giving her any additional negative information, but I also know that she is entitled to know that information and to incorporate it into her decision making. I discuss this situation with my supervisor and with the neuropsychologist.

When Rhonda returns for the next appointment, I tell her that I have been weighing all the pluses and minuses of all the options and ask her whether she has been doing the same. She relates that she has been so afraid that she has been using drugs again. She adds that she also has reduced the number of her sex partners and was able to convince two of them to use condoms. Throughout the session I focus on the positive aspects and the negative aspects of each action—and show her how these stack up on paper. I believe that it might help to simplify some of the issues by showing them to her visually. It is clear to see in this manner that if she continues in her present lifestyle with David, the negatives far outweigh the positives. She asks if I can get her into a residential treatment program. Fortunately, I have access to a residential drug treatment program for women and their children; this program is also equipped with a specialized HIV component. I have arranged a visit for Rhonda to check out the program. When she visits the program and talks to a number of the clients, she finds out that quite a few of them have the same issues and problems that she has. Later, she asks me if she could bring her children with her into the program. We then have one of the first discussions about the dangers of leaving the children with her mother.

Rhonda is afraid that if she leaves David he will harm the children. He knows the children are with her mother, and Rhonda fears he will threaten her mother, and he will physically abuse the children or even take them away.

I explain to her that she could have the children with her in the residential treatment program, if we get permission, but that it will take some time. I explain how I could contact child welfare and what the process would be like. Once she enters the drug residential treatment, the child welfare worker can meet with her and her counselor and begin the plans for weekend visits with the children. Rhonda asks me whether I would be willing to do all this for her. When I say yes, she begins to cry and agrees to let me begin the process.

Throughout this process I have felt the ethical tensions. Even when Rhonda agreed to enter the treatment program, the tensions continued. As we work out her leaving David, discussing her plans with her mother, and working with child welfare, it is clear that at any moment Rhonda could easily return to her old coping behaviors, decide against the positive choices, or be harmed by David before she entered the treatment program. When she finally enters, I feel great relief. Now Rhonda has an opportunity to change her life and reduce the risks to her life and health, and David and her other sex partners also have reduced risk from Rhonda. In addition, if she stays in the drug treatment program, she will have access to good medical care, vocational training, and parenting training within a safe environment.

REFERENCES

American Psychological Association. (1992). Ethical principles of psychologists and code of conduct. *American Psychologist, 47*, 1597–1611.

Beauchamp, T., & Childress, J. (1989). *The principles of biomedical ethics*. Oxford, England: Oxford University Press.

Bradley Center v. Wessner, 250 Ga. 199, 296 S.E.2d 693 (1982).

Dalton, H. (1993). Criminal law. In S. Burris, H. Dalton, & J. L. Miller (Eds.), *AIDS law today: A new guide for the public* (pp. 242–262). New Haven, CT: Yale University Press.

Decker, J. F. (1987). Prostitution as a public health issue. In H. Dalton, S. Burris, & the Yale AIDS Law Project (Eds.), *AIDS and the law: A guide for the public* (pp. 81–89). New Haven, CT: Yale University Press.

GA. CODE ANN., §16-5-60 (1997).

GA. CODE ANN., §19-13-4 (1997).

GA. CODE ANN., §24-9-47 (1997).

GA. CODE ANN., §24-9-47(j) (1997).

GA. CODE ANN., §31-2-1 (1997)

GA. COMP. R. & REGS. r. 90-5-48-.05 (1997)

Keppler v. Brunson, 205 Ga. App. 32, 421 S.E.2d 306 (1992).

Kritzer, H., Bogart W., & Vidmar, N. (1991). The aftermath of injury: Cultural factors in compensation seeking in Canada and the United States. *Law & Society Review, 25*, 499–543.

Lamb, D. H., Clark, C., Drumheller, P., Frizzell, K., & Surrey, L. (1989). Applying Tarasoff to AIDS related psychotherapy issues. *Professional Psychology: Research and Practice, 20*, 37–43.

Martin, J. M. (in press). Ethics in the treatment of human immunodeficiency virus infection and acquired immunodeficiency syndrome. In S. F. Bucky (Ed.), *The comprehensive textbook of ethics and law in the practice of psychology*. New York: Plenum Press.

Tarasoff v. Board of Regents of the University of California, 551 P.2d 334 (Cal. 1976).

10

THE MENTALLY ILL, HIV-POSITIVE CLIENT: THE CASE OF MILDRED

ROBERT A. WASHINGTON, KAREN STROHM KITCHENER, AND SCOTT BURRIS

ORIENTATION TO THE MAJOR ETHICAL ISSUES HIGHLIGHTED IN THE CASE

Clinicians whose clients are no longer competent to make their own decisions must deal with issues of confidentiality and duty to protect as well as issues related to their client's specific impairments and limited competency. The following case illustrates the challenges of dealing with someone who is actively psychotic, unable to self-medicate, and a potential threat to others.

CASE PRESENTATION (BY ROBERT A. WASHINGTON)

I am a psychologist working part-time in an outpatient day treatment program in Virginia for adults with serious mental illness. Most of the clients have spent years in and out of the state mental health hospital. The recent development of new antipsychotic drugs has enabled them to leave the hospital and begin productive lives in the community. The day treatment program uses behavior-reinforcing techniques to teach skills in daily living.

Our success rate has been above average; that is, most of our clients remain in the community and with vocational training are able to find meaningful work. Several live in group homes, and some have returned to their families.

Mildred, age 37, is an example of the program's success. She has been in the hospital for the past 9 years, on a ward for patients who are difficult to place in the community; when I met her, she was in her eighth hospitalization since age 19. However, the "wonder drug" clozopine has controlled her psychotic symptoms, and for the past 13 months she has been able to participate in the program and attend daily treatment sessions. She has off-grounds privileges and should be ready for discharge in about 3 months. Mildred uses her privileges to visit her mother, who appreciates having her home. They have a close relationship and spend time attending church, shopping, and watching television.

Mildred has a 20-year-old daughter, the result of a high school romance. Because Mildred was unable to care for her, she was placed in foster care. The two have recently begun to talk, and Mildred has apologized for not being available to her.

Mildred is very frightened. She remembers living on the street as an alcoholic and "street whore." She is just beginning to talk about those days, and a lot of her memory is vague. When she complained of "just not feeling right" and voiced her suspicions that she might have the "bug," I urged her to be tested for HIV, and she agreed. I spent considerable time counseling her prior to testing and after she learned of her positive status. She has accepted her status and even moved beyond self-blame. She recognizes that she has two illnesses—alcoholism and mental illness—and she appropriately blames them for predisposing her to behavior that led to HIV infection. She says she is glad she miscarried three times because she would not have wanted to place children at risk.

Six months ago, Mildred's viral load was well over 500,000. She was immediately placed on triple combination therapy, which included a protease inhibitor. It was not easy to find a medication regime she could tolerate, but since doing so she takes her medications for HIV as faithfully as she takes psychotropics. She understands that missing doses could result in resistance. She has been rewarded by a significant drop in her viral load. I applaud her attention to detail.

Recently Mildred and I have been working on disclosure issues. Mildred has told no one, including her mother, of her HIV status. She is afraid that the knowledge will disturb her newfound relationship with her daughter. She said she would never want anyone to know and pleaded with me not to include it in her record. She thinks that her church members, who have been supportive of her as a person living with a mental illness, would reject her if they knew she had HIV and had lived on the street. She maintains that her involvement with the church and her relationship with her daughter represent her new identity, the person she has become.

Today I learned that Mildred has decompensated and is now on a locked ward. Although she seemed somewhat agitated the last time we met, she did not let on that she had stopped taking psychotropics almost a month ago. She started being verbally abusive to her mother last Friday. She stayed out all night, so her mother telephoned the hospital. Police apprehended Mildred after a drunken brawl with a woman over a man. She had minor lacerations, which were treated in the local hospital emergency room. She was then transferred to the acute ward of the hospital where she has been quite belligerent.

When I visited Mildred, she was so heavily sedated that she was almost incoherent. She cried; she said she wanted to prove to everyone, including me, that she did not need (psychotropic) medications. She begged me not to disclose her HIV status because the daughter of one of her church members works as an attendant on the ward. At that point she became very seductive as though she were offering herself sexually to convince me to agree with her. I tried to emphasize her need for her HIV medication compliance—she had been without for at least 2 days. However, she simply was not coherent enough to engage.

PAUSE AND IDENTIFY YOUR PERSONAL RESPONSES TO THE CASE

I understand Mildred's mistaken belief that she could manage without psychotropics. Unfortunately but understandably, most clients have to try that. After all, it is difficult for people to think that they must always take these medications, which keep them sane but make them feel very restricted. I think Mildred will further understand and accept her condition following this incident.

I am much more concerned about Mildred taking the "cocktail" for HIV. I think the possibility of increased viral burden and disease progression is great. Yet she does not want anyone to know about her illness, and she is certainly not ready to respond to the questions she would be asked. I have no idea whether her church members would reject her, but I know her judgment has been good in the past, and her relationship with her daughter has just begun.

I am equally concerned about the potential danger that Mildred presents to others. If she is behaving seductively with me, she is likely to behave that way with others on the ward. The patients are unaware of her HIV status. Were she to have sex or a physical altercation, she could put others at risk.

Although Mildred is not a danger to herself in the traditional sense, it is not in her best interest to be without her medication. I wonder whether I am contributing to her possible harm or the harm of others by not breaking confidentiality. Furthermore, she is unable to think rationally and to act in anyone's best interest. Does that allow me to break confidentiality to prevent her from possible illness and death or possibly exposing others? If the nursing staff knew, they would give her the medication as prescribed. They might also feel the need to warn other patients, because her seductive behavior has become obvious.

Although I do believe that I am legally bound to protect Mildred or others, I certainly feel a moral obligation. I am not at all sure about the ethics of this situation.

REVIEW THE FACTS OF THE CASE

Mildred is dependent on medication to keep the proliferation of the HIV virus in check. Although sex is prohibited on the wards, Mildred is behaving quite seductively and was probably engaging in unprotected sexual behavior before her hospitalization.

There is every reason to believe that Mildred was taking her medication prior to her current decompensation. She currently is incapable of making rational decisions.

Mildred does not want the hospital staff to know of her HIV status; she is particularly concerned about one staff member, whom she knows from church. Thus far, I have honored that request.

Mildred would be furious (and perhaps even litigious) were I to disclose. More important, she would feel betrayed.

CONCEPTUALIZE AN INITIAL PLAN
BASED ON CLINICAL ISSUES

I will convene a team meeting that includes Mildred's physician. If he is unavailable or unwilling to attend, I will consult with him about the risk to Mildred of not continuing treatment and how that risk increases with time.

Without disclosing the subject of my concern, I will speak to the chief of nursing for the hospital to see if a way can be found to provide medications without the knowledge of a member of the ward staff. If so, I will explain that to Mildred as soon as I possibly can to see if she will agree to disclosure. I will also explain what her doctor has advised.

In the meantime I will obtain consultations about the ethical guidelines and the law, to see if I have an ethical obligation to make sure no one is potentially harmed should Mildred engage in sex on the ward.

CONSULT THE ETHICS CODE AND ASSESS THE ETHICAL ISSUES (BY KAREN STROHM KITCHENER)

The issues in Mildred's case have much in common with the other cases in this book regarding the duty to protect because she may be engaging in sexual activity with other patients on the ward who do not know about her HIV status. What makes the case different, however, is that according to Dr. Washington, she is presently incapable of making rational decisions. Furthermore, in addition to being a potential danger to others, she is a danger to herself because she is unable to take her medication to keep the proliferation of the HIV virus in check. If she does not do so, the possibility of developing a resistance to medication is high, and she clearly is jeopardizing her own life. At the same time, Dr. Washington is feeling pulled in multiple directions. In ethical terms his faithfulness to the promises he has made regarding confidentiality is being pitted against concerns about life-threatening harm both to Mildred and to others.

I will summarize for Dr. Washington the major issues that overlap with other cases in this book and then point out the differences. As with the prior chapters, I will begin with the American Psychological Association (APA, 1992) Ethics Code and then discuss what the foundational ethical issues add to the understanding of the case.

APA Ethics Code

The standards from the Ethics Code that are the most relevant in this case are the ones regarding confidentiality. Although Dr. Washington did not mention it in his description of the case, I am presuming that when Mildred was rational, he met the requirements of Standard 5.01, Discussing the Limits of Confidentiality; this standard requires that psychologists talk about these issues at the outset of treatment. Assuming that he did, she was informed that confidentiality might be broken when and if she became a danger to herself or others. On the other hand, Standard 5.02, Maintaining Confidentiality, notes that psychologists have a primary obligation to maintain client confidences, and Standard 5.03, Minimizing Intrusions on Privacy, obligates psychologists to limit those with whom they discuss confidential information. These obligations seem to weigh heavily on Dr. Washington's mind as he conceptualizes an initial treatment plan limiting as much as possible those with whom Mildred's HIV status is discussed. However, Standard 5.05, Disclosures, notes that when permitted by law psychologists can break confidentiality to protect the patient or others from harm. The same standard also notes that confidentiality can be broken to provide needed professional services for the patient or to obtain professional consultation. In this case, breaking confidentiality to discuss her issues with the chief of nursing would be covered by this standard, assuming such consultations were allowed under the law of the state in which Dr. Washington is operating.

The last standard that seems relevant in this and every case is Standard 1.14, Avoiding Harm. Here, the obligation is to avoid harm when possible and to minimize it when it is not possible to avoid. Aspirational Principle E: Concern for Others' Welfare reiterates the importance of minimizing harm when ethical conflicts occur.

The facts of this case suggest some obligation on Dr. Washington's part to break confidentiality both for Mildred's benefit and to protect the others on her ward. Considering how to minimize the harm that will occur to his relationship with Mildred seems to be a primary consideration in his treatment plan because he attempted to identify a way to provide treatment to Mildred without disclosing her HIV status to ward staff. On the other hand, because she is HIV-positive and may be engaging in sexual activity with other patients, he may decide that both staff members and patients must be informed. He could point out to the ward attendant the importance of keeping this information confidential even from Mildred's mother.

Foundational Ethical Principles

The issue of Mildred's autonomy is a critical one. Although respect for autonomy includes respecting other's decisions even if we believe them to be mistaken, it is based on the assumption that the decisions that others make are autonomous. As described in chapter 3, an autonomous decision must be intentional and must be based on adequate knowledge as well as the competence to comprehend knowledge and its implications. That does not seem to be true in Mildred's case. She is heavily sedated and is unable to think rationally and to make reasonable decisions about her own behavior and their implications for others. Her mental illness and her lapse in taking her psychotropic medication exacerbate this. One may conclude that her actions and choices do not appear to be autonomous at this point in her life. Furthermore, because other patients do not know of her HIV status, they cannot make reasonable decisions about engaging in sexual activity with her. If their mental status is compromised, even if they had the information, their ability to choose not to participate is limited.

On the other hand, when Mildred was rational she requested that Dr. Washington keep the information regarding her HIV status confidential, and the principle of fidelity would suggest that keeping that promise is an important one. That promise, however, was probably based on the caveat that if she became a danger to herself or others, Dr. Washington might be unable to maintain her confidence. His trustworthiness is also an issue under the principle of fidelity. If Mildred were rational and Dr. Washington broke confidentiality, she might see him as untrustworthy; however, she is not rational. Assuming she becomes so again, she may find some comfort in knowing that Dr. Washington is willing to set some limits on her ability to harm herself.

The principles of beneficence and do no harm should make Dr. Washington consider what can be done to help Mildred under the circumstances and to consider interventions that will both help her and do her the least amount of avoidable harm. He must consider the harm that might come to Mildred both in her relationships with her mother and daughter and with others in her church if he breaks confidentiality. On the other hand, beneficence strongly suggests that he do what he can to help Mildred resume her medication for HIV, a life-threatening condition. By talking about Mildred to the chief of nursing to see if she can get her medications without informing the staff, Dr. Washington is respecting her privacy; he is limiting the people to whom her status needs to be disclosed, thereby respecting her wishes while helping her and protecting her from harm.

He might also want to consider other similar alternatives that would respect her privacy and thus avoid harming her, as he evaluates how to protect other patients on the ward. For example, he might talk with Mildred's physician about taking her off the heavy sedatives, so that she might be more rational. If removing her from sedatives might allow her to make more reasonable decisions and would not harm her or other patients, Dr. Washington could talk with her about her seductive behavior and the importance of remaining celibate on the ward. If this is not possible, then he might consider alternatives like isolating her until her antipsychotic medication begins to take effect. Although her HIV status might have to be revealed to the staff, her privacy with other patients could be protected, and they would be protected from her acting out behavior. As noted earlier, if the staff were informed, he might talk to the staff member who has a connection to Mildred's church and remind that person of the importance of maintaining Mildred's confidentiality. Furthermore, beneficence and non-maleficence would require that if Dr. Washington decides that he must break Mildred's confidentiality, then he also follow up with Mildred to help her deal with the consequences of others finding out about her HIV status once she is rational.

As with other cases in which patients have been engaged in socially undesirable behavior, the principle of justice should lead Dr. Washington to ask whether his decisions are based on a fair evaluation of the data and not on preconceived beliefs about Mildred and her behavior. Dr. Washington states that he felt very proud of the gains that Mildred had been making in various realms of her life. Although he says that he understands her mistaken belief that she could make it without her psychotropic medication, he may resent her decision because it has now caused him additional work as well as placed him in a position of having to make a difficult decision. Justice would require that Dr. Washington consider whether his own feeling of disappointment is biasing his decisions.

Balancing the Ethics Code and Foundational Ethical Principles

Dr. Washington clearly has deep compassion for Mildred. The most difficult question that he has to answer is whether he can remain in a caring relationship with her in light of her decision to discontinue her antipsychotic medication. It would not be caring, however, if he did not help her to return to her triple combination drug therapy. If she does not return quickly to her medications, she may develop a resistance to these and other medications. The ultimate consequence may be death. Failure to act under these circumstances would not uphold the principles of beneficence or nonmaleficence and might even be seen as negligent. This is especially true because Mildred cannot make an autonomous decision about her own life. Failing to take some action to protect the other patients from her endangering behavior would be similarly hard to justify.

Moreover, assuming that Dr. Washington informed Mildred at the outset of treatment that he might need to break confidentiality if she endangered herself or others, she knew the possible consequences of her actions at that point in time. Although it is probably the case that she did not anticipate the consequences when she stopped taking her psychotropic medication, Dr. Washington would not be breaking an absolute promise to keep information about her HIV status confidential. Likewise, although it may be difficult for her to appreciate initially, there are consequences when she fails to take her antipsychotic medications or her HIV cocktail, and it is important for Mildred to know that. It may also be important for her to know that Dr. Washington is willing to intervene to prevent her from harming herself.

On the other hand, it is always best to honor promises, respect autonomy even when it is limited as it is in Mildred's case, and uphold the principles of beneficence and doing no harm. The best option is to make decisions carefully and to consider alternatives that can honor all of the principles to the extent that it is possible. As already noted, considering alternatives like isolating Mildred until she is rational and providing her HIV medication as confidentially as possible would be better than breaking her confidentiality with staff and patients. If that is not possible, Dr. Washington would be justified in breaking his initial promise to Mildred to maintain her confidentiality. He would, however, remain responsible for helping her deal with the consequences of that decision.

IDENTIFY THE LEGAL ISSUES (BY SCOTT BURRIS)

Dr. Washington is correct that he is under no legal obligation to take charge of this situation. Both Mildred's medical care and the regulation of her sexual conduct are now the primary responsibility of others. Nevertheless, Mildred is his patient, and he does have a general duty to provide her with care that meets professional standards. It may be useful to explain why his obligations are limited, because a better picture of the legal aspects of this situation may help him develop and implement his plan.

Mildred is under control, in a locked, observed ward where sexual activity is prohibited. This has two immediate implications. The first will be that, from the law's point of view, the primary duty-holder here is the hospital, which promises to provide a safe environment. Unless Dr. Washington has reason to know that the hospital cannot fulfill its duty, he can rely on this assurance until such time as he learns of facts that make clear the hospital cannot be trusted. Provided that he advises the hospital staff of Mildred's tendency to be sexually active (as discussed below), Dr. Washington does not have the special, unique knowledge of the risks and control over Mildred that might trigger for him a duty to warn or protect. The second implication is that there is no clear, immediate threat to others, again negating a *Tarasoff* sort of duty (*Tarasoff v. Board of Regents of the University of California*, 1976). I hasten to add, however, that any worry about a duty to warn here is academic only: In Virginia, where this case takes place, the Supreme Court has rejected *Tarasoff* and its broad duty to protect third parties (*Nasser v. Parker*, 1995).

That does not mean that it would be legally prudent for Dr. Washington simply to walk away from the case. Most of the time, the best legal course is to follow a sound professional one. Dr. Washington seems to think he should let the people in the ward know of the risk Mildred poses if she has sex with other patients, but he is worried that this would violate her rights to the privacy of her HIV diagnosis. Like many states, Virginia does have an HIV privacy law, which probably would not prohibit the disclosure that Dr. Washington wants to make, but I do not think he needs to disclose any HIV information to attain his goals of protecting other patients and securing good medical care for Mildred.

This case illustrates that disclosure of a person's HIV status is not always necessary to deal with a threat of transmission. The problem here is Mildred's seductive behavior, not just her HIV status. A competent hospital staff will not be unaware of the many risks, including sexually transmitted diseases, posed by sexual behavior by patients with a mental illness. Just as universal precautions are now the norm in hospitals, in settings like this everyone concerned should assume the risk of disease transmission in unprotected sexual activity. It should be sufficient for Dr. Washington to alert the staff that Mildred will probably try to have sex and that such behavior would be very destructive for her. In this way the issue of sex, and the possibility of a sexually transmitted disease, are flagged without disclosing her HIV status.

The other problem is Mildred's medical care for HIV. At least on the medical facts as we know them in 2001, this is the first of the cases we have examined in this book to present a situation that sounds like an emergency: Even an interruption of a few doses could instill resistance, undermining the efficacy of combination therapy. (Medical opinion may change, but we must operate on the information we have available today.) Dr. Washington feels an ethical need to do more than just stand by and watch, but what can he do?

Here, too, there is little or no legal risk to Dr. Washington if he chooses to disclose. There are at least two reasons why the Virginia HIV confidentiality statute does not prevent him from acting. First, the statute is narrowly written. Unlike many other state laws that cover all "HIV-related information" in the medical record (Burris, 1993), Virginia's HIV confidentiality law by its terms protects only HIV test results (Va. Code Ann., 1997). In other states, courts have split on whether such laws cover just the HIV test result itself (*Urbaniak v. Newton*, 1991) or should be read more broadly to cover disclosures that entailed the release of a person's positive results (*Santa Rosa Health Care Corp. v. Garcia*, 1998). More to the point, there is an exception to the confidentiality rule in Virginia that applies exactly to this situation: The statute allows release of information to a "health care provider for purposes of consultation or providing care and treatment to the person who was the subject of the test." I'm very confident that Dr. Washington can legally inform the hospital staff of Mildred's need for HIV care.

As with the sex issue, however, I do not think simply disclosing Mildred's condition really gets Dr. Washington where he wants to go. The issue here is not really Dr. Washington's legal or ethical responsibilities, but how he can get the rest of the important players to fulfill their obligations.

His idea of assembling the team—in our thinking if not in the office—is a good one. A sense of their legal obligations may help him in his work.

The big missing person in this case so far is the treating physician, who already knows that Mildred has HIV. HIV confidentiality law is no bar to Dr. Washington alerting the physician of Mildred's whereabouts, her lack of medications, and the special concerns about privacy that obtain.

The hospital itself—the current caregivers in the ward—also have an obligation to see to the medical as well as the mental health needs of the patient. Was a medical history taken? If this is the same hospital system in which she is receiving her medical care, have her records been acquired? For a medical facility to take no action to ascertain a patient's current health status and medication needs sounds like pretty serious malpractice.

The hospital also has an obligation under the state HIV confidentiality law to keep Mildred's diagnosis confidential. This obligation encompasses the employee Mildred knows (*Doe v. Flores*, 1996). Whereas it probably would not require the hospital to transfer or otherwise exclude this woman from the loop, the law certainly requires the hospital to make it clear to this employee that what she learns about Mildred's health cannot be revealed even to her mother.

Dr. Washington's most pressing concern is fidelity to Mildred and particularly helping her maintain her family and community relationships. It seems to me that the role he picks for himself in this is that of a facilitator, who brings together all the people who need to address Mildred's issues and deal with them well. He has a clear and reasonable plan and yet he may worry that his plan will expose him to legal liability. His legal risk, however, is very slight.

IDENTIFY AND ASSESS THE OPTIONS
(BY ROBERT A. WASHINGTON)

I am so glad that I was able to get good advice to assist my planning for Mildred. What felt like a terrible dilemma does not feel quite as bad. Although I remain concerned that Mildred may engage in unprotected sex while on the ward, protecting the other patients is the responsibility of the hospital staff. I feel freer to think exclusively about what is in Mildred's best interests. It is clear that two things mitigate against any legal or professional action if I decide to disclose Mildred's need for antiviral medication. First, she is currently unable to make rational decisions for herself. As such she is not autonomous. Second, the law allows me to release the results of her HIV test to a health care provider for purposes of treatment. I feel comfortable that one way or the other I must make this information known to hospital personnel. I telephone the chief of nursing and arrange for a meeting tomorrow.

Next, I talk to Mildred's infectious disease physician. He is unavailable to meet with me and the chief of nursing, but he does fax a note detailing the medications and dosage schedules. He also makes it clear that he is willing to talk with hospital personnel. He agrees that safeguarding Mildred's confidentiality, if at all possible, is extremely important because maintaining her confidence is key to her willingness to remain compliant with any medication regime.

The limited possibility of litigation does not necessarily make me happy; I regard ethics and law as considerations but not determinant factors. What concerns me more is my relationship with Mildred, because much of the value of therapy depends on that relationship. I had promised to keep her secret while working with her to be more comfortable with disclosure. Fidelity and trust are essential to the relationship, and I know that Mildred will feel betrayed when I tell her that I plan to discuss her condition with the chief of nursing. I am also acutely aware of the "out" I allow myself by telling clients about the limits of confidentiality. Of course, I can fall back on that as if to say "I told you so," but the truth is that neither of us anticipated this kind of situation when those limits were discussed. In the final analysis I am relying on my belief that Mildred knows that I care and the faith that that knowledge will sustain the relationship in spite of the perceived betrayal. If the relationship were not firmly rooted in a felt sense of caring, there would be much less reason to be hopeful.

CHOOSE A COURSE OF ACTION AND
SHARE IT WITH YOUR CLIENT

The next step is a visit with Mildred to explain what I plan to do. She is not at all happy, although she is a little less sedated and has begun to worry about taking her antiviral medications. I explain that I am going to meet with the chief of nursing to see if the medications can be dispensed without the knowledge of her mother's church friend. However, I also explain to her that once I disclose to the chief of nursing, I cannot guarantee that she will be as discreet as Mildred would like. I explain to her that it is the responsibility of all hospital employees to respect the privacy of patients; that includes the member of her church. Mildred is not mollified. I tell her that I will proceed with my plan because her well-being is extremely important and that there will be plenty of time to talk later. Right now the most important thing is to make sure she is able to get her medications. Mildred sulks.

IMPLEMENT THE COURSE OF ACTION: MONITOR AND DISCUSS OUTCOMES

The meeting with the chief of nursing is quite formal. I explain Mildred's situation to her and add parenthetically that I am certain that she would not want a lawsuit as the result of "Mildred's business becoming community property." She gets my drift. That day Mildred begins receiving antiviral medications as prescribed by her infectious disease physician. When I explain the results of the meeting with the chief of nursing to Mildred, she is disbelieving. I cannot say that I blame her. I am pleased that she does not "fire" me (I was prepared for that).

Mildred and I continue to meet following her discharge from the hospital. She continues to accuse me of telling her business, but it is clear that she is forgiving and even thankful that she continued to receive her medications while in the hospital. At first she averred that people in the church were looking at her differently, but now she no longer does. She wants me to guarantee that her mother and other church people will not find out. The discussions that followed about the repercussions of disclosing have been useful and have moved Mildred a step closer to sharing with her mother. They also allow me to reinforce the limits of confidentiality and the need to continue to take psychotropic medications; I tell her that when she decompensates, all bets are off. We talk about the need for the use of condoms when having sex. Mildred tells me that she is very aware of that need and reminds me that it is only when she has decompensated that she is not. Just one more reason, I add, that it is important for her to take her medications.

What impresses me most is Mildred's sincere concern for the safety of others. She once again talks about being glad that she did not have children while infected and says she could not stand the idea of infecting someone else. This strong conscience, derived from good upbringing and reinforced in her church, gives us a lot to discuss. Responsibility is something she must have for herself and for others, I remind her. Condoms are a symbol of that responsibility. She understands. One day she might understand that my protecting her has helped make it possible for her to protect others and, most importantly, protect herself.

REFERENCES

American Psychological Association. (1992). Ethical principles of psychologists and code of conduct. *American Psychologist, 47*, 1597–1611.

Burris, S. (1993). Testing, disclosure and the right to privacy. In S. Burris, H. L. Dalton, & J. L. Miller (Eds.), *AIDS law today: A new guide for the public* (pp. 115–149). New Haven, CT: Yale University Press.

Doe v. Flores, 236 Conn. 845, 675 A.2d 835 (Conn. 1996).

Nasser v. Parker, 249 Va. 172, 455 S.E.2d 502 (Va. 1995).

Santa Rosa Health Care Corp. v. Garcia, 41 Tex. Sup. Ct. J. 535 (Tex. 1998).

Tarasoff v. Board of Regents of the University of California, 551 P.2d 334 (Cal. 1976).

Urbaniak v. Newton, 226 Cal.App.3d 1128, 277 Cal. Rptr. 354 (Cal. Ct. App. 1991).

VA. CODE ANN., §§32.1–36.1 (Michie 1997).

11

THE ADOLESCENT AT RISK FOR HIV: THE CASE OF JAMES

ROBERT A. WASHINGTON, KAREN STROHM KITCHENER,
AND SCOTT BURRIS

ORIENTATION TO THE MAJOR ETHICAL ISSUES HIGHLIGHTED IN THE CASE

The following case involves issues related to confidentiality and the duty to protect an adolescent client who is abusing drugs and is having unsafe sex with older men. Primary issues for the therapist include confidentiality to protect the well-being of the adolescent client versus the duty to report suspected child abuse and the duty to protect others.

CASE PRESENTATION (BY ROBERT A. WASHINGTON)

I am a school psychologist in Maryland and have been called in by classroom teachers to assess James's declining academic performance and determine whether it is related to emotional problems. Although I do not know James well I recognize him as a star athlete with whom I have had occasional hallway conversations about sports. I have always been fond of him and felt that he was comfortable with me.

James, age 16, strikingly handsome, and African American, until recently has been an "A" and "B" student as well as a basketball and track star. According to his homeroom teacher James's grades began to slide after Christmas. He started getting mostly "Cs," and his teachers report that he seems depressed, distracted, and tired most of the time. In March, James decided to quit both the track and the basketball teams. He told his coach and his parents that he needed more time to concentrate on schoolwork in order to improve his grades and get into a "top-notch" college. His parents approved, because they believed that his grades required attention. It is now April and James's grades continue to decline, and he is increasingly absent from school because of "the flu."

During our first counseling session, James initially attributes his declining performance to a failure of discipline. When I comment that his teachers have reported that he has been sick a lot lately, he becomes agitated and looks worried. After some persistent pressure on my part, James "unloads." Through his tears James says that he has needed someone to talk to for a long time. He says that he is glad that I am his counselor because he "knows that I am cool and that I will understand." He then discloses that he has realized that he was gay since age 12 but that he has been very "closeted" at school and at home. He says that he really hates acting "straight" at school and that he has no intention of "coming out" because he has seen how "gay boys" get harassed and beat up. He goes on to say, "even if nobody bothered me at school my father would find out, and I'd kill myself if that happened." (I use this opportunity to explain to James the limits of confidentiality. I make sure that he understands that if he is in danger or a danger to others, I may feel compelled to share information he gives me in confidence.) James explains that his father is a 56-year-old marine sergeant who is a heavy drinker and prone to explosive outbursts when he is intoxicated. James's 54-year-old mother works as a senior administrative coordinator for a large computer company. Both parents are dedicated to their jobs and work extremely long hours. They regard their son as a "straight arrow" who needs little supervision because he "understands the meaning of responsibility and discipline."

As the story unfolds, I learn that last September James met Paul, a 23-year-old openly gay man who works at a department store in the mall. Paul introduced James to the clubs in the city and since then, as James puts it, he "can't get enough." He often sneaks out of the house after his parents go to sleep, sometimes staying out 3 or 4 nights a week until 4:00 am. He loves to dress in drag and successfully "walks" in competitions. Because he is young and good looking, he is appealing to older men.

After Christmas, James began going home with men that he met at the clubs. A new friend, Jerry, turned him on to "ecstasy" and crack cocaine. Jerry has continued to supply James with drugs, and he has offered to let James stay with him at his apartment. When James is high, he has unprotected sex. Occasionally, James has had sex with several men in one night. James stated that his major concern is that he is getting addicted to crack. He says that he has been partying too much and that he has not been feeling good lately. Although he states that he needs to get himself together, he also states that the only times he really feels good is when he is high with his friends at the clubs. He discloses that he has been thinking about quitting school, getting a job, and moving in with Jerry. When I remind him that he is an excellent student with good prospects for college, he says that he might get his GED and go to college later. At the moment he just wants to get away from school and get away from his parents so he can start being who he really is.

PAUSE AND IDENTIFY YOUR PERSONAL RESPONSES
TO THE CASE

My first emotional reactions to this case are self-protective. I experience feelings of impotence, anger at the system, and a grandiose defensive wish that the world could be run the way I see fit.

I find myself wishing that I did not have to confront the issues that this case presents, any one of which requires considerable thoughtfulness and care to resolve. I went into this kind of work to help children with the normal problems of youth, not with this particular variation on the theme. If I notify the police the matter would soon be out of my hands and my control (and probably out of control). An investigation would ensue. James says he would kill himself if his father were to find out. I do not think that is true, but I do not know him well enough to rule it out. I have heard that gay male adolescents are at much greater risk for suicide, and to make matters worse, he is using mood-altering drugs. Furthermore, he is adamant about not disclosing to his father, who has a volatile temper. Would doing the legally binding and ethical thing, which is designed to protect him, be the best thing for James, or would it place him in different jeopardy? When he says that his father is explosive, what exactly does he mean? An investigation would be extraordinarily disruptive of their family life. They would need to be prepared for it.

To date, the other staff and I have not tackled the elephant in the middle of the classroom—those students who are or may be identified by others as gay. We have not done what we could to make it comfortable for them to share their concerns before they become unavoidable crises. We kind of hope the issue will not come up even though we know some students are harassed (as James mentions). We have shirked our responsibility to these students because of our fear of public reprisals. The school board and the community would come down hard on us for reaching out to gay students. Eventually, this issue was bound to come to my door; I guess it is time for me to take my head out of the sand.

As I pause long enough to begin to think about James, I am despondent. He could be ill, deathly ill. The adults taking advantage of him are unscrupulous and should be held accountable for what I see as unscrupulous behavior on their part. Is he doing what a lot of gay teenagers feel they must do—make themselves available to reprehensible adults because there is no socially acceptable place to turn for sexual exploration?

REVIEW THE FACTS OF THE CASE

I consider James to be my client. I am not sure the school system would agree; the school system probably sees itself as my client. The explosive potential of this situation is such that I need to consult with those in higher authority. I must choose carefully because I want to work with someone who will be deliberate and thoughtful. And I must tell James whom I will inform.

He needs a good medical work up. That can probably be arranged without parental consent because he is 16.

From a developmental point of view, he seems ahead of his age group expressively and intellectually. I am more inclined to reason with him than to act quickly to protect him from continued danger. I know that Jerry has no legal custody or control of James, yet I wonder if a case for child abuse can be made because he is giving him drugs and offering him to others for sex. Certainly his actions are unlawful. I feel obliged to report this behavior. Fortunately, I have told James that I cannot maintain confidentiality if he is in danger or dangerous. I gave examples when we first met. Does he want me to put a stop to this situation? Are the specifics of this situation such that he does not think my guidelines apply? Does he think that I will circumvent my own rules? I need to find out which it is. He needs to know that I believe that he is in danger, and I need to clearly explain that to him.

More important, I hear and sense James's tremendous pain and recognize his agitation. It is his agitation that concerns me most because it could lead him to be impulsive. I am not aware of all the causes but I know he feels alone, which is why he acknowledged the need to talk to someone. He has chosen me, and I must honor that choice and not push him into further isolation. There is the possibility of using his trust in me to begin a healing process. That has to be the guiding principle for me.

CONCEPTUALIZE AN INITIAL PLAN
BASED ON CLINICAL ISSUES

I see James as a confused adolescent. On the one hand, he says that he feels like himself when he is high, and on the other he is very worried about addiction. He is quite agitated—afraid of disclosure yet wanting to be himself. He is alone—other than myself he has not disclosed his problem to anyone who might be responsible and who might advise him.

My first task is to make sure that James recognizes that I really do understand his plight by acknowledging the difficulty gay youth encounter and his felt lack of support at home. I will emphasize that I understand his sense of aloneness and his legitimate fear of social stigma.

Second, I want James to clarify what he expects of me.

Third, I will remind James of my discussion of confidentiality and dangerousness. I will then tell him that I hope we can agree on a course of action that ceases to place him in danger and engage him in conversation toward that end. I will suggest that he and I both get consultation from others with more experience with the issues related to gay youth from a gay youth center, if one exists, or an experienced counselor. I will tell him that I am compelled to seek legal advice but that I will not divulge his name. I will assure him that I will take no action until we have gathered more information and considered options.

Fourth, I will remind him that he could be ill, perhaps with HIV disease. I am sure he recognizes the possibility because AIDS awareness has been an integral part of his health curriculum. We will explore possibilities for a medical examination, including an HIV antibody test.

Finally, I will make sure James understands that in the not-too-distant future, I must share this information with school authorities. Although we will discuss this, the ultimate decision is mine. I cannot control what will happen then so I would like for us to have a plan in mind, one each of us can support.

CONSULT ETHICAL CODES AND ASSESS THE ETHICAL ISSUES (BY KAREN STROHM KITCHENER)

James's case presents a classical ethical dilemma where the psychologist must decide between two harms—the harm that may result if confidentiality is broken and the harm that may result if it is not. Unfortunately, although child abuse laws were designed to protect children from violence, psychologists often feel conflicted about reporting because they perceive the costs of breaking confidentiality to be high (Brosig & Kalichman, 1992; Kalichman, 1993). In James's case, this is particularly true because he has threatened to kill himself, and the consequences of revealing his homosexuality both at school and at home may also be very negative. It is no wonder Dr. Washington is feeling so conflicted.

Although the ethical issue that stands out in this case is confidentiality, James's age and the question of what is in his best interests complicate it.

The Ethics Code (American Psychological Association [APA], 1992) offers some guidance about appropriate courses of action, and the more general ethical issues identified in chapter 3 are also critical. Because Dr. Washington does not know whether James is HIV-positive, it is unclear whether he is exposing others to the HIV virus by having unprotected sex. If he is HIV-positive, the issues surrounding the duty to protect others are similar to the ones discussed in earlier cases and are not repeated here.

The APA Ethics Code

It is important to note that Dr. Washington did inform James when he entered treatment that there were limits to confidentiality. He even helped him understand the limits by providing specific examples. This is consistent with Standard 5.01 of the Ethics Code (APA, 1992), which requires psychologists who enter into a professional relationship to discuss with the clients the "relevant limitations on confidentiality." It is notable that he believes James is developmentally "old" for his age, which suggests that James had the competence to understand those limits. Informing him of the limits indicated respect for James's rights to make autonomous decisions about how much and what information to share with Dr. Washington and was consistent with aspirational Principle D: Respect for People's Rights and Dignity. Under the circumstances, Dr. Washington's question about whether James wants him to intervene seems reasonable.

Other ethical issues were raised, however, when James disclosed that he was frequenting gay bars, that one adult was supplying him with drugs, and that his father has an "explosive" temper. It is possible that James is being abused. Dr. Washington might wonder whether he can and should disclose this information, and if so, to whom he should disclose it. Standard 5.05 of the Ethics Code allows psychologists to "disclose confidential information without the consent of the individual only as mandated by law, or where permitted by law for a valid purpose, such as . . . to protect the patient or client or others from harm." In other words, the standard gives Dr. Washington permission to break confidentiality when it is required by law or if the law permits it and if there is potential for James to be harmed by his own actions or by others. Clearly Dr. Washington needs to consult with a lawyer regarding what constitutes child abuse in his state. On the other hand, what this standard acknowledges is that even though confidentiality is a primary obligation of psychologists (Standard 5.02), sometimes it is more ethical to break confidentiality than to keep it. This is particularly true when a life is at stake. This standard would allow Dr. Washington to break confidentiality if child abuse laws mandate it and if James is a danger to himself. As noted in previous cases, the Ethics Code does not mandate that Dr. Washington disclose the information, which underlines the difference between the Ethics Code and the law. It does, however, pose the question: Is a greater good served for James by breaking confidentiality than by keeping it?

Standard 5.03, Minimizing Intrusions on Privacy, should remind Dr. Washington that breaking confidentiality should not be done lightly and that if he decides to do so, it should be done in a way that minimizes intrusion on James's privacy. For example, Dr. Washington presumes he must consult with someone in "higher authority." He needs to question this assumption. If he does so, he should consider how much of James's story he needs to reveal and to whom he needs to report to protect James. For example, James seems most concerned that his homosexuality not be revealed at school and to his parents. Dr. Washington cannot report James's anonymous sexual partners, anyway. He could, however, report Jerry just for providing James with crack cocaine. Similarly, he may or may not have to inform the police. At a minimum, Standard 5.03 suggests he needs to question to whom and what he needs to report. In addition, Standard 8.03 recommends that if the demands of an organization, such as a school system, conflict with the APA Ethics Code, psychologists should clarify the nature of the conflict and make known their commitment to follow the code. It recommends that to the extent possible the psychologist should resolve the conflict in a way that permits adherence to the Ethics Code. In this case, it would imply the importance of maintaining James's confidentiality.

If Dr. Washington ultimately decides that it would be in James's best interests to consult with a "higher authority," he should, as he suggests, identify someone who is "thoughtful and deliberate." It may be that the child abuse can be reported without James's peers finding out that he is gay if he wishes to continue to remain in the closet.

Standard 1.14 of the Ethics Code also requires that psychologists avoid harming clients and "minimize harm where it is foreseeable and unavoidable." In this case, Dr. Washington is aware that breaking confidentiality has the potential for harming James; if he decides to do so, he must decide how to minimize the impact of that harm. In addition, aspirational Principle E: Concern for Others' Welfare, should remind him that one of his primary responsibilities is to contribute to James's welfare. Concern for James's welfare would mean that Dr. Washington needs to carefully assess James's lethality and whether his father is abusing him or whether he might if his homosexuality were revealed.

Foundational Ethical Principles

As noted in earlier cases, the rule of keeping information confidential in therapy is based on the ethical responsibilities associated with fidelity and the respect accorded to autonomous persons. In terms of fidelity, there are issues of trust and promise keeping. Because Dr. Washington did not promise to keep information absolutely confidential, he would not be breaking a promise if he revealed information about James to protect him. On the other hand, trustworthiness is a clinically tricky issue with adolescents. James may believe, despite the original conversation about the limits of confidentiality, that because Dr. Washington is cool he will not "rat" on him. Nevertheless, trustworthiness is also often associated with keeping one's word, and Dr. Washington did warn James about the need to break confidentiality under some conditions at the outset of treatment. Consequently, Dr. Washington's plan to talk to James about his expectations and to remind him about their discussions of confidentiality and dangerousness is particularly important.

Another rationale for maintaining confidentiality derives from autonomy because autonomous persons have the right to keep information about themselves private (see chapter 3). The issue of autonomy, however, is clouded in this case by James's age and decision-making ability. Although many investigators have concluded that 15-year-olds have a reasonable level of competence and can evaluate information well enough to make informed choices (Grisso & Vierling, 1978; Mann, Harmoni, & Power, 1989; Weithorn & Campbell, 1982), most of the data on adolescents' competence have been gathered in laboratory settings where the implications of the decisions are not as critical as they are in the real world (Kitchener, 2000). On the basis of what is known about older adolescents' competence, some argue that there is no justification for affording adolescents less of a right to confidentiality than is given to adults (Gustafson & McNamara, 1987). On the other hand, Sobocinski (1990) maintained that "in determining competence in adolescents engaged in behaviors that are immediately rewarding but possess the risk for long term negative consequences, one must carefully assess the youth's ability to comprehend and appreciate the personal relevance of risk-taking behavior" (p. 243).

Dr. Washington does not know whether James is HIV-positive. If he is not and continues to have unprotected sex, the consequences of his behavior could be life-threatening. In addition, James may be depressed, he is clearly stressed, and he has admitted to drug abuse. All may affect his competence. Furthermore, adolescents generally lack experience in making long-term decisions, particularly about such momentous issues (Melton, 1988). As a result, it may be reasonable to question James's competence. Under these circumstances, the criteria for competence must be stringent (Sobocinski, 1990). Because adolescents have the majority of their life ahead of them and because they have little experience with such life-endangering decisions, it is better to err on the side of "false negatives (competent adolescents judged to be incompetent) rather than on the side of false positives" (Powell, 1984, p. 67). If James is not competent and he and Dr. Washington cannot agree on a plan of action, Dr. Washington would be ethically justified in acting paternalistically, breaking confidentiality and informing one or both of his parents, assuming they would respond with his best interests in mind. Although in the short term such an action may be painful, it may be the most beneficent in the long run if it protects James from a life-threatening disease or from other serious harm. On the other hand, Dr. Washington might want to explore James's relationship with his mother. If James perceives his mother as potentially supportive, he may be willing to give Dr. Washington permission to talk to her directly. A result may be that they may be able to develop a plan that could both protect James and avoid breaching confidentiality.

The foundational principles of beneficence and doing no harm are also relevant. Because beneficence provides the foundation for Concern for Others' Welfare (aspirational Principle E) from the Ethics Code, it emphasizes Dr. Washington's responsibility to assess James's suicidal ideation as well as the possibility that James's father is abusive. It also supports the decision to help James get tested for the HIV virus. Furthermore, for gay adolescents, identity development is often a painful and difficult task because of negative stereotypes, the lack of positive role models, and the absence of appropriate opportunities to explore their sexuality (Barrows & Halgin, 1988; Gonsiorek, 1988; Troiden, 1988). As a result, Dr. Washington's support and understanding have the potential of being powerful, positive forces in James's life. Last, helping others depends on being competent (see also Standard 1.04). Adolescents pose particular challenges, and working with them requires understanding the literature on adolescent development. Thus, beneficence should remind all psychologists that they should not move into working with special populations without proper preparation and consultation. Because Dr. Washington is a school psychologist, he should have that background.

In this case, it may not be possible to do no harm. The arguments are strong for intervening in some way to protect James from self-inflicted harm or the abuse of others. On the other hand, this principle would emphasize thinking carefully about how to do the least amount of avoidable harm. If James can be involved in planning Dr. Washington's intervention, a balance between doing good and avoiding harm may be struck.

Last, the principle of justice should remind Dr. Washington to treat James fairly. In this case, treating him fairly means neither underestimating his competence because he is an adolescent nor overestimating it. It should also remind him to consider the consequences for James even though he would like to lash out at the "unscrupulous adults" who are taking advantage of him.

In addition, justice raises the issue of the fair treatment of gay adolescents in the school setting. James claims they are discriminated against in his school; consequently, they have to struggle with their identity issues virtually alone. Although Dr. Washington's immediate concern is James's welfare, the larger issue is how to tackle the "elephant in the room" so that homosexual students can receive fairer treatment. If he does so, other adolescents may avoid resorting to extreme choices, such as James has made, to feel accepted or to explore their sexuality.

Balancing the Ethics Code and the Foundational Ethical Principles

How should Dr. Washington weigh these issues as he makes decisions in this case? Dr. Washington clearly cares deeply about James and wants to avoid harming him further. Consequently, he needs to consider how to do the least amount of avoidable long-term harm. The arguments for intervening in some way to protect James are strong. James is involved in life-threatening activities, his competence to make decisions regarding those activities may be limited, and he has his whole life ahead of him; thus, there is a great deal to lose if no one intervenes. To decide what will do the least amount of avoidable harm, Dr. Washington needs more information regarding whether he must disclose to school authorities, whether James is HIV-positive, and whether or not James's father is abusive. After gathering this information, he should get legal advice about whether child abuse laws apply.

Because Dr. Washington has reason to believe that James can partici- pate in decision making regarding his own life when he is not using crack cocaine, involving him in the planning is also ethically sound. It respects his autonomy and allows him to help to determine how his welfare can best be served. On the other hand, should Dr. Washington determine that James's suicidal threats are serious, he should not hesitate to protect him in some manner. Whatever decision he makes, he needs to consider how to respect James's privacy to the extent that it is possible and to continue to support him through the next few difficult weeks. His compassion for James will help him identify the least-worst alternatives for him.

Although Dr. Washington's primary ethical responsibility is to James, aspirational Principle F: Social Responsibility, encourages psychologists to consider using their knowledge of psychology to contribute to the community in which they work and live. In other words, the Ethics Code suggests that the highest professional ideals would be served by Dr. Washington looking beyond James to how he can aid other gay adolescents in the school.

IDENTIFY THE LEGAL ISSUES (BY SCOTT BURRIS)

This is a good place to restate the reminder that not all information about a person who has or might have HIV is "HIV-related information" protected by HIV privacy laws. The possibility that James has or will become HIV infected is a major source of risk in the case, but for the moment Dr. Washington does not know that the boy is HIV-infected and cannot reasonably presume that he is. What we are facing is a case of a sexually active adolescent in danger from drug use and risky sexual behavior, but also from social homophobia and the potentially hostile attitudes of one or both of his parents. This would be difficult enough if James were a private patient; the situation is complicated by Dr. Washington's legal obligation to report abused or neglected children to the authorities. Given our uncertainty about whether or not James is infected, we can safely postpone discussion of any sort of *Tarasoff* (*Tarasoff v. Board of Regents of the University of California*, 1976) duty to warn and concentrate on how Dr. Washington might weave his way through the rest of the legal thicket.

The most urgent step is to get James into medical care. Dr. Washington is correct that James can get HIV testing and care without his parents' knowledge or consent (Health-General Article, 1997), but if he can pay for the care only with their insurance they will not be in the dark for long.

The next set of issues has to do with Dr. Washington's possible obligations to the child abuse and neglect authorities. Let's begin with how the law would classify James's sexual activity. A 16-year-old may be said to be above "the age of consent" for sex, in the sense that it is not rape for a person his age or older to have sex with him (Md. Code. Ann., 1997, § 464B). However, Maryland still has laws on the books prohibiting "sodomy" and "unnatural or perverted sexual practices" that have traditionally been deemed applicable to consensual homosexual sex and carry criminal penalties of up to 10 years in prison (Md. Code Ann., 1996, §§ 553–554). In the eyes of the law, James is not a young gay man struggling to come out in a homophobic environment—he is at best a victim and at worst a criminal.

All states have laws requiring psychologists and others who suspect child abuse or neglect to report to child welfare or law enforcement authorities. The obligation to report supersedes confidentiality rules, and these statutes confer immunity on the reporter. Dr. Washington is obliged, both as a psychologist and as a school employee, to report cases of child abuse and neglect to the local child welfare department (Md. Code. Ann., 1997, §5-704). James's case, however, falls between the cracks of the statute's language. Although part of James's problem is that he is being preyed on sexually by older men, for purposes of reporting *sexual abuse* is defined only to include conduct of people in the child's family or household or those who otherwise have custody or control over him (Md. Code Ann., 1997, §5-701). The law does not require reporting simply because a child is sexually active (*Planned Parenthood Affiliates v. Van de Kamp*, 1986).

The law also requires a report in cases of *neglect*, which is defined as "failure to give proper care and attention to a child by the child's parents

... under circumstances that indicate that the child's health or welfare is significantly harmed or placed at risk of significant harm" (Md. Code Ann., 1997, § 5-701). One could argue that James's parents have failed to provide an environment in which he could safely address his sexual identity, but given that he has been concealing his feelings and his activity, the argument is strained. How can a court rule that they are neglecting him when they cannot reasonably be expected to know what he is doing or the nature of the trouble he is having? Why should the state intervene before giving the parents a chance to act? I do not believe that Dr. Washington is obliged to report this matter, but he could do so, and provided his report is made in good faith, he is immune from liability (Md. Code Ann., 1997, § 5-708).

I find this to be one of the hardest cases in the book. The law, which carries deep social biases against sexual behavior among minors, let alone homosexual activity, is not a source of much insight into the rights and wrongs of this situation, let alone of rescue for James. At this point, I have to switch to my tactical mode, looking for some idea about how the law might be helpful to James.

Dr. Washington could think about using the law to get James's current adult friends off his back. Given the drug use and the "sodomy" that is going on, a threat from Dr. Washington to call in the police might scare off James's enablers (at least the current crop). That will not be much help if James does not find a way to get some safer structure back into his life, but at least it is something.

It is obvious that the response of James's parents is critical. If they can find a way to support him, all things are possible. If they react as he predicts, James's lot will be dire indeed. Legally, he will be subject to his parents' control until he is 18, unable to contract (to, say, sign a lease for an apartment) and probably limited in his access to benefits. Yet there is some hope in even the direst scenario. Many, many gay men have been rejected by their families and lived to tell the tale. If the only way out of this situation is for James to build a new life, Dr. Washington will probably be able to find some help in the community.

IDENTIFY AND ASSESS THE OPTIONS
(BY ROBERT A. WASHINGTON)

Although initially confusing, it was clarifying to consult with an expert on ethics and an attorney. I am surprised that the information from the ethics expert is less directive than that of the lawyer; I expected just the opposite.

Their words are thought provoking. I now must reconsider the four assumptions that underlie my original plan. The first addresses the need I have felt to tell someone of higher authority. Although there is no rule that I must inform school authorities, clearly this is a potentially explosive situation, and I would like to act in a manner that is respectful to all systems involved. There is the possibility of public attention.

More important, I had believed that law and the Ethics Code required reporting child sexual abuse to the Department of Social Services or the police. What a complex and at times conflicting set of injunctions this information presents. The Ethics Code gives me permission to break confidentiality if the law requires reporting or permits it. At 16, James is above the age of consent for consensual sexual activity, and the law does not define the adults with whom he is having sex as abusing him because they have no control over him. I believe this is a double bind. Yes, he may be able to make decisions for himself and understand the gravity of them, assuming he is free to do so. However, even in the best of all possible worlds, homophobia takes that freedom from him because it does not allow him to freely express his sexual urges. The "unscrupulous" men who have sex with him can count on his not telling because of his fear based on stigma; thus, they are able to exercise control over him. But the truth of the matter is that there is nothing to report because this sexual activity is with anonymous partners. To add insult to injury, I run the risk that he will be charged with sodomy. Nevertheless, I cannot rest knowing that these men will continue to take advantage of vulnerable boys like James unless something is done to stop them. Do I have responsibility for them? The Ethics Code suggests that I do have social responsibility. But I must forego these concerns until I know that James is safe.

Safety is the primary issue I will discuss with James. I will let him know that I believe he is in a dangerous situation because both drug use and participating in unsafe sex put him at risk for several complications. My major task will be to develop a plan with James to ensure that he is out of danger.

I will add to the plan an assessment of the degree of risk James's father presents. Has his father ever physically abused him? If so, how often, under what circumstances, and how forcefully? On the basis of his answers and his level of fear we must discuss how likely is it that his father will abuse him if he finds out that he is gay.

It is true that I think of James as competent because he seems mature for his years in terms of judgment. He is easy to engage in collaborative work toward therapeutic goals. He appears to catch on quickly to what I am saying about his situation, and his responses are clear and indicate that he comprehends the many issues that are at stake. I regret at this point that I did not focus enough on clarifying whether James has an awareness of his own vulnerability in the several high-risk situations in which he participates. He has expressed concern about becoming addicted, which is a good sign but may suggest that he already is. I am committed to determining what other immediate and long-term, social, and health risks he believes his behavior poses?

My current plan includes having a discussion with James with the following goals and strategies for achieving them.

- make sure that James recognizes that I understand the complexity of his plight. I understand that it is very difficult to be gay and in high school and that that difficulty is compounded by his not getting support from his parents and school officials. I will also reiterate James's concern about being addicted and agree with him that drug use presents the greatest threat to him. By paraphrasing his thoughts and reflecting his feelings, I will make sure that James recognizes my empathy.
- clarify James's expectations of me. I will simply ask James what he would like for me to do to help him. It is possible that he might not know, so I must be careful if it becomes necessary to suggest possibilities.
- assess James danger at home, including current and potential abuse at the hands of his father. I will inquire about any past acts of violence his father may have committed.
- assess James's risk for suicide should his sexual orientation become known to family and/or peers. We will discuss what he believes to be the consequences of disclosure.
- get a clear picture of the extent of James's drug use. I will take a drug history.
- arrange for James to have a comprehensive health examination with a pediatrician who is sensitive to the concerns of gay children. Because he has been ill, not because he may have HIV, I will get information about physicians from the local gay health organization and share it with James.
- make sure that James understands that I firmly believe that he is in danger. Drug use and unprotected sex and possibly an abusive home situation all place him in danger.
- develop a plan with James for getting him out of any and all danger.

CHOOSE A COURSE OF ACTION AND SHARE IT WITH YOUR CLIENT

James and I meet for the second time. He seems subdued and very unhappy. I wonder aloud how things are going for him and what he has thought about since our last meeting. He says that things are about the same and that he is less and less able to concentrate in school. He is afraid that he will fail. I tell James that that is a realistic possibility but not as life threatening as his continued drug use. Although James is usually verbose and articulate, he does not respond, which leads me to believe that there is some truth in the statement. I tell James that although we have many things to talk about during the meeting, I want him to understand that we have to find a way to get him off drugs. I would like for us to have a plan for doing so either by the end of this meeting but certainly no later than the next. When I get no response I ask James if he understands. He nods affirmatively.

I feel like I must convey firmness and commitment to reducing James's risk and at the same time communicate understanding and compassion. Both are necessary stances to take for James's welfare and the strength of the therapeutic alliance. I am becoming more and more convinced that James sees me as someone to put a stop to his activity. What I fear is that he believes that can be done magically, with little pain or effort on his part.

I tell James that there are things we began to discuss last time that I would like to hear more about. They include more about his father's angry outbursts, more about his statement that he would kill himself if his father finds out about his being gay, and more about his drug use. I ask if there are things he would like to add to the list. He adds that he continues to feel bad—that his cough does not go away even though he has been taking cough syrup and aspirin.

I ask James why he thinks he has this persistent cough. He says he does not know but he wonders if it is the result of smoking crack. I simply say, "Could be." I wonder if he is afraid he has done damage to his lungs and recognize that there are other possibilities for his cough. He says he does not know.

I tell James that I would like to arrange for him to see a physician through the school nurse, who can make a referral. He says that would be fine but he does not want her to "know his business." I tell him that we have to have a reason for referring him and ask what he thinks that should be. He seems bewildered. I tell him about the gay youth agency and suggest that he call there to see how they handle this kind of situation. I tell him he can do so anonymously. He agrees and I give him the number. I add that his cough could be related to his drug use, HIV, both, or neither. I tell him that he needs a thorough physical to determine what is wrong and what may be contributing to it. He nods.

I ask, "How often do you use crack?" He says he uses it every weekend and whenever he is able to slip out at night. He goes out on those nights when his father goes to sleep after having had several drinks. When his father has been drinking, he knows he will not wake until morning. I ask how many times each week does that happen. He says "only a couple." I ask how he is able to go out, use drugs, and still get to school in the morning. He says that the drug makes him speed and that he does not get sleepy until the next day about third period. Until that point he feels too jittery to sleep. It is during those early morning hours that he regrets the night before but during the night he is too busy having a good time. He says that Paul and Jerry really understand him, and he likes being with them although Paul does not like the fact that Jerry gives him drugs. Paul keeps saying that that is not what he had in mind and that they have a responsibility to help James.

I ask James if he realizes that Jerry could get into big trouble. He nods, and I ask why he thinks that could be. He says because Jerry is giving drugs to a minor. I agree and add that Jerry is giving drugs to a minor whom he then offers to other men for purposes of sex. I say, "James, do you know I could report your activity with Jerry to the police?" He nods affirmatively. Now that James knows that I have not done that which he most fears—disclosed him—I ask him why, if he knew I could, did he come to me with his concerns. He responds that he really does not know, but he recognized that he needed help because he does not like what he is doing but does not know how to stop. He feels that he can be himself when he is with his "friends," but he is afraid of continued drug use. He hates the jitters the morning after. He cries.

I tell James that I recognize how much he wants to stop using drugs and how much he wants to be free to be the gay young man he feels he is and that I want to help him with both. He is not the first gay teenager to feel alone and afraid. He is also not the first person to think that drug use will solve his problem, only to find out that it makes things worse. The drugs have stopped him from getting to know himself as a gay adolescent unless he believes that all there is to being gay is drugs and sex while using drugs. I reiterate the suggestion that he call the gay youth center and tell him that most of the young people who participate do so without their parents' knowledge. He says he will.

I then ask James how dangerous his father is (what is the worst he has done). James tells me about a time when he stayed out beyond permission, his father caught him coming in and shook him so hard that he "thought his brains would come out." He says that his father yells and screams a lot. I ask him why he is so afraid of his father knowing that he is gay, and he says that his father, when under the influence, has on several occasions said that "they never should have let those damn fags in the military" and that he would like to round them up and shoot them. James further says that he is sure that he would hurt him if he were to find out.

I ask how his mother copes with his father's drinking and anger. He says that she tends to avoid dealing with him, that he does not know why she stays with him, and that she could not be happy because they do very little together. He thinks she is afraid of his father, too. I wonder how she would react to the knowledge of his homosexuality. He says he does not know. He thinks she would be disappointed. "But I would always be her baby boy."

I then tell James that he knew all along that moving in with Jerry was not a reasonable option for him and he knew that I could never agree to his doing that. I tell James that he also knows that his drug use is already a serious problem that he is unable to control. I further tell him that I could attempt to begin the process of gaining control by reporting Jerry to the authorities but that I do not want to do that because I think that an official investigation would ensure that his father would find out. The only alternative I can think of is to involve his mother, because an assessment for drug treatment is essential and cannot be arranged without parental consent. He insists that he does not want her to know. I ask him for an alternative. He does not have one. I tell him that we can engage his mother's assistance or I will report Jerry to the police, but in either case I insist that we have a way of getting him what he needs—immediate drug treatment.

At that point James begins to insist that he can stop on his own. I tell him that I have trouble believing this. He asks for a week to prove it. I tell him he can have a week to think about either reporting Jerry or telling his mother but not a week to convince me that he can kick the habit on his own. I remind him of the number of times he had told me that drugging was his major concern and that he wanted to be different. If he could do it on his own, he would have done so by now.

A week later James returns. I am surprised because I thought he would stay away and test my resolve to take action to help him stop using drugs. He asks if we had to take either course of action and I said we (or I) must. I reiterate that I cannot allow him to continue on the dangerous course he had started. I tell him that I recognize how much he wants to be free from the psychic pain he feels and that I know that the drugs and sex free him temporarily; however, drugging created many more problems for him. I wait a while and then ask which alternative he prefers. He says neither but that he can handle it if I tell his mother.

We then discuss how to approach her. We agree that I will telephone and ask for a meeting with her and James to discuss the reasons for his recent school failure.

IMPLEMENT THE COURSE OF ACTION: MONITOR AND DISCUSS OUTCOMES

The meeting with James's mother is surprising. James is present yet quiet. He had informed me that he would not be able to speak but that he wanted the truth to be told. I explain James's homosexuality and drug use and, most important, his desire to stop. I tell her that the men giving drugs to him have also been having sexual relations with him. She acknowledges that she has known that something was wrong with her son but ignored it as she does so many things, hoping it would go away. She thanks me and tells James that she wants only the best for him and will always love him. She further says that for now she will not tell her husband. She places a call to Jerry and threatens him with arrest if he continues to supply her son with drugs and forbids him to have any contact with James. She puts James on a strict curfew and agrees to go with him to the doctor. (James had finally gone to the gay youth center and gotten the names of physicians.)

From time to time I see James, who fortunately is not infected with HIV. James and his mother have become quite involved at the gay youth center. He is very pleased with the support he has received from the center and from his mother. Now he goes out to be with other gay youth. James recognizes that he may have to attend summer school to repeat a couple of subjects. His drug use has stopped, but the physician and I both convince his mother to get him into counseling for substance abuse.

I was quite relieved to disclose the information to James's mother. I searched for a way that would present the least possible harm and ensure his safety. I assumed it was worth the risk when James let me know that his mother and father do not have a close relationship and that she would always see him as "her baby boy." Things certainly could have backfired, but the risk was better than not acting and putting James at further risk. James was almost certain to go downhill if no action were taken. He is not out of danger. It will take some time to understand the role of drugs in his life and alcohol in his father's.

Now that James is getting good supervision, nurturing, and counseling, I have decided to gather six staff, teachers, and other counselors to discuss ways that the school can be more sensitive and supportive to gay and lesbian and questioning youth. I will need fortification to change the system, and justice demands a systems change.

REFERENCES

American Psychological Association. (1992). Ethical principles of psychologists and code of conduct. *American Psychologist, 47,* 1597–1611.

Barrows, P. A., & Halgin, R. P. (1988). Current issues in psychotherapy with gay men: Impact of the AIDS phenomenon. *Professional Psychology: Research and Practice, 16,* 426–434.

Brosig, C. L., & Kalichman, S. (1992). Clinicians' reporting of suspected child abuse: A review of the empirical literature. *Clinical Psychology Review, 12,* 155–168.

Gonsiorek, J. C. (1988). Mental health issues of gay and lesbian adolescents. *Journal of Adolescent Health Care, 9*, 114–122.

Grisso, T., & Vierling, L. (1978). Minors consent to treatment: A developmental perspective. *Professional Psychology: Research and Practice, 9*, 412–427.

Gustafson, K. E., & McNamara, J. R. (1987). Confidentiality with minor clients: Issues and guidelines for therapists. *Professional Psychology: Research and Practice, 18*, 503–508.

Health-General Article, MD. CODE ANN. §§20-102 & 20-104 (1997).

Kalichman, S. E. (1993). *Mandated reporting of suspected child abuse.* Washington, DC: American Psychological Association.

Kitchener, K. S. (2000). *The foundations of ethical practice, research, and teaching in psychology.* Mahwah, NJ: Erlbaum.

Mann, L., Harmoni, R., & Power, C. (1989). Adolescent decision-making: The development of competence. *Journal of Adolescence, 12*, 265–278.

Melton, G. B. (1988). Adolescents and prevention of AIDS. *Professional Psychology: Research and Practice, 19*, 403–408.

MD. CODE. ANN., §464B (1997).

MD. CODE ANN., §§553-554 (1996).

MD. CODE ANN., §5-701 (1997).

MD. CODE ANN., §5-704 (1997).

MD. CODE ANN., §5-708 (1997).

Planned Parenthood Affiliates v. Van de Kamp, 226 Cal. Rptr. 361 (Cal. Ct. App. 1986).

Powell, C. J. (1984). Ethical principles and issues of competence in counseling adolescents. *The Counseling Psychologist, 12*, 57–68.

Sobocinski, M. R. (1990). Ethical principles in the counseling of gay and lesbian adolescents: Issues of autonomy, competence, and confidentiality. *Professional Psychology: Research and Practice, 21*, 240–247.

Tarasoff v. Board of Regents of the University of California, 551 P.2d 334 (Cal. 1976).

Troiden, R. R. (1988). Homosexual identity development. *Journal of Adolescent Health Care, 9*, 105–113.

Weithorn, L. A., & Campbell, S. B. (1982). The competency of children and adolescents to make informed treatment decisions. *Child Development, 53*, 1589–1599.

12

KEEPING SECRETS FROM THE HIV-POSITIVE ADOLESCENT CLIENT: THE CASE OF KAMAU

SANDRA Y. LEWIS, KAREN STROHM KITCHENER,
AND SCOTT BURRIS

ORIENTATION TO THE MAJOR ETHICAL ISSUES HIGHLIGHTED IN THE CASE

The role of the psychologist who works with an adolescent may conflict with his or her role and relationship with the client's parent or family. This conflict may arise when a young client directly asks the therapist for information that was disclosed in confidence by the parents. Such scenarios often arise in connection with the disclosure of HIV diagnosis to children and youth. These issues become even more crucial as children with HIV become adolescents and develop an interest in sex and a desire to plan for their future. The case of Kamau highlights this scenario and the complex nature of disclosure of diagnosis to adolescents who acquired HIV infection as infants or children. The case occurred in New Jersey.

CASE PRESENTATION (BY SANDRA Y. LEWIS)

Kamau is a 13-year-old African American boy whose mother died of AIDS about 1 year ago. None of his family members have formally told him that his mother died of AIDS. Prior to her death, Kamau's mother made plans with her sister Frances to care for her children (Kamau, an 11-year-old, and a 15-year-old) in the event of incapacitating illness or death. Frances accepted this responsibility and has been committed to caring for Kamau and his siblings.

Shortly after her sister's death, and at the suggestion of their pediatrician, Frances had Kamau and his siblings tested for HIV infection. Kamau was the only one of three children to test positive. His only risk factor was determined to be perinatal transmission of HIV infection. Thus, he had been living with HIV infection for more than 13 years. Although some adult family members are aware of Kamau's diagnosis, his aunt has not yet told him his diagnosis. She has simply told him that he has a lung condition.

Since his diagnosis, Kamau has attended an HIV care clinic once a month. During one visit both he and Frances talked with their care team (physician, nurse, and social worker) about his concentration problems, sleeping difficulties, and sadness. Kamau was given a psychotherapy referral. During my psychosocial assessment, Frances reveals to me that she is afraid Kamau would give up on living if he were told he has HIV infection. This prevents her from telling him his diagnosis, yet she acknowledges that she will eventually have to. Although we have discussed her disclosing the HIV diagnosis to Kamau, she says she is not yet prepared and consistently instructs the health care team not to tell Kamau anything about his HIV status. I have informed Frances that children and youth often begin to have questions about their health and that eventually we will have to prepare her to talk with Kamau about his diagnosis. Despite her resistance to disclosure, she supports Kamau's therapy sessions with me and brings him every week.

Kamau does well in school and has a few close friends. He has recently developed a keen interest in a young woman named Sonya. He has indicated to me that they are on the verge of having sex. During a therapy session, Kamau tells me that he wants to know what is wrong with him. He says he knows his aunt is not telling him the whole story about his lung condition. He asks me to tell him what is really wrong with him and then states that he believes he has AIDS. Kamau says he worries about infecting Sonya and that he worries that he is dying.

PAUSE AND IDENTIFY YOUR PERSONAL RESPONSES TO THE CASE

I feel caught between the client and the parent. I feel guilty about lying to Kamau because his Aunt Frances has not given me permission to discuss his HIV diagnosis with him. I feel some anger because Kamau has a right to know about his health so he can do the best job of planning for his future. I am worried he may have already had unprotected sex and may not be telling me because he is afraid to tell anyone. If this is the case, Sonya may have been exposed to HIV and may be infected. What is my obligation to her?

I am torn between these feelings and Frances's fear about possible health decline. This is a no-win situation in which I must lie to Kamau or violate Frances's confidence. If these feelings are prolonged, they may inhibit my ability to explore Kamau's and Frances's underlying concerns as well as family relationships and concerns. If I stay caught in these emotions, I will be unable to get a clear picture of Kamau's needs and actions. I will be unable to think of resources available to me and to the family.

I decide to say to Kamau that he has shared "a lot of scary and confusing feelings" and suggest that we go through each of his concerns. He confirms that he has not had sex with Sonya but wants to because everyone else is having sex, and he does not want her to think that he is afraid. However, he says if he really does have AIDS he could give it to Sonya, and he may also die soon. He got the idea he has AIDS because he overheard a family member saying his mother died of AIDS. At this point, my emotions are settled enough that I can talk with Kamau about planning a therapy session to talk with his aunt regarding his fears. I explain to him that many of the questions he has about his health have to be discussed in the presence of his guardian because she has responsibility for making sure he gets the health care he needs. I ask about any changes he has noticed in his body; there have not been any to date. I reassure him that I have regular contact with the medical team who referred him to me and that they have told me that he is doing quite well.

REVIEW THE FACTS OF THE CASE

Pediatric HIV infection is often a multigenerational family disease. Family members across generations may be HIV-infected, but even if they are not, all family members are affected by the changes HIV causes within relationships and roles. In Kamau's family, Frances's role changed from aunt to mother. She, Kamau, and his siblings are coping with the loss of the children's mother and simultaneously adjusting to their new family environment. They are likely still working on effective family communication strategies. Frances is concerned about Kamau's health and seems to want to protect him from what she perceives as undue stress.

Kamau is an example of a long-term survivor of pediatric HIV, and current advances in HIV treatment make it even more likely that he may live into his 20s. He has grown from a child to an adolescent with a chronic illness. His developmental needs have changed. His sexuality is developing, and he will need to make plans for his future as is appropriate during adolescence. The changes and vicissitudes of adolescence are heightened by the impact of HIV infection. Like all adolescents, Kamau needs safer sex education. Indeed, for him practicing safer sex may not only protect his partner but also protect him from complications caused by infections contracted through sexual contact. In addition, he may be more likely to practice safer sex if he is aware of his HIV diagnosis. Currently, he seems appropriately worried and wishes to take appropriate steps to find out about his health and protect his girlfriend. His impulse control appears adequate enough for him to delay sexual contact until he can get some answers to his questions. His reasons for wanting to have sex seem to be more externally motivated—"everybody's doing it."

CONCEPTUALIZE AN INITIAL PLAN
BASED ON CLINICAL ISSUES

Kamau's concerns about his health and the possibility of death are of primary concern. He has lost his mother and has overheard that she died from AIDS. He now fears that he is going to die, too. He is also at a time in his life when he is beginning to explore intimacy in relationships, career ideas, values, and other tasks associated with adolescence. Peer pressure plays an important role in his decisions. Initially, I explore his concerns about his health and what he would do differently if he had AIDS or if he did not. I make a plan for a family session in which he can talk more with his aunt regarding the conversation he overheard about his mother and his concerns about his health.

Before the family session, I will meet alone with Frances and let her know that he has some concerns about his health. I will emphasize to her that this is common in children and adolescents with a chronic illness and work with her to prepare her to talk with Kamau. It will be important to assess whether she has thought about how she will disclose Kamau's diagnosis to him. I will explain to her that parents and guardians often feel a sense of relief and improved communication after they disclose a diagnosis. It will be important to identify people—family members, members of the health care team, church members, or school officials—who will be sources of support to them once she discloses. Those who already know Kamau's diagnosis may be the most obvious support.

Frances's difficulty in disclosing the diagnosis to Kamau may be related to her feelings about the loss of her sister and her fears about losing Kamau. She may worry that an HIV diagnosis is too much for him to handle but may also feel she has difficulty handling the diagnosis. Some communication with Kamau's health care team may be useful in reassuring her about his current health status. It may also be true that Kamau has asked a member of his health care team about his having AIDS. If so, this may help Frances understand the need to be more open with him. I will suggest to her that sometimes circumstances can make us ready to confront a situation we felt unprepared to handle. Indeed, she has shown she can handle new circumstances in making a transition from being an aunt to being a mother to three adolescents.

CONSULT THE ETHICS CODE AND ASSESS THE ETHICAL ISSUES (BY KAREN STROHM KITCHENER)

As I read Dr. Lewis's report of her dilemma with Kamau, I am struck by how caught she feels between her responsibilities to Kamau and his aunt's request to keep his HIV status confidential. On one hand, she feels guilty, as though she is lying to Kamau because Frances has not given permission to honestly deal with his health status. She may also feel torn between Kamau's right to know and his guardian's fear about his possible health decline if he learns the truth. Cases like these can be perceived as no-win situations in which practitioners feel they must lie to the child or violate the parent's or guardian's confidence. In this case, Dr. Lewis's concerns are exacerbated by her awareness of Kamau's maturing sexuality and the possibility that he may infect his girlfriend Sonya.

APA Ethics Code

Sometimes stepping back and considering the ethical issues involved can help resolve some of a practitioner's confusion about how to proceed. The Ethics Code (American Psychological Association [APA], 1992) gives some guidance in Standards 4.01, Structuring the Relationship; 5.01, Discussing the Limits of Confidentiality; and 1.21, Third-Party Requests for Services. Both Standards 4.01 and 5.01 require that psychologists discuss with clients early in their relationship the relevant limitations of confidentiality. Standard 5.01 is explicit in requiring both minors and their legal representatives to be involved in the conversation about confidentiality. In this case, it would suggest that Dr. Lewis must clarify with Kamau's aunt the extent to which the information regarding his HIV status is confidential. Similarly, Standard 1.21a states "When a psychologist agrees to provide services to a person or entity at the request of a third party, the psychologist clarifies to the extent feasible, at the outset of the service, the nature of the relationship with each party." Section b of that same standard acknowledges that sometimes the psychologist may be called on to perform conflicting roles because of the involvement of a third party and that under these circumstances the direction of his or her loyalties must be clarified.

In Kamau's case part of the problem may be that Dr. Lewis is conflicted about her loyalties. The issue is this: Should her primary loyalty be to Kamau or his aunt? Here, it appears that Kamau is the client and, therefore, Dr. Lewis's first responsibility is to him. It is important to acknowledge, however, that because Frances is his guardian and brings him for treatment, maintaining a relationship with her that facilitates Kamau's treatment is critical. Furthermore, she may have a legal right to make decisions about his treatment. (Dr. Lewis ought to get legal counsel on this point.)

Aspirational Principle B: Integrity and Principle E: Concern for Others' Welfare are also helpful in thinking about this case. Principle E should remind Dr. Lewis that Kamau's welfare should be the primary consideration in any plan she makes. The plan should minimize harm to the extent that it is possible. This is further supported by Standard 1.14, Avoiding Harm.

Aspirational Principle B identifies another issue that psychologists need to consider in cases like this because it suggests that relationships between psychologists and their clients should be "honest, fair, and respectful." The foundational principle of fidelity helps clarify the implications of having integrity in relationships: The relationship with Kamau is a fiduciary one, meaning it is based on trust and confidence. The ability to help Kamau over the long run with all of these problems including his difficulty concentrating, his sleep difficulties, and sadness depends on his ability to trust Dr. Lewis. Without such trust, she cannot help him. In other words, Dr. Lewis must ask whether her ability to help Kamau therapeutically will be damaged if she lies to him.

In summary, the Ethics Code suggests that therapists must first clearly identify to whom they owe their primary loyalty and then, particularly when working with a minor, they must clarify expectations about confidentiality. In addition, they must use good clinical judgment to answer these questions: What is in the best interests of my client? Is there a way that I can join with the child's parent or guardian to make a decision about my client's best interests? Will I destroy my ability to help my client in the long run if I do not honestly answer his question about having AIDS?

It is important to acknowledge, however, that sometimes a decision may be made that does not completely satisfy all parties involved. In these circumstances, psychologists should try to act in a way that will promote the client's welfare to the extent that it is possible while doing the least amount of avoidable harm.

Foundational Ethical Principles

As Dr. Lewis develops a plan for working with Kamau, she must consider issues of autonomy. He is a maturing adolescent; thus, she must consider to what extent he is competent to be involved in decisions regarding his own life. Most data suggest that in a laboratory setting, the decisions of 15-year-olds are as competent as those of older adolescents who are considered to be legally competent and can provide independent consent to treatment (Grisso & Vierling, 1978; Mann, Harmoni, & Power, 1989; Powell, 1984; Weithorn & Campbell, 1982). Although Kamau is not 15, younger adolescents exhibit some characteristics associated with competence and understanding (Weithorn & Campbell, 1982). As a result, Kamau probably is capable of meaningful involvement in his own health-care-related decisions even if he is not fully autonomous. Furthermore, respect for his developing autonomy would mitigate against withholding from him crucial information that will affect his long-term life plans.

On the other side of this issue are the foundational principles of beneficence and do no harm. The foundational principle of beneficence may be helpful in clarifying the responsibility to contribute to his welfare. In this case, Dr. Lewis must ask, what is in Kamau's best interests, and what will harm him the least? Responding to this question is not an easy one because there are no clear-cut answers in this case. It is not clear whether confirming Kamau's beliefs that he is HIV-positive will be more beneficial than not telling him. This is a clinical issue that involves a therapeutic judgment based on knowledge of Kamau as well as the literature on adolescents and how they typically respond in similar situations.

Kamau's best interests are also the primary concern of his aunt. It is her belief, however, that his best interests are served by not revealing that he is HIV-positive. If Dr. Lewis can get Frances to participate in the decision making about what is best for Kamau by discussing with her the consequences of revealing or not revealing his HIV status, she may not feel so caught between Kamau's needs and his guardian's desires. In fact, this is exactly what Dr. Lewis is planning. This tactic is further supported ethically by Dr. Lewis's concern about protecting Kamau's potential sexual partners from harm.

As already noted, the foundational principle of fidelity is critical in this case both ethically and clinically. Earlier in treatment Dr. Lewis withheld information from Kamau regarding his HIV status. It may not have been in his best interests at that time to reveal the information because he may not have been ready to hear it. Now, however, he has explicitly asked whether he has AIDS. Dr. Lewis would be deliberately lying if she said he did not have the disease without qualifying her answer. Generally, deliberate lying is considered less ethically acceptable than withholding information if the person does not request it.

In fact, it is only a matter of time before Kamau learns the truth. With time, he will become more aware that he is getting treatment at an HIV clinic and that others at the clinic are HIV-positive, or the information will be leaked to him in some other way. By lying, Dr. Lewis, his aunt, and the health care team may undermine Kamau's trust in the ability of adults to help him. Because of his HIV status such trust may be critical in maintaining his health.

Issues of fidelity also arise, however, when Dr. Lewis considers her responsibility to Frances. Frances may believe that Dr. Lewis implicitly promised that she would not reveal Kamau's HIV status. Consequently, Dr. Lewis has an ethical responsibility to clarify her agreement with Frances. Furthermore, her ability to work successfully with Kamau may be undermined if Frances does not believe that she is trustworthy.

The foundational principle of justice similarly suggests that, from an ethical standpoint, Kamau should not be treated as a child when and if he is competent to be treated in a more mature way. On the other hand, it would also suggest that he should not be treated completely as an adult if he is not totally competent. Rather, fair treatment means considering his developmental status as a young adolescent.

Balancing the Ethics Code and the Foundational Ethical Principles

The aspirational principles from the Ethics Code and the foundational ethical principles support providing Kamau with honest information about his HIV status (assuming that clinically it is in his best interests to do so). He is old enough and appears mature enough to be involved in decisions about his own life. To honor Frances's wishes, Dr. Lewis would have to avoid telling Kamau the truth or lie to him if he inquires whether he is HIV-positive, and being trustworthy is critical to helping Kamau. Furthermore, failing to tell Kamau could lead to others contracting the HIV virus if he becomes sexually active and unknowingly exposes his partners.

Dr. Lewis's plan to meet with Frances and talk with her about Kamau's concerns is a good one. She needs to be honest with Frances and to let her know that Kamau believes he has AIDS and has directly asked about it. Furthermore, if Dr. Lewis believes it is in Kamau's best interest to provide him with honest information, she also needs to provide Frances with that information. She may also want to help Frances understand Kamau's changing developmental needs. Providing Frances with this kind of information would be respectful of her right to make more fully informed decisions about Kamau's health and her role in it.

Dr. Lewis's compassion for Frances is apparent in her plans to help her identify sources of support and to deal with her feelings of guilt and loss surrounding Kamau's disease. Her willingness to deal with Frances as another person about whom she is concerned is an example of the ethical virtue of care or compassion. Frances also has Kamau's best interests in mind, and this should be acknowledged and valued.

If, however, Frances maintains her stance of not wanting Kamau to be informed, Dr. Lewis needs to make a decision about whether to tell Kamau anyway. Because of the potential risk to Sonya if she and Kamau become sexually active and because of the truth-telling issues for Kamau, the ethical press falls on the side of breaking the promise to Frances and informing Kamau. Sonya has no reason to believe that she is at risk and thus to take precautions to protect herself. Furthermore, depending on her age, maturity, and knowledge, she may not be fully competent to make such decisions. If Dr. Lewis decides to inform Kamau without Frances's permission, she should tell Frances about her plan and allow her the opportunity to be involved in the process. She may mitigate some of the harm by explaining her reasons and respecting Frances's desires about whether she wants to be involved in the disclosure. She should continue with her plan to help Frances find support and deal with her feelings. To do so is both beneficent and caring.

In the short term Dr. Lewis should talk to Kamau about his own developing sexuality. This may both help him decide if he really wants to become involved sexually with Sonya and provide the opportunity to talk with him about using safer sex practices to avoid pregnancy and sexually transmitted diseases.

IDENTIFY THE LEGAL ISSUES (BY SCOTT BURRIS)

Dr. Lewis obviously believes that it is time for Kamau to learn the truth about his condition. She bases this conclusion largely on his mental health needs and his capacity to cope. Telling him gives full respect to his personhood and will presumably eliminate a serious risk of harm to Sonya. If telling Kamau is the best choice from the professional point of view, then my legal advice to Dr. Lewis is to do just that. I would be most worried if she went against her professional judgment merely to reduce her perceived risk of being sued. One thing is certain: If Sonya gets infected because no one told Kamau he was at risk, some people, including perhaps Dr. Lewis, are going to pay a lot of money and feel a great deal of shame, irrespective of the formal state of the law today. Fortunately, however, the plan Dr. Lewis has proposed will keep her litigation risk to a minimum.

Dr. Lewis comes into the case because Kamau became depressed and was referred to her for mental health care. Dr. Lewis is treating Kamau for depression. Her primary legal as well as professional obligation is to provide him with the care he needs in a way that meets professional standards. If she cannot take care of him without his knowing about his HIV disease, she either has to arrange for him to be informed or withdraw from the case, making clear to Frances and the rest of the care team her view that he should be told of his condition.

Trying to get Frances to see the need to disclose is a good idea. Although Dr. Lewis is forcing the issue of informing Kamau, using her professional status and expertise to get Frances's attention, she is not acting unilaterally. It seems likely that an open discussion among Dr. Lewis, Frances, and perhaps the physicians will yield a plan to inform Kamau. If Frances still refuses, however, and Dr. Lewis wants to continue to treat Kamau, she will have to inform him herself. Will this violate any laws or expose her to a lawsuit from Frances?

There is no HIV confidentiality issue. Kamau is the patient and the subject of the information. State HIV confidentiality laws (including the laws of New Jersey, where Dr. Lewis practices) uniformly allow release of HIV information to the patient.

Telling Kamau over Frances's objection would entail disregarding her legal authority to make health care decisions for him, including decisions about what information he can receive. In New Jersey, as elsewhere, unmarried people under age 18 are usually considered legally incompetent to make health care decisions (Arnold, 1992). For several reasons, however, I think it is safe to treat this requirement as a mere formality whose breach would not expose Dr. Lewis to a successful lawsuit by Frances. First, New Jersey law does allow minors to seek care, even without a parent's knowledge or consent, for "venereal disease" (N.J. STAT. ANN., 1997, §9:17A-4). Although HIV is not really classified as a venereal disease under New Jersey's disease control law (N.J. STAT., 1997, §26:4-27), one could argue that the intention of the statute is to allow minors to make health care decisions about sexual health matters that they would not want their parents to know about.

More important, Dr. Lewis has a compelling reason to tell Kamau. The stark reality of a responsible young man unwittingly infecting his girlfriend is likely to crowd Frances's formal legal claim to control right out of the picture. Finally, to actually make a claim and recover money, Frances would have to convince a judge and jury not only that it was wrong for Kamau to be informed and for Sonya to be protected, but that she (or Kamau) was harmed by the disclosure. (I should say that my advice depends on Dr. Lewis's confidence that Kamau will be able to handle the news. If he were to commit suicide or injure himself after being informed, the story Frances would have for the jury would be very different: an arrogant psychotherapist who thought she knew better than the boy's closest relative.)

Dr. Lewis could disclose Kamau's infection to him, if she wanted to, at minimal legal risk. Must she disclose to avoid incurring liability for failing to protect Sonya? This is a hard question if we look only at the law on the books in New Jersey. A state statute prohibits *Tarasoff*-style suits for failing to warn or protect unless the patient is threatening to carry out "an act of imminent, serious physical violence," which Kamau clearly is not (N.J. STAT. ANN., 1997, §2A:62A-16). If we consider how a judge or jury might react to the case, however, the risk to Kamau's caregivers is harder to discount. Although there is no case clearly addressing this in New Jersey, courts in other states have held that a physician does have some duty toward a sex partner of a patient to make sure the patient has accurate information about his having or being able to transmit a sexually transmitted disease (*DiMarco v. Lynch Homes-Chester County*, 1990; *Reisner v. University of California*, 1995). The *Reisner* case, described in chapter 8, is very analogous. Although the most likely defendants in such a case would be Kamau's physicians, Dr. Lewis could easily be swept in as well.

Telling Kamau is the most defensible legal course. Being careful to treat Frances with respect should further reduce any remote risk that she might resort to legal action.

IDENTIFY AND ASSESS THE OPTIONS (BY SANDRA Y. LEWIS)

Both the ethical and legal consultants seem to agree that the best course of action is to inform Kamau of his HIV diagnosis. The ethical consultant raises some critical issues and questions to consider when working with minors in this situation. Specifically, therapists must clarify to whom they owe their primary loyalty, determine what is in the best interests of their minor client, and look at ways to join with the guardian in order to address the needs of the minor client.

The ethical consultant asks whether I will destroy my relationship with Kamau if I do not respond affirmatively to his belief that he has AIDS. The consultant suggests that failure to do so amounts to lying to Kamau because he has revealed a concern that he has AIDS. I spent time exploring Kamau's health concerns and explained that his aunt, as his guardian, has responsibility for his health care and so it is best to have her present when we discuss the details of his health. Thus, I do not believe that there is a risk that he will feel that he cannot trust me or that I have lied to him.

Both consultants seem to feel that disclosing the HIV diagnosis is in Kamau's best interest and in the best interest of his girlfriend Sonya. Protecting Sonya and providing Kamau with the whole picture about his health seem central to their recommendations. They both agree that involving Frances in the disclosure process is important and that I should look for ways to work with her regarding disclosure to Kamau. However, both consultants suggest that if Frances resists this plan of action, I should inform her that I believe it is in his best interest to tell him, inform her of how I will proceed with the disclosure, and do so without her consent. The consultants give the impression that this would result in minimal, if any, ethical consequence or legal liability. The legal consultant implies there may be more liability related to failure to disclose in the event that Sonya were to become infected following sexual contact with Kamau.

Both consultants seem to see Kamau as the client and not his aunt, although she has legal responsibility for his health care, including some control over whether he continues psychotherapy with me. Furthermore, I believe that when minors are in therapy, family therapy is integral to the process. The ethical consultant acknowledges that a trusting relationship between Frances and me is important to Kamau's psychotherapy. However, the consultant implies that if violating Frances's trust is in Kamau's best interest, then that must take precedence.

CHOOSE A COURSE OF ACTION AND SHARE IT WITH YOUR CLIENT

The ethical consultant, the legal consultant, and I all agree that the most optimal plan is to involve Frances in the disclosure and to help Frances understand Kamau's changing developmental needs and the importance of sharing diagnosis with him given his most recent concerns and inquiries. However, according to the consultation, if this cannot be achieved, then the most ethical course of action is to disclose to Kamau under the best possible circumstances without his aunt's consent.

The consultants' advice seems consonant with my initial plan to have a family session with Kamau and Frances so that he can speak with her about his concerns. However, Frances will need to be prepared that Kamau has concerns; she should not be so taken by surprise that she shuts down and refuses to engage. Thus, I will need to meet with her alone before the family session with Kamau. During this session, I will explore her concerns and reassess her readiness to disclose to Kamau. Between sessions it will also be important to check with Kamau's health care team because they may have information crucial to the disclosure process.

During the next session, I share this plan with Kamau and inform him that I will meet with his aunt first to hear concerns and let her know he has some concerns he wants to discuss with her. Before Kamau and Frances leave the office, I arrange with her to attend the next session with Kamau.

IMPLEMENT THE COURSE OF ACTION: MONITOR AND DISCUSS OUTCOMES

Between sessions, I speak with Kamau's health care team social worker, Pamela, who informs me that Kamau has had more questions about his health and has revealed concerns about having AIDS to her. When Kamau and Frances arrive for their family session, I speak with Frances first and get her assessment of how Kamau is doing. She reports that he is sleeping better and seems interested in a girl. I inquire if Kamau has been asking her any more questions about his health. She says she has not noticed this, and I mention that both Pamela and I have noticed that he has more questions about his health and what is wrong with him. I explain that children and adolescents often begin to have more questions as they live longer or experience more medical interventions. I remind her of previous discussions we have had about disclosure of diagnosis to Kamau. She emphatically insists that she does not want to tell him he has HIV infection and that I am not to tell him his diagnosis.

I inquire what Frances would like us to tell Kamau when he asks questions about his health. She states that we should continue to tell him he has a lung condition and nothing more. She does not feel that this is lying to him because he does have a lung condition. She does not want to worry him with any more information. She still believes that he will give up on living if he knows he has HIV.

I ask Frances if she has any concerns about Kamau's health. She begins to cry and states that she cannot stand the thought of Kamau having AIDS and suffering with this disease. She remembers how sick her sister became, and she just cannot imagine that her "baby boy" may suffer that way. She does not understand AIDS, but she fears that it can cause very bad symptoms and pain. She cannot bear to answer questions about what will happen to him. She does not know what she would say to him, and she cannot talk to him about dying. She lost her sister, and she does not want to lose her nephew. She wants him to focus on living.

I acknowledge that Frances is right in many ways. A positive attitude is important to maintaining good health. I tell her that she has some very difficult and heartfelt concerns, particularly her concern about how she would help Kamau when he asks difficult questions about HIV, AIDS, or death. I tell her that she has the support of the medical team and me and that we have helped many parents and guardians who have the same concerns she does and that we will help her answer Kamau's tough questions.

I ask what she thinks she would say to him if he ever asked her more questions about his disease. She states that she tries to be positive and always talk to him about how well he is doing so he does not focus on questions. I note that he has had more questions for his medical team and me and that I agreed to help him share his concerns with her. I reassure her that we are willing to help her answer any questions he has but that he is getting older and disclosure will become more and more unavoidable.

She is still quite nervous and does not want to tell Kamau about AIDS or anything other than a lung condition. We continue to explore her concerns. She sticks to her position. I remind her that Kamau is reaching the age when young people become interested in sex and ask her if she has talked with him about sex, safer sex, girlfriends, and intimacy. She cannot imagine her "baby boy" could be interested in sex but admits that kids are faster these days. We discuss the importance of teaching Kamau safer sex practices not only to prevent the spread of HIV infection but also to protect him because he has a compromised immune system. She says aloud, "I wouldn't want any more children to have to suffer with this disease." I agree that nobody wants to see that happen and that is just one of the reasons to prepare Kamau to make healthy decisions about sex.

I ask her to listen to Kamau's concerns and agree to support them both through the tough questions and issues. Kamau comes in to the office and immediately notices that his aunt has been crying. He wants to know what is wrong. She reassures him that she is all right and asks him to tell her what is on his mind. He looks to me, and I ask him to share the story about what he overheard. He tells his aunt that he heard another relative saying his mother had AIDS. He wants to know if this is true. She tells him it is true. Then he asks, "What's wrong with me?" She tells him that he has a lung condition. He says, "Is that all?" She says, "No" and begins to cry. I comfort her and him and remind them that this is a difficult conversation and that they can take a minute to breathe and collect their thoughts. Finally, Frances looks Kamau in the eye and says she never knew what she would say to him about his illness. She only wanted to protect him from harm. He has already lost his mother; she feels that he has been through too much already. She just wants to keep him healthy. He says he knows that there is something else wrong with him besides the lung condition and asks if he has what his mother had. She confirms that he has HIV infection.

After a few moments, I ask Kamau if he has any questions. At first, he shrugs his shoulders. I tell him that he may not be sure what to ask right now but Pamela, his social worker, and I along with his doctor and nurse will answer any questions he has. I remind him he has been doing really well and we are going to keep helping his Aunt Frances get him the best care. I tell him HIV infection is what we consider a chronic illness because people can live quite a long time with it. Frances tells Kamau she will do everything within her power to keep him healthy. I tell them that if they have questions they cannot answer, they should speak with his medical team or me. I encourage them not to worry if their questions seem silly, because all of their questions are important and deserve answers.

I remind them that disclosure is a process and that they may have more questions over time. We agree to have at least two more family sessions to discuss any feelings or questions that come up. I inform them that I will let Pamela know about our discussion and that she will be helpful in identifying other people who could be of support to them. Frances says that she knows she has to tell the other two children about their mother and Kamau. I agree to help her with this task if she wants me to. She thinks she and Kamau will try it on their own first. Kamau agrees.

As Kamau continues therapy sessions with me, we discuss his questions about living with HIV. He reveals concerns about whether he will "ever be able to have sex" and expresses the sentiment "who will want me." We discuss his fears of being unable to have closeness or being unwanted. Over time, we talk about the many ways, including safer sex, that he can have closeness or intimacy. I make a point of helping him explore his self-image and develop a balanced view of himself. I work with his aunt and health care team to set up a support system of people, some relatives and professionals, with whom he can talk about his HIV diagnosis. Kamau reports that it helps him to know that there is always someone he can go to with his questions, thoughts, and feelings.

REFERENCES

American Psychological Association. (1992). Ethical principles of psychologists and code of conduct. *American Psychologist, 47,* 1597–1611.

Arnold, P. (1992). Betwixt and between: Adolescents and HIV. In N. D. Hunter & W. B. Rubenstein (Eds.), *AIDS agenda* (pp. 41–67). New York: New Press.

DiMarco v. Lynch Homes–Chester County, 525 Pa. 558, 583 A.2d 422 (Pa. 1990).

Grisso, T., & Vierling, L. (1978). Minors consent to treatment: A developmental perspective. *Professional Psychology, 9,* 412–427.

Mann, L., Harmoni, R., & Power, C. (1989). Adolescent decision-making: The development of competence. *Journal of Adolescence, 12,* 265–278.

N.J. Stat. Ann. §2A:62A-16 (1997).

N.J. Stat. Ann. §9:17A-4 (1997).

N.J. Stat. Ann. §26:4-27 (1997).

Powell, C. J. (1984). Ethical principles and issues of competence in counseling adolescents. *The Counseling Psychologist, 12,* 57–68.

Reisner v. University of California, 31 Cal.App.4th 1195, 37 Cal. Rptr. 2d 518 (Cal. Ct. App. 1995).

Weithorn, L. A., & Campbell, S. B. (1982). The competency of children and adolescents to make informed treatment decisions. *Child Development, 53,* 1589–1599.

13

THE HIV-POSITIVE DISABLED CLIENT: THE CASE OF MIKE

BOB BARRET, KAREN STROHM KITCHENER, AND SCOTT BURRIS

ORIENTATION TO THE MAJOR ETHICAL ISSUES HIGHLIGHTED IN THE CASE

Often over the course of treating a client with HIV disease, the psychologist may encounter situations that generate safety concerns. Clients who are in advanced stages of HIV may suddenly become weak and unable to perform normal activities. Sometimes dementia may be observed first by the mental health practitioner. The ethical principle requiring respect for the client's autonomy may clash with the duty to protect both the client and the public. Consultation with medical personnel may help alleviate these situations, but often more direct action may be necessary.

CASE PRESENTATION (BY BOB BARRET)

Mike has been my client for the past several years. He initially presented shortly after learning that he was HIV-positive, and I have watched as he adjusted to his changed life and faced significant challenges. He has solid social support from both his family and friends, and he has done well despite fading health. He continues to be as active as he can, attending a support group and some social events and coming for counseling regularly. Presently he lives in South Carolina with his mother, who has a full-time job.

Over the past several months he has declined rapidly, mostly due to wasting; his body weight has dropped from 150 to 100 pounds, and he is no longer optimistic. Initially both of us had hoped that he might respond to new medical treatments, but he failed on three different combinations and now is merely hanging on as his condition worsens. His mental status has also been affected; he has noticed that he gets confused. He tells me that he went to the grocery store and when he came out he could not remember what kind of car he had. He had to call his mother to ask her before he was able to find it. On another occasion, he was driving and could not remember where he was going, so he just turned around and went home. Later he realized that he had missed lunch with a friend.

Driving is really important to him. He states that as long as he can get in his car and go places he knows he is still alive. He fears that once he is unable to drive he will go nuts and die. "I've given up almost everything I enjoy already. I am so glad I can still get around," he tells me. Last week he started using a cane because he was afraid of falling. My impression is that he is failing rapidly.

In the present session he has talked about dying. He is afraid he is going to die, but he does not want to go back to the hospital, and he is not sure his mom is comfortable taking care of him at home. His main concern, however, seems to be that giving up another activity will signal that death is near. He clings to his driving as a source of reassurance that his death is not imminent. We talk about how he might know when to quit driving. He says that when the time comes, he believes he will know, and then he moves on to other subjects. The session has gone well, but I am acutely aware of his lack of energy and the effort he makes to interact. As he struggles to his feet before leaving, I ask casually who drove him to the clinic. He responds, "I'm still driving. It's kind of hard. I had to use my cane twice to push on the brake pedal. I just didn't have enough strength in my leg to stop the car."

Startled, I ask him to sit down and begin talking about the risk involved in his driving. He says that his physician has not mentioned driving as an issue and that his mother seems unconcerned as well. I believe that, given his lack of strength and his inability to get out of his chair unassisted, he has no business driving but am unsuccessful in convincing him. I go over the possible danger to others and express my concern that he could hurt himself, but he is not responsive to my arguments. I point out how weak he is and remind him of the times that he had become disoriented and confused. He says that I am overreacting and that he gets around OK. I am afraid to let him drive himself home and feel sad that he now has to face another loss. Unsure about how to proceed, I ask him to stay put for a moment while I step outside the office to think.

PAUSE AND IDENTIFY YOUR PERSONAL RESPONSES TO THE CASE

My own sadness over Mike's deteriorating condition is very obvious. I am annoyed that neither the medical staff nor his mother has been paying close attention to his deterioration at least as far as driving is concerned. In previous conversations with Mike's mother, I concluded that she was distancing herself from his situation and would not be a resource. Although there is a chance that he might be able to get himself home without getting in an accident (after all, he drove himself to the clinic without incident), I can see that he is very weak. Driving the car would not be easy for him, and if he did not hurt himself or someone else in an accident, I am not convinced that he would not get lost on his way home. I worry that his mother is not getting involved in his driving ability, as she appears unable to face what seems to be happening. I feel protective toward Mike and know he would not want to hurt anyone, and the idea of him driving around lost repels me. Telling him that he cannot drive home is not going to be easy because he is so afraid of losing that freedom. I hate to be the one to take away this symbol of his independence, and I am afraid that if I push too hard he will get angry and feel that I have abandoned him just like his mother has. I could call a taxi or take him myself if he would let me, but once he goes out the door I really cannot control what he does. As long as he has his car keys, he is likely to attempt to drive. However, he has given me a release to speak with his mother and his physician, so I know I can call his mother to see if she might come to pick him up. I am going to have to make a quick decision because others are waiting to see me.

REVIEW THE FACTS OF THE CASE

When he drives, Mike presents a danger to himself and others, but he is unwilling to acknowledge his limitations, and others who are close to him, like his mother and his physician, have chosen not to intervene. I worry that I could be held liable if he did cause an accident or hurt himself. However, if I have to force him to hand over his keys, I run the risk of alienating him as a client at a time when he needs more support and understanding.

CONCEPTUALIZE AN INITIAL PLAN
BASED ON CLINICAL ISSUES

It occurs to me that one thing I can do immediately is to ask a colleague to see Mike; she has expertise in functional assessment of people with disabilities. I seek out my colleague in the clinic and tell her my concerns, and she agrees to see Mike then and there. After I have introduced the two of them, I step outside so I can get in touch with his physician and his mother to see if they are aware of his condition. I will also use this time to let my next client know that I am running late. If my colleague agrees with me that he is unable to drive, I will ask his mother to pick him. While we are waiting on her arrival, I will explain to Mike what I have done and attempt to maintain his confidence.

My associate agrees that Mike should not be allowed to drive, and she tells him that. Mike's physician comes over to see what is going on and also agrees that Mike should not be driving. When I sit down with Mike in my office, he says he does not want his mother involved, and he agrees to take a taxi home. He also agrees to bring his mother in the next day to speak with the physician. In the interim I decide to discuss this situation with an ethicist and a legal expert, mostly to reassure myself that I am acting properly.

CONSIDER THE ETHICS CODE AND ASSESS THE
ETHICAL ISSUES (BY KAREN STROHM KITCHENER)

As I consider Dr. Barret's dilemma, I am immediately aware of the deep and abiding concern he has for the client, coupled with his awareness that Mike may be a threat to others as well as himself as he continues to drive. I consider the case from the perspective of the American Psychological Association (APA, 1992) Ethics Code and then from the perspective of foundational ethical principles.

APA Ethics Code

The two standards from the APA Ethics Code that are most relevant are Standard 1.04, Boundaries of Competence, and Standard 1.14, Avoiding Harm. Without knowing Dr. Barret's experience in working with clients like Mike, it is not quite clear whether Standard 1.04b or 1.04c applies in this case. Standard 1.04b focuses on whether the clinician is competent to practice in a particular case, and Standard 1.04c focuses on how to be competent in areas that are new for the profession: "In those emerging areas in which generally recognized standards for preparatory training do not yet exist, psychologists nevertheless take reasonable steps to ensure the competence of their work and to protect patients, clients, students, research participants, and others from harm." In either case, the therapist needs to consider whether he is competent to assess the client.

In this case, Dr. Barret had to decide whether Mike was able to drive without endangering himself or others. Because he was aware of his own limited ability to make functional assessments, Dr. Barret took reasonable steps to ensure the competence of his decision by consulting with another professional who could confirm or disconfirm his own assessment of Mike's competence. Rather than making an incautious and impulsive decision to call Mike's mother, he stepped back and asked for a colleague to confirm his evaluation, thus assuring to the extent possible that his evaluations of Mike's driving ability were reasonable and fair.

Standard 1.14 states, "Psychologists take reasonable steps to avoid harming their patients or clients, research participants, students, and others with whom they work, and to minimize harm where it is foreseeable and unavoidable." This standard reiterates the importance of carefully considering any action that might hurt Mike and minimize that harm when it is foreseeable. Again, Dr. Barret seemed to be very aware of the potential consequences of his actions to destroy the last vestiges of freedom that Mike associates with driving and the potential damage that the intervention might cause to their therapeutic alliance. By talking with Mike and explaining his position, Dr. Barret tried to minimize the damage to their therapeutic relationship.

Three of the aspirational principles of the APA Ethics Code are also relevant: Principle D: Respect for People's Rights and Dignity, Principle E: Concern for Others' Welfare, and Principle F: Social Responsibility. Principle D emphasizes the importance of respecting the rights and dignity of all people. Particularly pertinent in this case is the reminder to respect the autonomy and self-determination of all individuals. This principle, however, also notes that these rights must be balanced with legal or other obligations. This is, of course, the crux of the problem in Mike's case: Dr. Barret must balance Mike's autonomy with other obligations. The question is how to do so.

Principle E: Concern for Others' Welfare provides another reminder to contribute to the welfare of clients like Mike and to minimize harm when conflicts occur in ethical obligations. As already noted Dr. Barret attempted to do this. Once his assessment was confirmed and he made the decision that he would not allow Mike to drive, he talked with Mike about his concerns in order to minimize the potential that his decision would spoil their therapeutic relationship. Furthermore, he allowed Mike to exercise his remaining autonomy by choosing whether to take a taxi home or call his mother. Dr. Barret's actions both respected Mike's limited autonomy and fulfilled his responsibility to the community, which is emphasized in Principle F: Social Responsibility.

Foundational Ethical Principles

The foundational ethical principle of autonomy offers further clarification in this case. It is important for Dr. Barret to remember that basically autonomy means self-rule on the basis of a plan that the person has chosen for himself or herself (see chapter 3). It presumes that the individual making those decisions has adequate knowledge as well as the capacity to understand the information and use it in a reasonable way. It would not be ethical to restrict Mike's driving if he is competent and is capable of making an autonomous choice (assuming that he is not endangering others), but that is not the case. According to Dr. Barret, there is evidence that Mike's mental competence is deteriorating. His inability to acknowledge his physical incompetence only exacerbates the issue. In this case, it would be more unethical to treat Mike as though he were fully able to make autonomous competent decisions than to ignore his growing incompetence, because his understanding of the situation appears limited or inaccurate and the consequences of driving could involve harming others or further harming himself.

That is not to say that Mike is totally incompetent. He may be capable of making autonomous decisions in some situations and not others. He is apparently lucid enough in Dr. Barret's office to participate in making a decision about how to get home. By allowing him to do so, Dr. Barret is respecting the limited autonomy he has. Furthermore, he apparently gives Dr. Barret no reason to believe that he would not follow through on his decision to take a cab; thus, there was no reason for Dr. Barret not to trust his decision.

By refusing to allow Mike to drive home independently, Dr. Barret acted on the principles of beneficence and doing no harm; he operated on what he thought was in Mike's best interests and the best interests of society. As he thought through the case, he tried to balance the good consequences of intervening with the harmful ones, which is one of the requirements of beneficent action. He seemed to be aware that, despite Mike's psychological pain at giving up driving, he would not be doing Mike any favors by allowing him to believe he could continue to drive. If he were to harm someone or seriously damage himself, his pain and suffering might only be exacerbated. In this case, both the potential magnitude of harm and the probability of harm (see chapter 3) are high enough that an intervention seems ethically justifiable.

Dr. Barret seems concerned about issues of fidelity. Is he being unfaithful to his relationship with Mike? Will he be perceived as untrustworthy?

Although Mike's reactions cannot be totally predicted, Dr. Barret did attempt to help him understand the problem and why he should not drive any longer. In some respects Dr. Barret's actions can be seen as both very honest and trustworthy. Mike can trust Dr. Barret to help him understand his own boundaries, even if he does not like them, and to be honest with him, even if it hurts. Those are often characteristics of a deep therapeutic relationship as well as an ethical one. Dr. Barret has approached his client in a respectful, caring manner, and this may help Mike face this new loss without abandoning his therapeutic support.

Dr. Barret's actions in no way seem unjust. He has not singled Mike out because he is HIV-positive, which would be irrelevant to the question of whether he is competent to drive a car. Rather, his decision has been based on characteristics that are relevant to the issue at hand; the fact that Mike is no longer physically or mentally competent to drive. Furthermore, he has consulted with a colleague to ensure the fairness and accuracy of his assessment.

Balancing the Ethics Code and the Foundational Ethical Principles

Dr. Barret seems to be following an ethical course of action under the circumstances. This is not to say that his decision is an easy one. Sometimes ethical choices leave us feeling regretful that we cannot find a perfect solution that will uphold all of the ethical principles (see chapter 3). In this case, Mike may feel hurt because Dr. Barret confronted him about his competence to drive, but the alternatives would be far worse. If Dr. Barret finds that Mike has resumed driving at a future point, he would be justified in taking stronger action, such as talking to Mike's mother directly or asking Mike to leave his keys with him.

IDENTIFY THE LEGAL ISSUES (BY SCOTT BURRIS)

This consultation is in the nature of a postmortem: The deed has already been done. But it gives me a chance to praise my client, and in so doing to reinforce one of the most important legal messages I can give: Do not let the law become a reason for not following your own professional instincts. With Mike waiting in the next room, Dr. Barret was under pressure. He had a general sense that he had a "legal duty" to prevent harm to third parties under some circumstances and that a patient could sue under some circumstances for a breach of confidentiality. He had no time to talk to an attorney. He did several things to help himself legally. Most important, he kept his professional head. He took what time he had, and made a little more, to work through the problem in a professional manner. He took his instant impression that Mike could not drive and tried to build it into a professionally defensible assessment. He evaluated the facts he had and called in a colleague to independently test his impression. He then returned to the client, confronting him in a way that was useful therapeutically but also squarely identified the issue of risk to others and placed it in the patient's zone of responsibility, too. Then he followed up, to make sure that others with responsible roles understood the need to act. Well done!

Had he called me, I would have been able to reassure him that this course of action was also legally prudent. Once again, we have a situation that might fall into the broad compass of a duty to warn or protect, although, as in most of the cases we have seen, once we look at the facts in detail it looks like the duty would probably not be triggered or would be satisfied by the actions that the psychotherapist's own professional standards seem to dictate. Actually, South Carolina, where this case takes place, has rejected the notion that a psychotherapist has a duty to protect third parties at all (*Sharpe v. South Carolina Department of Mental Health*, 1987).

There is a good argument to be made that Dr. Barret would not have had an obligation to act on these facts even in a state that recognized a duty to third parties. The duty is generally based on the special knowledge a psychotherapist has of the risks the patient poses and his or her special capacity to control the patient (primarily through commitment) or warn the proper parties. These conditions do not necessarily obtain here. Dr. Barret is helping Mike adjust emotionally to his health status; Dr. Barret is not treating his HIV, and he has no special knowledge or competence to decide whether Mike can safely drive. He did not prescribe a medication that has impaired Mike's ability to drive. It is not clear that he even has unique knowledge about Mike's driving problems or general physical debilitation. Nor does Dr. Barret's position as a psychotherapist give him special control over Mike: He cannot have him committed merely for being a poor driver. Although there are cases in which psychotherapists have been held liable for driving injuries, the cases in which liability has been imposed generally involved a stronger connection between the patient's danger and the treating professional's expertise and responsibilities (*Hasenei v. United States*, 1982; Pettis, 1992; Pettis & Gutheil, 1993). Had Dr. Barret physically restrained Mike, he would have been liable for battery. Had he taken Mike's keys, he might have been sued for false imprisonment. He might win such suits by showing the necessity for the action, but my point is that these would have been drastic measures that we cannot really be sure were justified.

Does that mean just letting a person like Mike walk out the door? If he had decided to drive, I probably would not have advised Dr. Barret to bodily restrain him. Rather, I would have suggested that Dr. Barret fulfill his moral (and any legal) duty to address this risk by taking steps to flesh out the factual picture and to involve other interested parties. First, I would have suggested a consultation with Mike's physician. (The physician is aware that Mike has HIV, so there would be no question of an HIV confidentiality problem; nor, in voicing his concern for Mike's physical capacity to drive, would Dr. Barret really be disclosing therapeutic secrets.) If the physician shared Dr. Barret's concern, the case for action would be stronger. It seems very unlikely that Mike would have insisted on driving in the face of the pressure from both of his primary caregivers. If he did, Dr. Barret and Mike's physician could consider notifying the state driver's license authorities that Mike is no longer capable of driving. Nothing provides for reports in South Carolina law, but the authorities could revoke Mike's license if they determined that he was no longer physically capable of driving. There is no immunity from a breach of confidentiality suit based on a disclosure of this kind, but there is no need to actually reveal any private medical information about Mike. It does not matter why he cannot drive, only that he is presently unable to do so.

IDENTIFY AND ASSESS THE OPTIONS (BY BOB BARRET)

I feel so affirmed by the comments from Dr. Kitchener and Mr. Burris. They supported my actions and helped me understand what I might do in the future. I knew that I was doing the right thing when I had my colleague look at Mike. Still, I worried that I did not let his mother know what was happening.

A week later when I next see Mike, he seems weaker. He speaks about his deteriorating condition and his determination not to die in the hospital. For most of the session I follow his feelings about his approaching death, and both of us are engrossed in that aspect of his life. As the end of the session approaches I ask how his consultation with the physician had gone, and he mentions that they cancelled the appointment because his mother felt that his driving was fine. He goes on to tell me that he had driven to the clinic and that he had trouble but got there ok. When I ask what kind of trouble, he says that he ran two stop signs when he was unable to push on the brakes with sufficient pressure. I find myself back where I had started but armed with much more information.

My options are the same as they were the week before. I can let Mike drive home and hope he does not have an accident, or I can call his mother and ask that she come to get him. However, neither is likely to solve the problem because his mother seems unwilling to intervene. I can also get in touch with his physician, who may be in the clinic, and let him make an assessment. In effect, if I can get the physician in I can turn Mike over to his authority.

As I sort through the five foundational principles I struggle with the notion of depriving Mike of his autonomy. One of my most fundamental values about the counseling relationship is to work toward empowering the client, to continually value her or his autonomy. Taking away his ability to determine whether or not he can drive safely clearly deprives him of his own authority. The principles of beneficence and fidelity are entwined in my struggle to decide what to do. I want to be kind to Mike and not to dishonor the relationship that I value so deeply. I also want to make sure that my actions do not cause him to distrust me, especially as his death seems near. Abandoning him at a time when he may need my support would not be professional or humane. Would he understand that my concern about his ability to drive derives from feelings of beneficence and fidelity? There is no guarantee of that. Still, I can recall a healthier Mike who would not want to harm anyone and who would be able to recognize that driving while impaired was not a good thing. The principles of do no harm and justice lead me to act to protect the larger community.

Of the five principles, autonomy is the one that has been stopping me. The other four point in the direction of an intervention to stop him from driving. I believe that Mike's driving may cause potential harm to himself and others and that in order to be sure no harm is done and that justice prevails, it is time, at least temporarily, for him to give up the privilege of driving. Of course, helping him understand this is difficult because of his mental state at this time. Still, having known Mike over a period of time I recognize that in not allowing him to drive I am honoring the relationship we used to have; the person he used to be would not want to place others at risk. I hope that we will find a way to maintain our trust. I do not like what I plan to do. I am angry with his mother for not being more supportive and concerned about what I will do if his physician does not back me up; I do not want to come out looking like the bad guy to Mike.

CHOOSE A COURSE OF ACTION AND SHARE IT WITH YOUR CLIENT

With Dr. Kitchener's and Mr. Burris's perspectives in mind, I decide to involve Mike's physician in persuading Mike to give up his keys. If that fails, I can call the police and have him stopped before he gets too far out of the parking lot.

I explain to Mike that I simply cannot let him drive himself home because he might hurt himself or others. I tell him that I am going to call his physician and set up an emergency appointment and that we will abide by the physician's recommendation. The physician does a systematic evaluation of Mike's physical and mental state and tells him that he cannot drive and, because of his deteriorating medical condition, needs to be in the hospital. Mike becomes very distressed, insisting that he wants to go home. At first, he refuses to be hospitalized and is very angry with me. He tells me that I have betrayed him and that he does not want to see me again. I spend some time alone with him to see if there is some way he might understand that this decision is best for him. We discuss his many losses and his fear that this might be the end. I keep the focus on the importance of his being in a safe place, not harming others, and receiving the kind of care that will give him the best chance of living longer. Finally he agrees to enter the hospital when I assure him I will come by before I go home for the day.

I am relieved by his compliance. When I call his mother to let her know where he is, she says that she knows he is near death and that she cannot "take it." She asks me to let him know that she will be at the hospital in the morning. As the day wears on I worry about Mike being alone and sick, and I worry about how I will tell Mike that his mother is not coming to see him that night. I know that he might die quickly and cannot figure out how to arrange for someone to be with him if that time comes.

I get to the hospital after 6 p.m. and stop at the nursing station. The nurses tell me he is getting weaker and probably will not live through the night. I enter his room quietly, prepared to give him whatever reassurance I can. As I approach his bed I realize that he had just died. I sit with him for several minutes, holding his hand and telling him what an important person he had been to me and how much I would remember him.

I am left pretty much alone as I try to sort this out. I wonder if I did the right thing; he wanted to die at home, and I feel that I deprived him of that. Still, as sick as he was I know that he might have killed someone if he had attempted to drive. Even had he been at home it is unlikely that his mother would have been by his side. She was relieved that he had died in the hospital. I worry about just how faithful I had been to Mike. Had I let him down? Or had I really supported him in a way no one else would? My action had led to his being in the hospital and to his having people nearby as he died. In one sense he did not die alone. My presence just after his death might have been a comfort to him. It certainly was one expression of my honoring him. Later, I ask his physician if she had known how weak Mike was. She tells me that my attention had gotten Mike the kind of medical care he needed as he approached death. She had realized that it was likely he would die quickly, and she is glad that he died in the hospital.

I carefully document what I had done in Mike's chart before I send it to be filed. I know that what I did was best under the circumstances and hope that Mike would understand that as well. I have not faced a similar challenge since. One reason may be that the experience with Mike alerted me to the importance of bringing up certain issues early in the relationship. Now, as I see someone getting weaker I am much more likely to talk about the issue of driving and to let my client know how I would intervene if I were concerned. Mike has definitely helped me work more responsibly in these situations. Sometimes I think of him sitting by my side as I am involved in these complex discussions with other clients.

REFERENCES

American Psychological Association. (1992). Ethical principles of psychologists and code of conduct. *American Psychologist*, *47*, 1597–1611.

Hasenei v. United States, 541 F. Supp. 999 (D. Md. 1982).

Pettis, R. W. (1992). Tarasoff and the dangerous driver: A look at the driving cases. *Bulletin of the American Academy of Psychiatry Law*, *20*, 427–437.

Pettis, R. W., & Gutheil, T. G. (1993). Misapplication of the Tarasoff duty to driving cases: A call for a reframing of theory. *Bulletin of the American Academy of Psychiatry Law*, *21*, 263–275.

Sharpe v. South Carolina Department of Mental Health, 292 S.C. 11, 354 S.E.2d 778 (S.C. Ct. App. 1987).

14

THE SUBSTANCE-ABUSING, HIV-POSITIVE CLIENT: THE CASE OF ANGELA

JOHN R. ANDERSON, KAREN STROHM KITCHENER, AND SCOTT BURRIS

ORIENTATION TO THE MAJOR ETHICAL ISSUES

The introduction of new drugs for the treatment of HIV and the creation of potent combination medication regimens have restored a needed sense of optimism and progress in the struggle against AIDS. Treatment with combination therapies can result in inhibition of viral replication and reduction of virus load to undetectable levels in the bloodstream. However, research has shown that the benefits from combination medication regimens can be sustained only if rigorous adherence to precise dosing schedules and other dosing requirements is maintained. Interruptions in treatment allow the virus to resume rapid replication and to generate resistant mutant strains (Rabkin & Chesney, 1999).

Because poor adherence can lead to mutant strains that are resistant to anti-HIV drugs and thereby compromise a patient's potential for responding to treatment, mental health providers often are asked to assess whether a given patient is capable of adhering to a complex medication regimen. The following case demonstrates the clinical and ethical complexity of this type of request.

CASE PRESENTATION (BY JOHN R. ANDERSON)

Angela is a 19-year-old with HIV. She occasionally exhibits HIV-related symptoms such as fever, night sweats, thrush, and recurrent vaginal infections. Her CD4 cell count is 400 cells/mm3, and her viral load is greater than 130,000 copies/mL.

According to her physician, Angela is street smart but childishly innocent. She does not understand the full import of the virus that she carries, believing that it requires only a "minor adjustment in her everyday life." Angela has dreams of big things in her future: a fabulous house, a flush savings account, and a career as a funeral director.

According to her medical records, Angela had a difficult childhood. While her mother used drugs and was in prison, she was shuttled between an aunt's home and foster care. When her mother got breast cancer, Angela dropped out of the 12th grade to take care of her. Her mother died late last year.

Through her Medicaid coverage, she can afford the costly new drugs that might halt her progress toward AIDS. However, Dr. Jones, her doctor, is unsure whether to follow current treatment guidelines that call for combination therapy because he does not trust Angela's capacity to stick to a complex dosing schedule. Dr. Jones maintains that poor compliance with the drug-taking regimen could spell disaster because she might develop cross-resistance to an entire class of drug treatment and because she could become a significant public health problem if she engages in unsafe sex practices and infects others with a viral strain that is resistant to many drugs.

Since Angela started seeing Dr. Jones, she has missed three appointments and kept three. During this period, Angela has also become pregnant. During the past 15 weeks, while considering an abortion, Angela has not consistently taken the prescribed prenatal vitamins. She admits that in the recent past, she occasionally had a few drinks and smoked a joint or two.

During her last visit with Dr. Jones, Angela enthusiastically stated, "I decided to have my baby, so I think it's time for me to get my stuff together and get started on that new drug cocktail so my baby will have a healthy mother." Dr. Jones referred Angela to me and asked that I assess her appropriateness for initiating a new drug regimen involving two nucleoside reverse transcriptase inhibitors (NRTIs), AZT and 3TC, and one protease inhibitor, indinavir (Crixivan). Although Dr. Jones did not explicitly state it in his referral, I knew that if my evaluation revealed that Angela needed a substantial amount of assistance with treatment adherence, Dr. Jones would either withhold combination treatment or expect me to provide the assistance that Angela needed. In the public clinic where I work, the mental health professional who conducts the evaluation is typically the one who is expected to address the psychological and psychosocial issues identified during the evaluation.

PAUSE AND IDENTIFY YOUR PERSONAL RESPONSES TO THE CASE

I feel trapped. On one hand, I believe no one should be denied treatment, and thus part of me wants to say that Angela should be informed of the consequences of nonadherence and be given combination treatment. On the other hand, I share Dr. Jones's skepticism about her judgment as well as his sense of moral responsibility to withhold treatment if providing treatment at this time will compromise her capacity to benefit from treatment at a later date, when she might be better able to adhere to the treatment regimen. Yet I also feel strongly that the evaluation of Angela's capacity to adhere to the treatment regimen should be based on systematic assessment techniques instead of the snap judgment of Dr. Jones, whose recent comments suggest that he is fed up with Angela and thus may be inclined to be punitive.

I worry about the lack of widely established assessment methods for determining whether someone has sufficient capacity for adherence to justify moving forward with combination treatments. I know that I am not an adherence assessment expert, and I am not sure who is. I keep wondering how I should approach this referral. Unfortunately, I live in a small community, and there is no other professional in the area with more experience than me.

I also notice that Angela's pregnancy has affected my thinking. That Angela finds hope and empowerment in the prospect of having a baby makes me feel more inclined to recommend moving forward with combination treatment. On the other hand, what if I am wrong and the baby develops some kind of resistant strain? I try to put my worries aside and concentrate on conducting a thorough and thoughtful assessment of Angela.

REVIEW THE FACTS OF THE CASE

The referral requires that I assess Angela's capacity for adhering to a complex regimen involving about 14 pills each day to be taken at different times and different dosages, with the Crixivan requiring lots of fluids to prevent kidney stones as well as ingestion with an empty stomach. Angela has a history of poor treatment adherence and substance abuse and tends to underestimate challenges and overestimate her capacity. Although previously ambivalent about her pregnancy, Angela is currently excited about the prospects of giving birth and sees her child as a major source of motivation for staying healthy. I want to support her hope about the future and her optimism about her capacity to take care of herself better for the sake of her baby.

CONCEPTUALIZE AN INITIAL PLAN BASED ON CLINICAL ISSUES

I plan to identify those involved in research on adherence and consult with them on strategies for assessing adherence. I want to interview Angela to determine her understanding of her illness, her treatment, and the consequences of nonadherence. I will ask her what strategies she has for making sure that she takes pills properly, and I plan to conduct standard assessments of substance use, depression, anxiety, and intelligence. As I prepare to move forward, I am nagged by various questions:

- What criteria will I use for determining whether Angela is appropriate for this type of regimen?
- If Angela does not meet the criteria I establish for this regimen, what is the extent of my obligation to help Angela develop the skills necessary to meet the criteria?
- Once I am satisfied that Angela meets the criteria I establish for this regimen, what is the extent of my obligation to assess her ongoing treatment compliance?

Because these questions continue to trouble me, I decide to contact an ethics expert for a consultation.

CONSULT THE ETHICS CODE AND ASSESS THE ETHICAL ISSUES (BY KAREN STROHM KITCHENER)

Dr. Anderson is dealing with the kind of ethical dilemma that faces any psychologist working on the cutting edge of a field. On one hand, he knows that neither his training nor his experience enables him to make the kinds of decisions called for in Angela's case. On the other hand, very few people are knowledgeable, and there are few resources on which he can draw. His recommendation—whether Angela should take the new drug therapy—will have life-threatening implications for both Angela and her unborn child. Furthermore, he must deal with nagging ethical questions, such as the extent of his obligation to do more than he has been asked to do.

APA Ethics Code

As was true in chapter 13, the most relevant standard from the American Psychological Association (APA, 1992) Ethics Code is 1.04, Boundaries of Competence and particularly the sections on practice in new or emerging areas. Section b requires that when psychologists are moving into new areas, they do so only after undertaking appropriate study, training, supervision, or consultation. Section c notes that in emerging areas where standards of practice do not exist, psychologists should take reasonable steps to ensure that their work is competent and to protect their clients from harm. (See also Standard 1.14, Avoiding Harm.) Furthermore, Dr. Anderson needs to consider the standards regarding assessments. Several could be cited, but Standard 2.04b, Use of Assessment in General and With Special Populations, seems particularly important: "Psychologists recognize limits to the certainty with which diagnoses, judgments, or predictions can be made about individuals."

Dr. Anderson recognizes that he has limited expertise in this area, but he is also aware that he is the only one in the community to whom Angela's physician can turn, so he feels compelled to help. What advice do the above standards give him under the circumstances? First, the standards suggest that he must determine whether anyone has expertise in adherence. A careful literature search may help him identify who has expertise in the area as well as whether there are standards for competent practice. AIDS organizations in the surrounding area might be able to put him in touch with people with more expertise on adherence issues. In other words, taking reasonable steps to ensure the competence of his work implies that Dr. Anderson must become knowledgeable about the information that is available regarding the factors that might predict adherence. His plan to seek out those involved in research on adherence is clearly consistent with the requirements of the Ethics Code.

Because Dr. Anderson's ultimate recommendation has high potential for harm, he has a strong ethical obligation to gather as much information as possible before he proceeds. Furthermore, because of limited information about the ability of psychological tests to predict adherence, he needs to be particularly cautious when making predictions about Angela's behavior and inform Dr. Jones about his reservations (Standard 2.04b).

The Standards section of the Ethics Code offers little guidance regarding Dr. Anderson's questions about his obligation to help Angela meet any criteria he identifies for the treatment regimen or his obligation to assess her treatment compliance. This implies that if he does a responsible assessment using up-to-date information about adherence, he will have met minimal ethical standards as far as the APA Ethics Code is concerned. On the other hand, aspirational principles, which are designed to guide psychologists toward the highest ideals of the profession, set higher goals. In particular, Principle E: Concern for Others' Welfare and Principle F: Social Responsibility seem particularly important. Principle E suggests that ideally psychologists should try to contribute to the welfare of those with whom they work. In this case, it would probably involve helping Angela develop the skills she needs to comply with the new drug regimen, if that is what Dr. Anderson recommends. Because aspects of the patient–provider relationship can also be critical in promoting adherence to AIDS treatment, it may also imply making an intervention with Dr. Jones to help him develop a more supportive, less punitive stance toward Angela.

The second relevant aspirational principle, Principle F: Social Responsibility, reminds psychologists to be aware of their responsibilities to society. In this case, the principle implies that ideally Dr. Anderson should be concerned about the social consequences if Angela tries the new drug therapy and fails. As Dr. Jones points out, failure would be disastrous for Angela and might also create a public health risk if it led to a drug-resistant virus strain. The principle underlines the ethical importance of developing measures to support Angela's compliance if she begins treatment and to monitor her treatment compliance.

Foundational Ethical Principles

Throughout the case description, Dr. Jones and Dr. Anderson question both Angela's judgment and her sense of responsibility. She does not have a history of making highly competent decisions. Respect for autonomy in Angela's case might suggest that in addition to using an interview to assess Angela's understanding of her illness and the difficulty of complying with the treatment regimen, Dr. Anderson should consider whether she is competent to make a decision to follow the regimen and how he might enhance her understanding. For example, he might provide her with information about drug therapy and the implications of noncompliance for both herself and her unborn child. He also might suggest that she talk to Dr. Jones about trying a "dry run" during which she could take empty gel capsules on the prescribed schedule and with the necessary dietary requirements (PI Perspective, 1997) and then help her realistically evaluate her own potential for compliance. Furthermore, Dr. Anderson may discuss with Dr. Jones the availability of alternative treatments if he does not use one of the combination drug therapies, so that Dr. Anderson understands them and can help Angela understand them.

Evidence suggests that Angela's past decisions may have been based on poor understanding and knowledge; thus, they may not have been autonomous. Just interviewing Angela about her understanding of her illness, treatment, and the consequences of nonadherence may not provide sufficient evidence of her competence to comply if she does not understand the relevant information. Respect for Angela would imply that Dr. Anderson has some responsibility to enhance her ability to make reasonable decisions by making sure that she has good information and understands it. Once she does, Dr. Anderson may then be able to assess whether her plans for adherence are realistic. In fact, she may decide that a drug treatment that requires a less rigid compliance schedule may be better for her and her baby in the long run.

Two foundational principles, beneficence and do no harm, are critical in Angela's case; in essence, Dr. Anderson is trying to decide which alternative will be the most helpful and do the least amount of harm to Angela and her unborn child. As he suggests, the fact that she is carrying a child who has no choice regarding treatment makes the decision even weightier. Doing a competent assessment and drawing conclusions from it that are based on an up-to-date understanding of the literature on compliance is the first step in helping to decide whether Angela might be a reasonable candidate for a combination drug therapy. This must be a realistic assessment. There is no question that recommending the combination drug therapies could lead to harmful consequences for both Angela and her child if there is good evidence that she does not have a clear view of what to expect or how to manage the complex schedule.

In addition, acting in Angela's best interests could imply going further and helping Angela develop the skills necessary to meet the criteria or assess her ongoing treatment compliance. Dr. Anderson asks whether he is ethically obligated to do so. That is a complex question because beneficent acts may or may not be obligatory. For example, if a psychologist is hired to assess someone, doing a competent assessment is ethically obligatory because it is part of the implicit professional contract. To do an incompetent assessment might harm the client. Thus, beneficence requires competence. If the client were very poor and ill, bringing her food would also be beneficent. It would be a good moral thing to do, but it is not an ethical obligation. Unfortunately, the line between what is obligatory and what is not is often very thin. In this case, however, it does not appear that he has an ethical obligation to help Angela develop compliance skills.

The foundational principle of fidelity typically refers to issues of trust, truthfulness, and promise keeping between two or more people who enter into some kind of a voluntary relationship. When a professional like Dr. Anderson agrees at the request of a third party to see a client, that relationship has defined parameters. In this case, the parameters involve assessing

Angela's competence and with her consent reporting that information back to the physician. Dr. Anderson is at minimum bound by the principle of fidelity to keep his promise to fulfill his obligation. Other things being equal, he also needs to honestly report to Angela and Dr. Jones his conclusions and the reasons for them. Because issues of fidelity arise when people enter into a voluntary relationship, if Dr. Anderson is considering going beyond the defined parameters of the original relationship, he should consider whether Angela would want him to do so and if Dr. Jones would welcome his help. In other words, Dr. Anderson may decide he would be willing to help assess Angela's treatment compliance, but she or Dr. Jones might be unwilling to let him.

The question this case raises is this: Do psychologists have deeper obligations to clients that go beyond their agreed-upon contract? Feelings of compassion or concern about Angela and her child might compel a positive answer. The principle of fidelity would suggest that, at a minimum, Dr. Anderson should not promise something he cannot provide. Thus, he should not recommend Angela for a combination drug therapy based on the assumption that he will follow up on her compliance and then fail to do so because he is not truly committed or because Angela will not allow him to help. In other words, he needs to be clear about his contract and both his willingness and Angela's to go beyond it.

Because the foundational principle of justice involves the fair distribution of goods and services, it too is relevant in Angela's case. It suggests that the decision regarding whether or not she is a good candidate for drug treatment should not be affected by irrelevant biases. Dr. Anderson's commitment to do a fair assessment of Angela rather than respond to Dr. Jones's frustration with her seems a step in the right direction. Justice would imply that the decision regarding whether she is a reasonable candidate for treatment should be made as impartially as possible. Although her past behavior is a relevant issue, it should not be the only one on which the decision is made.

Balancing the Ethics Code and Foundational Ethical Principles

Angela's case raises one of the most difficult questions for health care professionals: When is one obligated to go beyond the ethical minimum and act on ethical ideals? Unfortunately, neither the Ethics Code nor the foundational ethical principles can answer this question. They can tell Dr. Anderson to be fair, to be competent in his assessment, and to promote Angela's autonomy by helping her understand her treatment alternatives. They can tell him that in a case like Angela's, which involves life-and-death issues and has potential social consequences, he is obligated to become more informed about adherence issues before he does an assessment. They can also tell him not to promise what he cannot give. They cannot tell him when to cross the line and become an ethical "hero," offering to do more than he is asked to do.

On the other hand, of all the cases considered in this book, Angela's seems to imply the need for an extraordinary effort both for her sake and society's. Estimates of the proportion of people who fail to adhere to the complex regimen required by the new combination drug therapies ranges from 15% to 90%, with an average of 50% (APA, Office on AIDS, 1997). If the consequences of nonadherence are as severe as Dr. Jones suggests they are, then someone needs to take responsibility to help patients enhance adherence. Because the probability of noncompliance is so high, failing to provide the guidance necessary to use the drugs effectively is probably harmful. On the other hand, the people primarily responsible for assuring that Angela takes the medication correctly are Dr. Jones and Angela. It is part of Dr. Jones's ethical obligation as the physician to help ensure that the treatment he is providing is competent and that involves supporting compliance with the treatment regime. Although it is to his credit that he is seeking consultation about the issue, his moral responsibility probably does not end there. That is, however, an issue for a medical ethics book.

Dr. Anderson asks about his own ethical obligation to go further. On the basis of the ordinary moral standards established by the Ethics Code and the foundational ethical principles, he would probably not have a professional, ethical obligation to do so. However, another level of moral activity (which Beauchamp & Childress, 1994, referred to as *supererogatory*) goes beyond the moral minimum required of all professionals. We might think of such morally meritorious or praiseworthy actions as involving moral excellence because they involve doing more than is required.

This is where the aspirational principles of the APA Ethics Code come in. They suggest that ideally psychologists should place the welfare of the client first and should act in ways that benefit society. By making these principles aspirational, however, the Ethics Code recognizes that psychologists cannot always meet these ideals and should not be considered blameworthy if they do not.

On the other hand, Dr. Anderson may not feel the actions to be morally optional. He may feel some personal sense of ethical obligation to do more than provide an adequate, responsible assessment. His feelings of compassion and care for Angela and her unborn child may motivate him to do more than is required as a professional. He may assume a sense of personal responsibility to help her with compliance. If he does so, he is performing a beneficent action that is not professionally obligatory. On the other hand, he should also be aware that compassion can cloud judgment and can lead to paternalism. Angela may not want his help. Furthermore, he should not let his feelings of compassion get in the way of a fair and competent assessment of Angela, lead him to cross professional boundaries, or promise something that he cannot really provide. If he cannot offer her the support himself, if Dr. Jones appears unwilling or unable to do, but if he feels compelled to help in someway, Dr. Anderson may need to consider whether there are other ways that Angela can get the support she needs and help her identify them.

IDENTIFY THE LEGAL ISSUES (BY SCOTT BURRIS)

American legal thinkers have long recognized the powerful role of the legal system in maintaining existing relationships of inequality in power and social status (Galanter, 1974; Kairys, 1998). Empirical research in the area of HIV supports the view that judges as a group tend to favor the legal positions of "haves" (like Dr. Anderson) over those of "have-nots" (like Angela), of institutions over individuals, and of parties seeking to preserve the status quo over those asking for a substantial expansion of legal rights or protections (Aiken & Musheno, 1994; Musheno, Gregware, & Drass, 1991). Thus, the law mirrors the stark differences of class (if not also race and gender) that provide the moral tension in Dr. Anderson's reflection and Dr. Kitchener's ethical opinion. Angela is powerless. Her social status defines her as irresponsible and incapable of self-efficacy. The social stereotypes inhabiting the minds of the professional classes resonate with this sense of Angela as the hopeless (and therefore enormously frustrating) Other. And just as she is outside the bounds of rational and competent living, so she is beyond (or beneath) the protection of law: She has no right to health care or the basic conditions of life necessary for health; it is her own fault that she cannot get it together enough to access the fine care we would like to give her.

Of all the cases in the book, this one most clearly illustrates the degree to which the law is unconnected to the needs of poor and otherwise alienated and marginalized people in our society. Her doctor can deny her life-saving treatment because he's irritated with her. Likewise, Dr. Anderson can pretty much do what he likes with her, and the chances of her being able to get a lawyer, much less to sue and then prevail, are infinitesimal.

I hope that Dr. Anderson will see that what I have given him is something other than "no advice." Law, like ethics, has its aspirational aspect. It provides a vocabulary for speaking about what ought to be. In these terms, I feel strongly that Angela has a basic human right to be treated as a worthwhile individual, a right not to be viewed only through a lens of social stereotypes and behavioral generalizations. She has a right to the basic conditions of income, education, housing, and physical safety that are the practical foundation of healthy choices. If she came to me for help, I would have a hard time finding the cubbyhole in which I could fit these claims under American law, but even as we think about this, dozens of talented AIDS lawyers around the country are trying to develop legal theories that could be used to protect poor people from being routinely denied access to combination therapy. They will try out these theories in cases that involve institutional defendants (large public clinics, Medicaid HMOs) that display a pattern of denying care in many cases. They will argue that imperfection in observing rigorous medication schedules is actually the norm for people with chronic conditions and that adherence cannot be well-predicted by looking at sociodemographic factors, including drug use and homelessness (Bangsberg, Tulsky, Hecht, & Moss, 1997). They will point to pervasive racial differences in the provision of health care, including HIV treatment (Moore, Stanton, Goplan, & Chaisson, 1994). They probably will not succeed in establishing any broad new rights, but the lawyers will aim for, and probably attain, some changes anyway: The threat of litigation, but also the political potency of ideas like equality and justice, will influence at least some physicians and health care institutions to reexamine their practices.

It is in that spirit that I have given Dr. Anderson my social sermon, which he probably did not need. The legal system places no obligation on him to take responsibility for helping to provide the conditions in which Angela can be healthy, but I hope he will do so in that spirit of excellence Dr. Kitchener evoked. All this notwithstanding, the fact that Angela has been the victim of social injustice does not change the practical imperative that she contribute to her own salvation. It may indeed be that Angela is just not a person who will stick with a tough regimen, but I would rather see Dr. Anderson come to that conclusion after helping her take a fair shot than simply to write her off at the start.

IDENTIFY AND ASSESS THE OPTIONS
(BY JOHN R. ANDERSON)

The ethical and legal consultations have helped me realize two things. First, I recognize how the role of the evaluator in my clinic is quite problematic. I now see clearly how the unspoken rule for evaluators ("if you find it, you fix it") has the potential for influencing both the interpretation of assessment findings as well as the recommendations that flow from those interpretations. I plan to discuss the general obligations and role of the evaluator at our next staff meeting. Second, I realize that in the specific case of Angela, conducting a competent assessment is not enough. Although neither the ethical standards of my profession nor the law require me to help Angela develop the skills to comply with the recommended drug regimen if my assessment indicates that she does not possess such skills, I feel a strong moral obligation to do so. If I cannot help her myself, then I feel a strong sense of personal responsibility to make sure that she gets the help from someone else.

Clarity about my sense of personal responsibility to help Angela makes me recognize that I need to clarify a number of things with Dr. Jones prior to conducting the assessment. What are the precise dosing, frequency and timing, storage, and dietary requirements of the treatment regimen he proposes? Are there less complex but equally efficacious treatment alternatives to the one he proposes? What are the differences in efficacy between his proposed regimen and less complex alternatives? What does Dr. Jones plan to do with the information derived from my assessment? If my assessment indicates that Angela is likely to have difficulty taking medications as prescribed, will Dr. Jones be willing to help her, or will he simply decide to provide her with some simpler but inferior regimen? If Dr. Jones is willing to work with Angela to ensure her success with combination therapy, what is he willing to do? Will he or one of his nurses provide the education and skills training that Angela needs in order to be successful? Will he or one of his nurses systematically monitor Angela's adherence and help her develop workable strategies when problems arise? Does Dr. Jones (or do his nurses) possess the knowledge and skills required to help Angela succeed?

My discussion with Dr. Jones results in good and bad news. The good news is that there is a less complex and equally efficacious treatment alternative. The AZT-3TC combination is offered in tablets that include both compounds (i.e., Combivir; each tablet contains 300 mg of AZT and 150 mg of 3TC). Thus, Angela can be placed on a much simpler regimen that would require a total of only 8 pills (i.e., one tablet of Combivir twice a day plus two tablets of Crixivan every 8 hours). The bad news is that neither Dr. Jones nor his nurses have the time or the training to help Angela improve her capacity for treatment compliance if my assessment indicates that she is likely to have difficulty adhering to combination therapies. Dr. Jones and his nurses are unfamiliar with adherence assessment or intervention, and as I anticipated they expect me to take the lead.

It is quite clear to me that this case may require much more work than I had originally planned, and yet I feel committed to helping Angela if she needs it. I am acutely aware of Dr. Kitchener's cautionary note about not promising more than I can competently deliver. After careful consideration of my current obligations, I resolve to devote the time it will take to educate myself and follow through with helping Angela even though her Medicaid coverage is likely to pay for only a small portion of the time that it will take. Mr. Burris's "social sermon" and my profession's aspirational principles serve as both anchors and inspiration for me as I think through my next steps.

Although I plan to identify those involved in adherence research and ask them for consultation about strategies for assessing adherence, Dr. Kitchener's consultation clearly indicates that I have "a strong ethical obligation to gather as much information as possible" before I proceed. That obligation suggests that I not only must learn a great deal about strategies for assessing adherence, but that I must also learn about strategies for enhancing adherence should Angela need the help. After obtaining and reading relevant information about adherence from the Project Inform and University of California at San Francisco Web sites, I call the Project Inform National HIV/AIDS Treatment Hotline and through that call I am able to identify a number of experts on HIV/AIDS adherence issues. Subsequent calls and email messages to these experts enable me to obtain a number of adherence assessment instruments, several background articles on adherence interventions, and numerous practical suggestions for assisting clients.

Dr. Kitchener's consultation indicated that respecting autonomy in Angela's case means helping her understand her illness, her treatment options, and the implications of noncompliance for both herself and her unborn child. According to Dr. Kitchener, respecting autonomy also means helping Angela realistically evaluate her own potential for compliance. By respecting Angela's autonomy in these ways I am also acting in ways that promote adherence. According to the literature, higher levels of adherence are associated with the following patient variables: understanding of the disease and the treatment regimen, perceived need for treatment, beliefs that treatment will be helpful, trust in providers, and social support for treatment adherence.

CHOOSE A COURSE OF ACTION AND SHARE IT WITH YOUR CLIENT

Given the foregoing considerations of autonomy as well as research findings, which indicate that adherence can be substantially influenced by patients' beliefs, knowledge, expectations, social support, and behavioral skills, I decide to approach Angela in a way that frames my adherence assessment as one part of a multistage process designed to help her maximize her success in adhering to a very complicated and demanding treatment regimen. It is now clear to me that I could not have framed the adherence assessment in this way had there been no prior agreement between Dr. Jones and myself with respect to assisting Angela with adherence. It is also clear to me that Angela would be unlikely to respond truthfully to questions about adherence if she believed that honest responses could result in the withholding of treatment.

According to the literature (Rabkin & Chesney, 1999), there is no consistent relation between adherence and age, sex, social class, ethnicity, marital status, or personality characteristics. Thus, one of the best ways to assess a patient's capacity for adhering to a complex drug regimen is to conduct a dry run, instructing the patient to take empty gel caps on the prescribed schedule while sticking to the prescribed dietary requirements. I decide to begin with an assessment of her understanding of her illness, her treatment options, and the implications of noncompliance for both herself and her unborn child. I then plan to help Angela evaluate her potential for compliance by conducting a dry run and by administering standard assessments of substance use, depression, anxiety, and intelligence. I plan to follow the period of assessment with a period of collaborative brainstorming sessions designed to address issues and problems identified during the assessment phase.

In presenting my plan to Angela, I emphasize the importance of truthful reporting and the relationship between her honesty and her medical team's ability to help both her and her baby remain healthy. To my delight, Angela responds enthusiastically to my plan and engages it with a level of enthusiasm that far surpasses my expectation.

IMPLEMENT THE COURSE OF ACTION: MONITOR AND DISCUSS OUTCOMES

Interviews with Angela reveal that she has an inadequate understanding of her illness, her treatment options, and the implications of noncompliance. It soon becomes apparent that her medical team had reviewed key information with her on numerous occasions but that they never paused to assess her understanding of what they told her. By slowing down the educational process, by breaking the information into manageable bits, by requiring Angela to write down key information in her own words, and by asking her to present the key information back to me, she develops a much better understanding of her medical care, and she becomes more invested in it.

The dry run experience helps Angela realize how difficult it is to successfully adhere to the proposed treatment regimen, and it helps her focus on potential trouble spots. She acknowledges that she has difficulty remembering to take her medication when she smokes pot or drinks alcohol. She also has difficulty taking her medication as prescribed when she is nauseated, when she is away from home, and when she has to take care of her nieces and nephews. She discovers that she often fails to plan ahead, as evidenced by her tendency to forget to bring pills with her. Situations that evoke feelings of anxiety or sadness also interfere with her capacity to remember her medical regimen.

Over the course of many weeks, Angela and I continue to monitor and discuss her adherence to the regimen of gel caps and pregnancy vitamins.

She learns to count out her pills in advance and to use pill containers with separate compartments for each time and for each day. She learns to establish daily routines and to integrate her treatment regimen into her routines. Over time, Angela develops a sense that she can succeed with the real thing.

Prior to initiating the combination therapy protocol, I worked with Dr. Jones's staff to help them develop a system for monitoring Angela's compliance and assisting her with problems. I stressed the importance of spending time with Angela and highlighting her successes. Eventually the responsibility for Angela's adherence shifted to Dr. Jones and his staff. During the period of transition, I continued to act as a consultant to both Angela and her treatment team.

I am pleased to report that both Angela and her baby are doing quite well. Not only did Angela learn to take her medication with very few "slip-ups," she also learned how to be more organized in other arenas of her life. It seems that the coordinated effort of the treatment team in connection with Angela's adherence produced a number of more generalized effects. Angela felt "cared for" and "believed in." She responded well to both the attention and the instruction. She took pride in her accomplishments, and her adherence successes seemed to lead to a more generalized sense of competency and self-efficacy. True to her word, Angela "got her stuff together" and became the healthy, competent mother that she wanted to be.

REFERENCES

Aiken, J. H., & Musheno, M. (1994). Why have-nots win in the HIV litigation arena: Socio-legal dynamics of extreme cases. *Law & Policy, 16*, 267–297.

American Psychological Association. (1992). Ethical principles of psychologists and code of conduct. *American Psychologist, 47*, 1597–1611.

American Psychological Association, Office on AIDS. (1997). *Combination drug therapy for HIV: Review of basic, clinical and behavioral science and a role for psychologists.* Washington, DC: Author.

Bangsberg, D., Tulsky, J. P., Hecht, F. M., & Moss, A. R. (1997). Protease inhibitors in the homeless. *Journal of the American Medical Association, 278*, 63–65.

Beauchamp, T., & Childress, J. (1994). *Principles of biomedical ethics* (4th ed.). New York: Oxford University Press.

Galanter, M. (1974). Why the "haves" come out ahead: Speculations on the limits of legal change. *Law & Society Review, 9*, 95–160.

Kairys, D. (Ed.). (1998). *The politics of law: A progressive critique* (3rd ed.). New York: Basic Books.

Moore, R. D., Stanton, D., Gopalan, R., & Chaisson, R. E. (1994). Racial differences in the use of drug therapy for HIV disease in an urban community. *New England Journal of Medicine, 330*, 763–768.

Musheno, M. C., Gregware, P. R., & Drass, K. A. (1991). Court management of AIDS disputes: A sociolegal analysis. *Law & Social Inquiry, 16*, 737–774.

Project Inform. (1997, Aug.). *Adherence to HAART.* [On-line]. Available: http://www.projinf.org.

PI Perspective. (1997, July). *Adherence to HAART: Project Inform.*

Rabkin, J. G., & Chesney, M. (1999). Treatment adherence to HIV medications: The Achilles heel of the new therapeutics. In D. G. Ostrow & S. C. Kalichman (Eds.), *Psychosocial and public health aspects of new HIV therapies* (pp. 61–82). New York: Kluwer Academic/Plenum.

University of California at San Francisco Web site. (1997, May). Hope to hold. Deborah L. Shelton, *American Medical News* [On-line]. Available: http://hivinsite.ucsf.edu.

University of California at San Francisco Web site. (1997, June). Strategies to establish and maintain optimal adherence. Margaret A. Chesney, *HIV Newsline* [On-line]. Available: http://hivinsite.ucsf.edu.

15

MULTIPLE ROLES WITH A DYING CLIENT: THE CASE OF PAT

TOM EVERSOLE, KAREN STROHM KITCHENER, AND SCOTT BURRIS

ORIENTATION TO THE MAJOR ETHICAL ISSUES HIGHLIGHTED IN THE CASE

Being involved with a client whose physical situation steadily deteriorates can be stressful for the therapist. At times, home and hospital visits generate a kind of intimacy that does not exist in a treatment office. Family members and friends may become part of the relationship, and at times, the therapist may feel the urge to become more of an advocate for the client or may want to stop by for a visit to provide support or some other type of care giving (Eversole, 1997; Winiarski, 1991). During home visits, therapists are often faced with a variety of unanticipated requests. For example, clients who have been lying in bed for hours may request a back rub or assistance in getting to the bathroom. On a routine home visit, therapists may find that clients need someone to run an errand or take them to the doctor or hospital for some urgent reason. Some clients may ask their therapists to assist as advocates in legal disputes involving disability, reasonable accommodation, or wrongful termination; to officiate at their funerals; or to assume custody of their children or power of attorney in medical decisions. Situations like these challenge therapists to make professional, reasonable, ethical, legal, and humane choices (Jue & Eversole, 1996).

CASE PRESENTATION (BY TOM EVERSOLE)

Pat was tested for HIV as part of a 7-day detoxification and drug treatment program for heroin and cocaine addicts. He was referred to me for psychotherapy upon discharge from the drug treatment program, and therapy began by addressing his commitment to sobriety in light of his recent news that he was HIV-positive.

At this writing, I have worked with Pat over a 3-year period and have watched as he gave up all substance use. I have admired the way he went back to work and attempted to create more effective relationships with his family. He lives with his two sons, ages 16 and 18, but has almost no contact with other family members. They and their grandmother, who lives across town, are the only people to whom Pat has disclosed his HIV status. Their mother left years ago and does not communicate with them. Other than their grandmother, there is no one to supervise them. Their relationship with Pat has not been easy. Pat was largely absent during his drug-using days, and his sons resent his wanting to take over now that he is sober. They are absent much of the time either at work or on the street and have little to do with him.

Pat has encountered many health problems during the past 2 years, and he now is unable to work. Our sessions moved from my office to his home during a period when he was nearly immobilized by neuropathy. I assisted in connecting him with a caseworker, who arranged for an AIDS service volunteer and home health care. Although Pat now has every service available to people with HIV in our area, the gaps in the service delivery system are readily apparent when I visit with him during our weekly sessions in his home. On a couple of occasions, he called prior to the session and apologetically asked if I would pick up a few things at the store on the way over because he had not eaten all day and there was no food in the house. I went to the grocery store and bought with my own money soup and crackers and a few other things.

Pat characteristically responds to my offers of tangible support (e.g., put the clothes in the washer, take the trash out, pick up a couple of things at the store) by saying things like, "Please don't put yourself out. I will be fine." However, it has been easy for me to take care of what needed to be done, and there was no one else around to do it. I called the home health care office several times, but their services and staffing are limited. Pat's volunteer from the AIDS service organization does what he can. I also contacted Pat's brother and encouraged him to help, but nothing has changed.

I am often aware of the differences between Pat's racial and ethnic background and my own. In Pat's experience, people learn to do without many of the things I take for granted. People who care about each other often look after each other in ways that I typically associate with family. At times, there has been tension between Pat and me when I wanted particular things to happen that did not even seem noticeable to him. Two things are very important to Pat: his funeral and the welfare of his sons after he is gone.

Last week, Pat was very sick, and he told me that his next hospitalization will be his last. He does not expect to survive another serious illness, and believing this, he made several requests. He asked if I would check on his sons after his death and make sure that they were all right. He asked if I would assume the power of attorney for medical decisions because he does not want his life to be prolonged by artificial means. He also asked me to help him organize his funeral, at which he wanted me to read "Crossing the Bar," the poem he read at his grandmother's funeral.

I have been worrying about what to do ever since. I do not want to get into a fight with Pat's brother, who believes that no costs should be spared in keeping Pat alive but that little should be spent on a funeral that "doesn't matter that much anyway." I believe that Pat's final wishes deserve to be honored, but I am unsure of what my role should be in terms of the medical power of attorney, the funeral, or looking after his sons.

PAUSE AND IDENTIFY YOUR PERSONAL RESPONSES TO THE CASE

Pat's requests have made me very anxious. I feel an urgency to give Pat an answer, but I am concerned about entering into the dual (therapeutic and personal) relationships he requests. I am aware that a strong personal relationship has developed in addition to the therapeutic relationship we have, and "boundary issues" have come into play. I am concerned that the personal relationship will impair my ability to select a course of action that best serves my client. It might also influence Pat's relationship with his family.

I feel sadness and grief at the impending death of a long-term client. At times I question my proficiency at and comfort with facilitating the tasks of grieving (Worden, 1982) and the mental health aspects of a client's death process. I also feel sad and angry that Pat has very little family support and no extended family.

Although I am comfortable working with people with AIDS and addictions, I realize my own anger toward an epidemic that has taken such a toll on the least fortunate in society. Although Pat and I are different, I identify with him and his fears related to mortality. I wonder and worry whether state laws prohibit a client's psychotherapist from holding durable power of attorney for medical decisions.

REVIEW THE FACTS OF THE CASE

The most salient facts in this case for me are the following:

- Pat and I have a therapeutic relationship of 3 years' duration.
- He is clean and sober, and he believes that he has end-stage HIV disease.
- He has little if any support from his brother, his sons, or his sons' grandmother.
- I see Pat at his home, sometimes bringing food or helping with household needs while I am there.
- He is using all the AIDS services available in our area.
- He and I have different cultural worldviews and experiences.
- He has requested three things of me: that I assume his power of attorney for medical care, that I help arrange and read a poem at his funeral, and that I check on his sons after he dies.

There are several questions and issues that I face:

1. How proficient am I in cross-cultural counseling and in facilitating substance abuse recovery? To what extent do I understand what it is like for a person of another race to have AIDS (in the context of his or her community, culture, and family)? How can I be empathetic?
2. What are dual relationships? Is there a difference between making a home visit, changing a bedpan, bringing food, eulogizing a client, and being a legal agent as far as dual relationships are concerned? Do I make home visits for all clients? Should I engage in client advocacy and arrange for a visiting nurse for my client? What is the role of the personal relationship in therapy?
3. Should I attend a client's funeral? What would I say to my client's bereaved parents and family if they asked me about their estranged child/father/brother? Do I understand the significance of funeral rites in my client's culture? What are my own unresolved issues about death, dying, grief, and loss?
4. Should I execute durable power of attorney for a client? Do I have the time and expertise to make medical decisions for my client should he need that? Could I execute the decisions I believe he would make if he were able? Would I be willing to advocate for Pat if his physicians were not following advance directives for his medical care?
5. Pat has not asked me to accept guardianship of his sons but simply to "check on" them after he dies. What is his expecta-

tion of me in that regard, and do I have the time and capacity to do that? Who actually will be legal guardian of the sons, and will he or she allow my visits?

6. If I agree to Pat's requests, will I compromise my therapeutic relationship, ethical obligations, or legal statutes?

CONCEPTUALIZE AN INITIAL PLAN BASED ON CLINICAL ISSUES

Pat has made several requests of me, and I do not believe that it would be fair to him or to me to give him a quick and final answer. There is more I need to know and to consider before choosing my course of action. Addressing this ethical dilemma will engage both our therapeutic and personal relationships.

Pat's requests are an honor, and I will acknowledge that. I will let Pat know that I cannot commit to agreeing to his wishes before I determine the following:

- his expectations of me regarding "checking in" on his sons,
- whether a legal guardian has been appointed for his sons,
- the accuracy of his understanding of his prognosis for life,
- whether or not he has signed advanced directives outlining his medical wishes,
- whether or not he has a will that includes a codicil allowing me to make funeral arrangements,
- the ethical or legal considerations (if any) that prevent me from agreeing to his wishes,
- my own assessment of my ability to do the things he requests in light of the work and time entailed.

In addition to the above information, I will review the goals of our therapeutic work together as they apply to this time in Pat's life. I must discern whether agreeing to his requests enables him to avoid issues, especially those relating to family, relationships, end of life, grief, and loss (Worden, 1982) that might be addressed in therapy.

CONSULT THE ETHICS CODE AND ASSESS THE ETHICAL ISSUES (BY KAREN STROHM KITCHENER)

Pat's case raises several ethical issues for his therapist, Mr. Eversole; some are related to his ongoing treatment, and some are related to the decision to assume power of attorney for medical care, speak at his funeral, and check on his sons after his death. Mr. Eversole seems primarily concerned about the multiple-role relationships as well as the issues that arise because Pat is a member of a difference race and culture than he is, so those issues will be dealt with here.

APA Ethics Code

As Mr. Eversole recognizes, being competent in the service of clients is critical in fulfilling the ethical responsibility to contribute to the client's welfare as defined by aspirational Principle E: Concern for Others' Welfare (American Psychological Association [APA], 1992). Similarly, as noted in chapter 8, the Ethics Code recognizes that treating individuals of a different race or culture may require specific knowledge about that particular group. Standard 1.08 (APA, 1992) reiterates the importance of obtaining specialized training, consultation, or supervision in order to ensure competent service and requires psychologists to make referrals when they cannot treat clients competently because of their differences. Consultation with mental health professionals of similar cultural background or with greater familiarity with the culture might help Mr. Eversole avoid making assumptions about the nature of family and friendships that could be critical when making decisions about such matters as whether to speak at Pat's funeral.

Although the ethical responsibility to be competent in the treatment of clients is straightforward, the issues involved in deciding whether to assume Pat's power of attorney or speak at the funeral are more difficult in this situation because Pat is estranged from his family and apparently has no friends who might help. The ethical standard that appears most relevant is Standard 1.17 regarding multiple relationships. On the other hand, aspirational Principle E: Concern for Others' Welfare, and Standard 1.14, Avoiding Harm, should remind Mr. Eversole that whatever decision he makes, not harming Pat and acting in his best interests should guide his decisions.

Standard 1.17 acknowledges that in many communities and situations, it may not be feasible or reasonable for psychologists to avoid social or other nonprofessional contacts with patients or clients. On the other hand, it notes that psychologists must always be sensitive to the potential harmful effects of other nontherapeutic contacts on their work with clients and on other people with whom they have a professional relationship. According to Cantor, Bennett, Jones, and Nagy (1994), the Ethics Code forbids therapists from entering into multiple-role relationships if it appears likely that the relationship might impair their objectivity or otherwise interfere with effectively performing their functions as psychologists. Furthermore, multiple-role relationships should be avoided if they might harm or exploit the other party.

From some perspectives, Mr. Eversole has already blurred boundaries in his relationship with Pat. By conducting therapy in Pat's home and doing little favors for him like helping him with laundry, picking up things at the store, and helping him with his toileting needs, he has entered into a relationship with Pat that might in some circumstances be sanctionable by ethics committees and licensing boards. The question that they would have to ask is whether these activities, which are not typically seen as part of the contract between a therapist and a client, were likely to have affected the therapist's objectivity or effectiveness or harmed or exploited Pat. It is unlikely, however, that cases like this one would lead to the filing of a complaint or the finding of a violation if one were filed.

Consequently, this standard identifies two critical elements that Mr. Eversole must consider when making the decision about whether to comply with Pat's wishes. First, he must consider whether accepting these roles may adversely affect Pat as well as others with whom he deals; second, he must consider whether the nontherapeutic roles might impair his objectivity about treatment or his ability to function in his role as a psychologist. Thus, Standard 1.17 and Standard 1.14 both suggest that Mr. Eversole must consider whether harm might occur if he agrees to accept Pat's power of attorney and to participate in his funeral as well as whether it is likely that his effectiveness or objectivity as the therapist will be undermined. As already noted, consultation with someone from Pat's racial or ethnic group or a psychologist who has dealt with similar requests might help with this decision.

It might also be helpful for Mr. Eversole to consider the meaning of dual or multiple-role relationships and the reasons for their prohibition in many cases. In essence, the idea of role conflict is one that has been recognized in social psychology for many years (Deutsch & Krauss, 1965; Getzels & Guba, 1954; Secord & Backman, 1974). Because roles carry with them certain expectations and obligations, failure to operate consistently with expectations that are typically associated with the role may lead others in the relationship to feel frustrated, angry, surprised, or disgusted. When a psychologist operates as a friend and a therapist, both the counselor and the client may become confused because the roles carry different obligations. As an example, friends are not obligated to maintain confidentiality whereas therapists are, friends engage in activities together whereas therapists typically do not do so with clients, and so on. In other words, role theory suggests that multiple-role relationships are ones in which a person is playing two or more roles with another person either simultaneously or sequentially. When the different roles are accompanied by different expectations or obligations, conflict can occur (Kitchener, 1988). When the conflict is severe, harm may result. At minimum, the therapist's objectivity and effectiveness may be negatively influenced.

As suggested earlier, Pat may already be somewhat confused about the blurred boundaries between a professional and a personal relationship. Because Mr. Eversole has already done some things for Pat (e.g., buying him groceries) that are more typically done by friends than therapists, he may have begun to see Mr. Eversole as more of a friend. Consequently, he may be more comfortable asking him to participate in other activities appropriate to friends, like speaking at his funeral.

Because harm occurs so often when therapists become sexually intimate with their clients, the profession has decided that these multiple-role relationships are always unethical. On the other hand, the profession has had almost nothing to say about relationship boundaries with homebound, dying clients. Changing a bedpan or buying groceries for a client who is incapacitated, hungry, and dying is probably more beneficent that harmful. Therapists are, however, obligated by Standard 1.17 to at least consider the possibility that they might be harmful or that they might negatively affect their objectivity and effectiveness as a psychologist by addressing such questions as these: How will these acts affect my professional relationship with the client? Is the client manipulating me? If I agree to the requests, will I end up resenting him and hurting him in the long run? Is there any chance that agreeing to the requests will reduce my effectiveness in working with this (or another) client? What are the chances that agreeing will impair my objectivity? In situations like this, therapists must balance the potential for harming the client with the realities of whether the therapist personally needs to help with daily necessities. Although helping in this way might negatively affect the therapeutic relationship, it might also allow Mr. Eversole to be more therapeutic.

Standard 5.02, Maintaining Confidentiality, should alert Mr. Eversole to another issue that should be considered. This standard points out that psychologists have a "primary obligation . . . to respect the confidentiality" of their clients. Typically, the information that a client is engaged in therapy is considered confidential. In this case, at a minimum, Mr. Eversole should point out to Pat that participating in the funeral might involve revealing that they were engaged in therapy together. If Pat still wants him to participate, Mr. Eversole should get his permission, probably in writing, to break confidentiality surrounding that aspect of their relationship. Because Pat's children, brother, and grandmother will probably attend the funeral, Mr. Eversole should also help Pat consider the impact that knowledge of the therapeutic relationship might have on them. If Pat does not give permission, then Mr. Eversole should consider whether he can participate in the funeral and maintain Pat's confidentiality.

In addition, the psychologist must consider the impact of participating in Pat's funeral on other clients. Will speaking at the funeral blur boundaries with other clients? Will others similarly expect him to speak at their funerals, and will this place a burden on him that he is unwilling to accept? Each of these issues needs to be weighed when considering the likelihood that therapeutic effectiveness or objectivity will be negatively influenced or whether harm will occur. Similarly, when deciding whether to accept the responsibility that accompanies power of attorney, he should consider whether this might in some way cloud his objectivity about treating Pat before he dies or otherwise interfere with his psychological responsibilities to Pat.

The ethical standards and aspirational Principle E provide considerable guidance in this case, and additional help in decision making is provided by aspirational Principle B: Integrity, and aspirational Principle D: Respect for People's Rights and Dignity. Principle B should remind Mr. Eversole that Pat should be treated with respect and that interactions should be marked with honesty, and he needs to be aware of his own value system and the impact that his values have on his work with Pat. Principle D underlines the importance of respecting Pat's dignity and fundamental worth. When faced with death, patients may be able to remain hopeful only about the possibility that they will die with dignity.

Foundational Ethical Principles

In addition to the explicit guidance in the APA (1992) Ethics Code, the foundational ethical assumptions identified in chapter 3 provide additional understanding of the issues identified by the APA Ethics Code. For example, the responsibility to benefit and to not harm clients underlines the importance of balancing the potential outcomes of responding positively to Pat's requests. Mr. Eversole must ask, What is the probability of helping him and what is the probability of harming him if I agree to speak at his funeral, accept his power of attorney, and so on? The foundational principles should remind Mr. Eversole that decisions that initially may appear to be beneficent can lead to harm in unexpected ways if therapists are not cognizant of the implications of their work. Beneficence should also remind him that even though the client's life is coming to an end, intervention through ways that can help the client die with integrity and dignity may be possible. Even if Mr. Eversole decides that participating in the funeral will not harm Pat or impair his own objectivity, a more beneficent action may be to see whether reconciliation with family or friends might be established. If so, they may fulfill the functions that he has requested Mr. Eversole to assume as well as allow Pat to die feeling supported by them. For example, it might be more meaningful to both Pat and his family if one of his sons reads the poem. The principle of beneficence would also support Mr. Eversole acting as an advocate for Pat and, as he suggests, attempting to arrange for home nursing care. As was noted in chapter 14, in the case of Angela, his professional relationship would not obligate him to agree to Pat's requests.

The responsibility to respect Pat's autonomy underlines the importance of involving him in decisions about the need to waive confidentiality if Mr. Eversole speaks at his funeral. In addition, the principle of fidelity should remind him to be honest with Pat about his own limits. Even if Mr. Eversole decides that it would be ethically acceptable to check in on Pat's sons, he should decline to do so if he does not want to take on the responsibility or does not believe he has the time or energy to do so. He should not make promises that he cannot keep after Pat dies.

As with the other cases involving clients with AIDS, the principle of justice means he should help ensure that Pat is treated fairly by those institutions with which he must deal. Furthermore, his own work should not be based on stereotypes regarding Pat's cultural background or socioeconomic status.

Balancing the Ethics Code and the Foundational Ethical Principles

Mr. Eversole recognizes the importance of going slowly and getting answers to several questions in order to treat Pat effectively and to decide whether to attend the funeral and to accept his power of attorney. In addition to the issues he lists, he should consider consulting with a member of Pat's culture to ensure his competence to deal with the decisions surrounding Pat's death. In deciding whether to participate in Pat's funeral, accept his power of attorney, or look in on Pat's sons, Mr. Eversole must ask how accepting these roles will affect others as well as Pat and whether they will impair his objectivity. In particular, he must ask what kind of harm might occur from taking on multiple roles and whether confidentiality will be affected. Standard 1.17 in the APA Ethics Code does not prohibit multiple-role relationships in all circumstances; rather, it requires that psychologists consider whether their actions are likely to impair their objectivity, decrease their effectiveness, or harm or exploit the client. If they are likely to do so, the new role is prohibited. He must also consider his own limits and give Pat an honest answer about his willingness to look in on his sons after he dies. Last, Mr. Eversole should not forget the importance of maintaining an attitude toward Pat that sustains caring (Noddings, 1984). Being with Pat in a caring relationship may be the most important gift that Mr. Eversole can give him as he faces the final days of his life.

IDENTIFY THE LEGAL ISSUES (BY SCOTT BURRIS)

Mr. Eversole is under no legal obligation to undertake any of the roles that Pat has asked him to fulfill. His legal duty consists only of providing mental health services that meet professional standards. As things now stand, the only legal risk he faces is getting so involved in his ancillary roles that his professional judgment becomes impaired, and he fails to fulfill the obligations of his psychotherapy role. His concern with this possibility is obvious, and I am not worried that he will make a mistake.

Nothing in the law bars Mr. Eversole from helping out informally with the funeral and the children, or taking on, in a more formal legal way, the power of attorney for medical decisions or guardianship of the minor child in the two remaining years before he is, for legal purposes, an adult. For everyone's sake, however, Mr. Eversole must take very seriously any promise to take on these duties, including keeping an eye on the potential pitfalls on the path.

First, consider Pat's end-of-life issues and the use of two different types of document: the power of attorney and the advance directive or living will. The law is clear that what care to get or refuse should be Pat's decision, not his brother's or his doctor's. The first and most important step to self-determination for Pat is clearly to articulate and formally record his wishes. The use of living wills specifying the patient's desires with respect to life-sustaining treatment is an increasingly familiar part of health care. According to the Supreme Court's decision in *Cruzan v. Director, Missouri Dep't of Health* (1989), people have a right to refuse life-sustaining care, but states (and hospitals) may require "clear and convincing evidence" of the patient's wishes. The living will is designed to provide that clear evidence of intent. The required form and procedures for advanced directives are dictated by state laws. The federal Patient Self-Determination Act of 1990 requires hospitals and nursing homes to advise incoming patients of their rights to refuse treatment, and institutions will provide patients with living will forms on request.

A living will is supposed to speak for Pat when he is no longer able to speak for himself, but experience suggests that it is a good idea to have a human spokesperson to make sure that the living will is followed and to deal with questions the will does not answer. Pat wants to give Mr. Eversole a power of attorney to make medical decisions when he no longer can. Generally, a power of attorney is a legal document in which one person (the "principal") gives another (the "agent") the authority to make decisions on his or her behalf. The document can grant as little or as much authority as the principal wants to grant and so may cover financial as well as medical matters. It can be limited to a specific period of time or extend indefinitely. A durable power of attorney remains in effect even if the principal becomes incapacitated and so is a vehicle to allow the agent to make health care decisions for the principal. A health care proxy or health care surrogate is a power of attorney exclusively for health care decisions. Pat does not need a lawyer to fill out a health care proxy, models for which can probably be obtained from a doctor or local hospital. By the same token, however, the effectiveness of the documents depends largely on the willingness of one's physicians and hospital to give them effect. Such directives are often ignored in practice, particularly in an emergency, so it is important for all members of the care team to be aware of the patient's wishes, and know the substitute decision maker, before a crisis. Pat should send copies of any documents he executes to his doctor. (For a full discussion, see Crockett, 1997.)

For Mr. Eversole, the biggest problem to watch out for is not that he could be liable for making a "wrong" decision, but that he will not feel comfortable in his ability to make the decision Pat himself would have made. This is particularly true on the question of "heroic" measures to keep him alive. Indeed, the hospital may not accept Mr. Eversole's substituted judgment if the course he requires will lead to Pat's death. Anyone undertaking the role of surrogate medical decision maker should discuss the future course of treatment with the patient and make sure the patient completes a valid living will.

Despite the problems and limitations associated with substituted judgment and living wills in the hospital, dealing with them could be a big help to Mr. Eversole in working through this situation. Filling out the forms provides an opportunity for Pat to get his children and brother together and to talk about his end-of-life wishes, including his funeral and the care of the children. Mr. Eversole may want to consider working with Pat in therapy to prepare him to use this opportunity to come to some clarity and agreement with his family, so that they will respect his wishes even if they do not agree with his choices.

Like the therapeutic relationship, the role of an attorney or a guardian is one of trust, in which one of the greatest risks (legally and morally) is mixed motives. Mr. Eversole is motivated by concern for Pat, but he can cover himself legally by making sure that there cannot be even a perception of self-interest in any formal legal role. He should make sure that he in no way stands to gain financially from Pat's early death or benefit in any way from the distribution of whatever property Pat has. Because Mr. Eversole is a psychotherapist, he would be particularly liable to a claim that he had manipulated Pat in his last days. I do not see a major risk here, but I want to attune Mr. Eversole to the importance of maintaining an appearance of propriety.

IDENTIFY AND ASSESS THE OPTIONS (BY TOM EVERSOLE)

As a solo practitioner in private practice, it is sometimes easy for me to overlook the need for consultation and ongoing professional development. This dilemma has afforded me an opportunity to seek professional assistance, and the consultation I received regarding my ethical concerns was both instructive and thought-provoking. In addition to helping me better serve Pat, consultation has prompted me to step away from the case somewhat and review my professional practice. My initial plan was to get more information. In light of input from the ethical and legal consultation, I am convinced that the plan was a good one. Consultation has reduced my anxiety somewhat and given me clarity on how to proceed.

The consultation also leads me to consider again whether or not I have adequately addressed Pat's lack of friends and family support in therapy. Have I done all that is appropriate to facilitate Pat's movement on relational issues? Would more work on these issues resolve the dilemma and better serve Pat than agreeing to all his requests at this point? Although we have worked on these issues in the past, it is possible that Pat may want to reconcile his estranged relationships at this new point in his life. My revised plan is to readdress this theme in therapy.

Pat and I have worked together for 3 years. My training and experience with diverse clients lead me to feel confident in my abilities at transcultural counseling. However, I have consulted with a leader in Pat's faith community about the appropriateness of my speaking at a funeral. She informed me that, in her (and Pat's) racial–ethnic community, funeral services are important occasions honoring the deceased person's life, that those significant to the deceased person are expected to be present, and that it is usual for service professionals to be present, especially if they are known to the family. This perspective is very different from my own family tradition, and I am glad I asked. It adds to my belief that Pat's request is not manipulative but consistent with his faith and community tradition. Thus, I feel it is appropriate to continue to consider this action as an option.

The next part of my initial plan was to acquire more information from Pat and to make a decision about the three requests that he has made of me. Pat gave me written permission to consult with his medical provider, who affirmed that Pat quite likely would not survive hospitalization for another severe illness. She was not aware of any advanced directives from Pat regarding life support and resuscitation. Because I told Pat that I would consult with others and needed more information from him, we were able to enter a discussion of the specific questions identified in my initial plan. During our session, Pat indicated that addressing these issues directly was empowering for him and that it had given him food for thought.

End-of-Life Issues and Pat's Funeral

Pat does not have a will, so there is no codicil that would allow me (as opposed to a family member) to make funeral arrangements for him.

There is no law or ethical rule that absolutely prohibits me from organizing Pat's funeral or speaking during the service. My remaining concerns fall into two categories: confidentiality and countertransference.

As far as confidentiality is concerned, I practice in a rural community and am the only practitioner known to see clients for HIV-related issues. This fact is well-known in the AIDS community. I need to get Pat's written consent to speak at his funeral. Part of informing Pat will involve a discussion of the potential effects of my presence there, especially effects on the confidentiality of his treatment. The consent will include a statement that he is aware that my presence and participation may indicate to some that he was in therapy with me and had AIDS. I also wonder what precedent or expectation this might set among other clients; I will need to address their expectations in an ethical manner as well.

As for countertransference, I need to evaluate my motivation to accept Pat's request. Is it to benefit my client, or is it motivated by my feelings toward a family that has not supported him in his declining years? Could my willingness to accept be motivated by a need to grieve this client's death?

Issues Regarding Pat's Sons

Pat would like me to "check" on his sons. Upon further exploration, Pat indicated that he would like me to visit them from time to time to "be sure that they were coming along OK and to serve as a role model for them." No guardian had been appointed for Pat's younger son. He was not aware that a guardian might be appointed by the state and that the guardian might determine who could visit the minor son. There is no law or ethical rule that would absolutely prevent me from serving in these capacities after Pat's death as long as doing so does not impair my objectivity, diminish my effectiveness, cause harm, or result in exploitation of Pat.

Although I am honored that Pat would consider me a role model for his sons, I have growing concerns about the time required and the duration of this responsibility. I wonder whether agreeing would serve the sons well or might actually pull the sons out of relationship with their family. As a result of previous family sessions and my home visits, Pat's sons know me; however, I am not sure that they see me as their role model. Furthermore, I could promise Pat to see his sons, but if the court appoints a guardian, I may not be allowed to follow through.

Issues Regarding Power of Attorney

Pat has not executed a document assigning power of attorney for medical or financial purposes. He has the option of executing a health care proxy, which will allow a surrogate to make his medical decisions if he cannot. Dr. Kitchener's ethics consultation indicates that certain dual roles are not allowed. However, neither the code nor the law explicitly prohibit me from accepting power of attorney or serving as Pat's health care proxy. Again, I need to ensure that doing so will not result in loss of objectivity, diminished effectiveness, harm, or exploitation. To put things in place to manage the end of his life, Pat needs a number of case management services. My course of action will include assisting Pat in getting these things done. Although I may need assistance from other specialists, we may be able to meet Pat's needs within the scope of my counseling practice. Pat is my client, and I am compelled to uphold the standards of professional practice.

I am concerned about my ability faithfully to serve Pat over what could be a prolonged course of dying, involving many meetings and possible confrontations with hospital staff. During those times, could I continue to provide psychotherapy at Pat's bedside separate from my role as his medical proxy?

CHOOSE A COURSE OF ACTION AND
SHARE IT WITH YOUR CLIENT

Part of me was hoping to find clear ethical rules or laws that would relieve me of this dilemma. Short of that, the deliberation I have outlined has helped me do the best job I can to reach a decision that I feel is ethically sound and legally defensible. In my records, I have documented my sessions with Pat as well as my consultations. I also documented my decision-making process as outlined below. I recognize that other therapists may not have made the decisions I made.

In preparation for communicating my decision and course of action to Pat, I reviewed the information I had gathered and my decision-making process.

Decision-Making Process

Monitoring my personal responses

I am aware that dealing with Pat's request has made me anxious and that at times I wanted to find a quick, easy, and safe "fix" for this ethical dilemma. In addition to peer and expert consultation, I decided to resume my own therapy to explore my own issues that resonate with Pat's as well as my issues around death, grief, and loss. This work has helped me retain objectivity in Pat's therapy and has opened new insights for me around my own issues. After this careful process of deliberation, I do not believe that my personal reactions to this case are impairing my decision.

Applying the ethical standards

Dr. Kitchener's ethics consultation was very helpful. Even though the code did not indicate one right answer for me, explanation of the code and the parameters under which I have leeway to make ethical decisions based on the specifics of the case (including my abilities) lent support for my ultimate decision. A clearer understanding of the code gave me a guiding standard that my decision must uphold. It must not impair objectivity, decrease my therapeutic effectiveness, cause harm, or result in exploitation. I do not believe that my decision will prevent me from upholding the ethics code of my profession.

Applying the foundational ethical principles

Dr. Kitchener raised many good questions in this regard. I weighed the probability of helping Pat and not harming him if I speak at his funeral, agree to mentor his sons, and assume medical power of attorney. I think there is great potential for harm if I agree to the last two requests.

Balancing the foundational ethical principles

I believe that agreeing to speak at Pat's funeral maximizes his autonomy because it allows him to be effective in planning his own funeral. My doing so benefits Pat and would do a minimal amount of harm to Pat or others. Agreeing to speak does not preclude further work to reconcile family relationships and allow Pat to choose other speakers. It is a course of action that is faithful to our therapeutic and personal relationships, and I would consider doing this for other clients. I do not believe that speaking at Pat's funeral will blur my boundaries with other clients. Although the principles are potentially in conflict, a decision to speak balances the five principles, doing the most good while doing the least amount of avoidable harm. On the other hand, Pat asked me to check in on his sons, but he expects much more. Accepting this responsibility and being unable to perform it has a high potential for harming his sons and leaving them without any real mentoring or parenting. For me, the potential for maleficence and the inability to be faithful to Pat's intentions outweigh all other principles. The same is true for Pat's third request, accepting power of attorney.

Using the legal consultation

Mr. Burris's advice reassured me that the risk of legal action against me was minimal in agreeing to all three of Pat's requests. Lacking a clear law to which I should defer, it put the dilemma squarely back on my shoulders! It did, however, highlight aspects of my decision that must prevail if I accept: sound therapeutic judgement and clear lack of self-interest or exploitation. I do not believe that speaking at Pat's funeral serves any self-interest or is likely to result in any financial gain. It is possible, however, that the licensing board in my state could have the opportunity to take issue with my decisions. In that case, documentation of my expert, peer, and legal consultations as well as my discernment process would be very important.

Integrating the ethical and legal consultations

Fortunately, the legal and ethical consultations were not in conflict. The law set the minimum requirements for my response, and the Ethics Code gave me clarity on the higher standard my profession requires. The Ethics Code provided leeway for me to move forward in ways that were best for my client, although I had to discern which of the conflicting principles would prevail. My personal abilities to adequately meet Pat's requests ultimately determined which of these three allowable functions I would perform for him. Both consultations prompted me to think of additional solutions that would serve my client well while relieving the ethical dilemma. My decision supports Pat's goals in therapy: maintaining his recovery from addictions, retaining personal authority in his life (living and dying with dignity), and strengthening relationships with his family.

Decisions Reached on Major Issues

In session, I will communicate the following course of action to Pat.

End-of-life issues and Pat's funeral

I will agree to speak at Pat's funeral and to help him arrange his funeral. I will not agree to arrange his funeral after his death.

I will tell Pat the ramifications that my appearance at his funeral might have regarding confidentiality and will get his informed consent as a condition for agreeing to accept this request. I have met Pat's sons and their grandmother. They know he has AIDS, and they are aware that he is in therapy with me. I do not believe that providing this service will impair my ability to perform my functions as a therapist. I do not believe that Pat's expectations of me in this role conflict with his expectations of me as his therapist. I understand that other clients may expect me to participate in their funerals. I am prepared to discern whether that is ethical on a case-by-case basis.

For some clients it is therapeutic to discuss how they would like their funeral to be and how they would like to be remembered. This could be helpful if I am to help Pat plan his own funeral, and it also might afford an opportunity to reengage his family members. It may be that there are relational issues he is willing to address in this context. Should relationships improve and family members become more involved, Pat may ask me to step aside at a later date. If it is acceptable to Pat, his sons may be able to read the poem at his funeral.

Issues regarding Pat's sons

I will not agree to check in on Pat's sons.

Although Pat's request that I remain involved with his sons is an honor, it entails much more than "checking in" on them. If I accept but cannot sustain the commitment to Pat's sons or meet their needs, it could in fact be harmful to them and other family members. It is also possible that I might not be allowed to keep such a promise to Pat, if an appointed guardian disallows it. I am not able to provide the mentoring Pat has told me his sons need; they will need more than casual visits. I will encourage Pat to arrange for guardianship of the younger son and a mentor for the older son, and I will communicate to Pat's sons that I will be available on a professional basis, should they want to see me for counseling or referrals. Addressing family and guardianship issues with Pat may be both practical and therapeutic.

In therapy, Pat and I will explore how he thought his sons would benefit by my guardianship and mentoring as well as his ability to provide some of that now or his feelings about not being able to do so. I plan for us to reexplore family relationships and potential community resources for fulfilling his wishes for these young men. We will discuss how Pat feels about my decision.

Issues regarding power of attorney

I will not accept Pat's durable power of attorney for medical decisions.

I will facilitate Pat's decisions about advanced medical directives and drawing up a will, and I will help him communicate his intentions to his medical proxy and physician. I will remain attentive to any changes in his wishes as we explore informing the family about his plans; they may not appreciate how near to death he is, and this may be an opportunity to improve his relationships with them if he is willing to involve them.

From a therapeutic perspective, it is important for Pat to find things in which he can realistically hope. Pat is an addict in recovery. He has told me that he does not want to "die like a junkie" especially in light of the life changes he has made over the past 3 years. It is important that he die with dignity and respect and that he retain some measure of authority over his care. The hospital should treat him fairly and adequately manage his pain. He needs a medical proxy and advocate. Although services in my rural area are limited, staff at our local agency for disabled and senior services have experience assisting in this area.

It is important for me to do a good job for Pat as his therapist throughout his life, and I believe that accepting responsibility for his end-of-life decisions would impair my ability to do so. The extraordinary demands of this role could challenge my ability to maintain an attitude of caring. I am concerned that in a time of fatigue and potential pressure from family members and medical personnel, I might not be faithful to Pat's end-of-life wishes. Thus, I will not accept that responsibility. It is important for Pat to have advanced directives and a medical proxy in place, and I will assist him in achieving that.

IMPLEMENT THE COURSE OF ACTION: MONITOR AND DISCUSS OUTCOMES

I anticipate that Pat will not be pleased with all of my decisions. Although I explained the limits of my professional relationship with him when we started therapy 3 years ago, I also know that Pat sees many interpersonal relationships from a different cultural worldview than I do (Dilley, 1989, Eversole, 1993a, 1993b). I will monitor the change my decisions may bring about in therapy and address it as is beneficial to the client. I will continue to see Pat and, if necessary, I will make frequent home or hospital visits. End-of-life and family issues are part of everyone's experience, and so I expect I will resonate with Pat's feelings of sadness and anger.

When I tell Pat of my decisions, he is sad and angry with me for not agreeing to look after his sons or administer his end-of-life wishes. Crying, he tells me, "I trusted you. I thought you knew me better than that." In therapy we work on his feelings of abandonment by me and his family and why others sometimes had not met his expectations. As part of my agreement, I facilitate Pat's own decisions about planning his funeral. Identifying why components of the funeral are important to him leads him to review his life during our sessions. He is able to grieve relationships that never were and to begin reconciliation with his sons. The person who provided the cultural consultation is able to assist Pat in finding a suitable guardian for his younger son. The guardian is an elder in Pat's community and agrees to be available for both young men as necessary.

POSTSCRIPT

Within 6 weeks Pat's health declined further, and he was admitted to our local hospital. The chaplain's office assisted Pat in drawing up advanced directives for his health care. His son's guardian assumed power of attorney.

Pat's AIDS service volunteer facilitated execution of his will, including a codicil allowing the guardian to conduct the funeral according to Pat's wishes. At Pat's funeral, his younger son wanted to read "Crossing the Bar," but he did not want to read it alone. We read the poem together, alternating verses.

I am satisfied that the decisions I made served Pat and his family, to the best of my ability, even though several parties were not pleased with my response. Knowing that I performed ethically and effectively in a difficult situation has helped to sustain me in this work.

REFERENCES

American Psychological Association. (1992). Ethical principles of psychologists and code of conduct. *American Psychologist, 47,* 1597–1611.

Canter, M. B., Bennett, B. E., Jones, S. E., & Nagy, T. F. (1994). *Ethics for psychologists: A commentary on the APA Ethics Code.* Washington, DC: American Psychological Association.

Crockett, P. (1997). *HIV law: A survival guide to the legal system for people living with HIV.* New York: Three Rivers Press.

Cruzan v. Director, Missouri Dep't of Health, 492 U.S. 917, 109 S.Ct. 3240 (1989).

Deutsch, M., & Krauss, R. M. (1965). *Theories in social psychology.* New York: Basic Books.

Dilley, J. W., Pies, C., & Helquist, M. (1989). *Face to face.* Berkeley, CA: Celestial Arts

Eversole, T. (1993a). *HIV and communities of color.* Washington, DC: American Psychological Association.

Eversole, T. (1993b). *HIV and persons with chemical dependencies.* Washington, DC: American Psychological Association.

Eversole, T. (1997). Psychotherapy and counseling: Bending the frame. In M. G. Winiarski (Ed.), *AIDS mental health practice for the 21st century* (pp. 23–38). New York: New York University Press.

Getzels, J. W., & Guba, E. G. (1954). Role, role conflict, effectiveness. *American Sociological Review, 19,* 164–175.

Jue, S., & Eversole, T. (1996). *Ethical issues and HIV-related mental health services.* Washington, DC: American Psychological Association.

Kitchener, K. S. (1988). Dual role relationships: What makes them so problematic? *Journal of Counseling and Development, 67,* 217–221.

Noddlings, N. (1984). *Caring: A feminine approach to ethics and moral education.* Berkeley: University of California Press

Patient Self Determination Act, 42 U.S.C.A. § 1395 (a)(1) et seq. (1990).

Secord, P. F., & Backman, C. W. (1974). *Social psychology*. New York: McGraw-Hill.

Winiarski, M. G. (1991). *AIDS-related psychotherapy*. Elmsford, NY: Pergamon Press.

Worden, J. W. (1982). *Grief counseling and grief therapy. A handbook for the mental health practitioner*. New York: Springer.

16

SUICIDE AND CONFIDENTIALITY WITH THE CLIENT WITH ADVANCED AIDS: THE CASE OF PHIL

BOB BARRET, KAREN STROHM KITCHENER, AND SCOTT BURRIS

ORIENTATION TO THE MAJOR ETHICAL ISSUE HIGHLIGHTED IN THE CASE

Clinicians routinely report that one of the major challenges they face in working with clients with HIV disease is knowing when to take suicidal thoughts seriously and whether to intervene once the decision to commit suicide has been made. This situation is particularly complex when ending life seems rational and extending a life that will be filled with suffering seems unjustifiable. Case law that addresses this issue has not been made, and society seems mixed in its attitude toward physician-assisted suicide when death is imminent.

CASE PRESENTATION (BY BOB BARRET)

Phil is a 37-year-old African American who is at the end stage of HIV disease. He has been in and out of the hospital four times in the past 6 weeks, and he is losing strength rapidly. His physician has told him that although he may lose his mobility, he could live for "some time" or he could die at any moment. Phil lives with his mother and younger sister and her three children, and he has a thoughtful and loving relationship with his family. Over the past 4 years, I have been impressed with his ability to use his illness as a springboard to understand himself and his family relationships more fully. He has been a volunteer speaker for an HIV/AIDS service organization and has served as a role model for many who live with HIV. He has been with others as they died and has often expressed a wish to die a peaceful death. He speaks easily about the many ways HIV has enriched his life. I have been impressed with his courage and find myself eager to give him support as his health declines.

Six months ago, Phil was unable to take the latest treatment, a combination of drugs that seemed to work with others with HIV. Phil was crushed when he was finally told he could not continue in the clinical trial, and shortly after that his health began to deteriorate.

Over the past several months he has accumulated a supply of pills "just in case" he wants to "check out." Most of our conversations about his possible suicide do not suggest an immediate danger. I had him take the Beck Depression Inventory (Beck, 1975) and he falls within the normal range. Still, I have told him that I cannot assist him and that he must "discharge" me as his therapist if he decides to kill himself. I told him that if I believed he was going to end his life I would probably have to try to stop him.

In our last session he tells me that he plans to take the pills in several days because he can see no sense in draining his family's strength when he is going to die anyway. I review with him the reasons that he has made this decision, ask him to tell me about the part of him that wants to continue living, probe into the status of his will and medical power of attorney, and explore his reaction if he tried to die and ended up still alive. He tells me that the pain has not been too great since his doctor prescribed medicine. We spend lots of time reviewing his relationship with his mother and other family members. They are very supportive of him and have consistently encouraged him to fight his illness. He also explores his feelings about being a burden to them. He knows that their financial and emotional resources are pretty low, and to some extent he does want to spare them additional distress. Mostly he says that he feels like his time has come, that he has had a rich experience and can see no purpose in the kind of emotional suffering that is ahead. He says he wants to die when he is conscious and still has his dignity. He agrees to think about all the things we have discussed, and we make an appointment for later in the week. I leave the session convinced that he is ready to die and that from a medical perspective the outlook is for a fairly rapid decline that will leave him bedridden and totally dependent on others. I have met with Phil's mother at the hospital on several occasions, and I told Phil and his mother that I would be available in the event of an emergency.

Two days later Phil's mother calls and asks me to come to the home to talk about Phil's plan to take his life. On the telephone she seems supportive of his plan, but she wants to be sure they have thought of "everything." I am distressed by Phil's suffering and agree to meet with them and to see if I can help. When I visit with the two of them I assist them in clarifying the decision and attempt to provide as much support as possible. Phil is in a great deal of pain, his body has deteriorated, and his mother is afraid that she will not be able to provide the kind of care he needs. She is not able to leave her job and knows that he cannot be left alone. They have met with a hospice worker but do not qualify for services because there is no one at home with Phil during the day. There was a chance an uncle would be willing to come over every day, but when the time came for him to make a commitment, he backed out. She and Phil first talked about the possibility of suicide 5 years ago when he was very sick. Since then the subject has come up from time to time, and his mother has consulted with other family members about this possibility. She seems comfortable about what he wants to do, and she is willing to assist him as he dies.

We talk about our experiences watching others die, and both his mother and I assure him that we are willing to be with him to the end if that is what he wants. I have seen many clients think that suicide is the best alternative and then change their minds as death approached, and I know that life ends differently for each person. Watching someone die is never easy, but knowing that the individual's wishes have been honored has given me a sense of peace in many tough moments. Still I am not sure I feel totally comfortable with my level of risk. Suppose he fails and ends up in the hospital? Suppose he tells others that I agreed with him or even that I did not challenge him? Maybe more medical information would help, or maybe a new treatment will come along. At the same time I have watched him suffer, and I have seen many die in terrible situations. He does not seem depressed, but he may simply be in a temporary slump.

I leave the session with an understanding that no decision has been made. Phil and his mother have agreed to let me think about alternatives before we meet again.

PAUSE AND IDENTIFY YOUR PERSONAL RESPONSES TO THE CASE

As I walk away from Phil's house I feel very conflicted. I worry over his suffering and feel helpless to do anything about it. I am sad that he seems to be getting closer to death, but I also am keenly aware of the strength and many insights I have gained from knowing him. I am anxious that I could be liable if he did try to take his life and either succeeded or failed. I do not think he is acting out of depression, but I am not sure. Typically when there has been a setback he talks easily about being sad but he fairly quickly reorients himself and moves forward. I personally believe that his life is his own and that he deserves the right to make a decision about living or dying. He has done a great job of inspiring others and in taking care of their complaints. He is not so comfortable being needy himself.

REVIEW THE FACTS OF THE CASE

The facts are not altogether clear in this situation. Phil is deteriorating and his physician has told him there is no further treatment available. He is bedridden, and there is no one at home to assist in his care on an ongoing basis. The Beck Depression Inventory did not indicate significant depression but that may have changed recently. Phil does have a supply of pills that may or may not bring about his death. His mother is aware of his thinking and seems to be supportive. As far as I know his physician has not been consulted, nor do other family members know what is being considered. Phil is capable of taking his stash of pills at any time.

CONCEPTUALIZE AN INITIAL PLAN
BASED ON CLINICAL ISSUES

Phil, his mother, and I assemble a team of his support system: his physician, a consulting psychologist, and his older brother. At this meeting we review all aspects of his situation. The physician says that there is nothing else she can do for him and that death could come at any time. The psychologist administers several assessment instruments and reports that Phil is not suffering from dementia or even excessive depression. His mother and his brother agree to support him in whatever he wants to do. The physician gives Phil a new prescription that will relieve his pain but could also be used by Phil to end his life.

Phil indicates that he is ready to end his life but he assures me that he will not act on that desire, at least until after our next appointment one week from now. It was agreed that during the intervening week he would assess whether the new medication reduces his suffering, and I will consult with knowledgeable colleagues about how best to proceed.

CONSULT THE ETHICS CODE AND ASSESS THE ETHICAL ISSUES (BY KAREN STROHM KITCHENER)

When a client like Phil expresses the desire to end his life, many therapists presume that ethically they must intervene to attempt to prevent the suicide; however, the issue is more complicated than it initially appears, as Dr. Barret seems to understand. Historically, the decision to break confidentiality and intervene with a suicidal client was based on Christian doctrine that suicide is immoral and the belief that suicide is not a rational decision, and thus, could not be based on autonomous choice (Mayo, 1993). Since psychologists have begun to work with clients who have serious illnesses like AIDS, discussions of rational suicide have begun to appear in the psychological literature (Rogers & Britton, 1994; Smith, 1989; Snipe, 1988; Werth, 1992; Werth & Liddle, 1994). In fact, Werth and Liddle found that 80% of psychologists believed in rational suicide in some cases. In the following section, these issues are considered from the perspective of both the American Psychological Association (APA, 1992) Ethics Code and the foundational ethical principles. References to pertinent issues in other case histories are made for the reader's benefit.

APA Ethics Code

Some psychologists may believe that the APA Ethics Code requires them to break confidentiality when clients become suicidal. Dr. Barret seems to imply this when he initially tells Phil that he may have to stop him from trying to end his life. Standard 5.05, Disclosures (the most relevant part of the code on this issue), permits psychologists to break confidentiality to protect the patient or client or others from harm when it is mandated or permitted by law. As noted in other cases, however, this standard grants permission for psychologists to break confidentiality when clients are at risk for harming themselves, but it does not require it (Canter, Bennett, Jones, & Nagy, 1994). On the other hand, many textbooks seem to presume that psychologists' primary responsibility is to prevent suicide at all costs. For example, Pope and Vasquez (1991) quoted a clinician as saying, "The overwhelming priority is to help the client stay alive" (p. 155). In addition, most clinicians have been trained to prevent suicide, and in most situations that is a sound ethical stance (Heyd & Bloch, 1981). However, Phil's case raises the question of whether the prevention of suicide is always the most ethical stance.

The majority of psychologists have little experience or training in considering the circumstances in which nonintervention with a suicidal client might be a reasonable alternative. The Ethics Code in Standard 1.04c, Boundaries of Competence, requires that when "generally recognized standards for preparatory training do not yet exist, psychologists nevertheless take reasonable steps to ensure the competence of their work and to protect patients, clients, . . . and others from harm." Being competent in working with Phil at this point in his HIV disease and particularly around an issue as sensitive as suicide is critical. The literature on suicide, AIDS, and rational suicide may not be an area with which the practitioner is familiar when in fact that literature may be useful to consider (see chapter 2 for a review). For example, suicidal ideation later in the disease process is often tied to despair, fear of dependency and physical deterioration, and observing the deaths of others who have AIDS (Kalichman & Sikkeman, 1994). Providing information on pain management and hospice care may give clients alternatives they have not considered (McIntosh, 1993).

Furthermore, several authors (APA, 1997; Siegel, 1986; Werth, 1995) have described criteria for rational suicide: The patient has made a realistic assessment of the situation, decision making is unimpaired by psychological illness, the decision is not coerced, the decision has been considered over an extended period of time, loved ones are involved in the decision, and the basis for the decision would be understandable to objective observers. Knowing these criteria could be very important in making the decision about whether to intervene in Phil's case. Furthermore, consulting with others who have worked with clients in the end stages of HIV disease may help evaluate the extent to which Phil's decision is substantially rational or is due to irrational beliefs about death, the extent to which it is based on accurate information, and so on.

In other words, Dr. Barret must ask whether he has provided competent services to Phil or whether he has reacted out of limited information and training with this population. In this case, Dr. Barret seems aware of his own limits. By consulting with others including Phil's physician, another psychologist, and Phil's support system, he can be more assured that his work with Phil has been adequate.

Standards 1.08, Human Differences, and 1.09, Respecting Others, are also relevant. They remind Dr. Barret to remain sensitive to ethnic and racial differences and to respect Phil's right and the rights of his family to hold values different from his own. In this case, Dr. Barret needs to ask whether his own cultural or religious values are interfering with his willingness to allow Phil to make a decision that is consistent with his own values.

The aspirational principles from the Ethics Code give little additional guidance. Principle E: Concern for Others' Welfare, reminds Dr. Barret to make Phil's welfare his primary concern and to minimize harm. Principle D: Respect for People's Rights and Dignity reminds him to respect Phil's rights to privacy, confidentiality, self-determination, and autonomy. Issues of autonomy are addressed in the next section.

Foundational Ethical Principles

The issue of whether Phil's decision is autonomous seems paramount because strong ethical arguments can be made that breaking confidentiality is warranted if his decision is not autonomous. As noted in prior cases and in chapter 3, an autonomous choice has three characteristics: It must be intentional, it must be based on adequate understanding of the issues involved, and it must not result from controlling influences (Beauchamp & Childress, 1989). Understanding involves both adequate knowledge and the competence to process it. The autonomy of decision making is at the core of the criteria for rational suicide described above. It should be noted that at least one physician has contended that all suicides, even with patients who are in the end phases of HIV disease, are a result of mental disorders and are substantially nonrational (Glass, 1988). On the other hand, Phil's pain is now being treated, he has considered the decision over several months, he has discussed the decision with his mother and his brother, and Dr. Barret has helped him explore the reasons to continue to live. Furthermore, Dr. Barret has involved another psychologist to help evaluate the extent to which Phil's decision may be the result of a mental disorder. The psychologist concluded that Phil is not suffering from dementia or extreme depression. These facts argue for Phil's competence to choose.

The other question that needs to be answered involves whether his decision is based on adequate knowledge. The facts of the case seem to support the belief that Phil has little time left to live, he has exhausted medical resources, and he has few alternatives. Because the decision has been discussed with his physician and Dr. Barret, they have considered alternatives like hospice care. Consequently, assuming that his choice to commit suicide is rational, the principle of autonomy would suggest that Dr. Barret would be ethically justified to allow Phil to take his own life. Werth (1992) further suggested that practitioners should help clients to explore suicide as a real and viable option. According to Faberman (1997), psychologists should not try to control the decision in cases like Phil's in which a client may seek to hasten his own death, but they should help ensure that the patient is free of pain and that the decision is rational, well reasoned, and voluntary. In this case, it does not appear that Phil's decision is being coerced by any one in his support system or by medical professionals.

Beauchamp and Childress (1989) suggested differentiating between assisting suicide and nonintervention or allowing suicide to occur. Assisting suicide typically includes helping the person make the decision or actually carrying out the decision. (Assisting in a suicide has legal implications that are discussed below.) Nonintervention implies that the therapist takes no active role in the suicide or suicide decision but does not attempt to stop the client even when there is a high probability that a suicide will occur. In Phil's case, Dr. Barret would be choosing not to intervene. If he decides not to intervene, Dr. Barret is implicitly placing a higher value on allowing the client to decide what is in his best interests and on the quality of life than he chooses to live than on the value of life in and of itself. If he makes this decision, others may strongly disagree and may pursue their disagreement through legal channels such as malpractice suits, although that seems un-likely in Phil's case.

The principles of beneficence and do no harm (as well as Standard 1.14, Avoiding Harm) are difficult to apply in Phil's case because it is unclear whether a greater harm or benefit would occur if Dr. Barret allowed Phil to die or if he intervened. An intervention might involve forcibly hospitalizing Phil, removing him from his family, and taking away from him the little control he has over his life. On the other hand, it might also allow him to share a few more moments of joy and sorrow with his family. Choosing to hospitalize Phil would be strongly paternalistic, and it would be hard to rationalize in light of Phil's apparently rational manner and his ability to make his own decisions.

The foundational principle of fidelity should remind Dr. Barret of the importance of remaining trustworthy and fulfilling his promises. It appears that Phil considers him to be so because he shares with him his plan to take his own life. Dr. Barret again needs to consider the impact on his client if he chooses to break that trust and breach confidentiality.

Last, the foundational principle of justice should lead Dr. Barret to examine whether Phil's poverty (his only source of income is Supplemental Security Income) and African American ethnicity may be influencing his decision. Would he fight this decision more if Phil were White and middle class? Sometimes health care professionals may not treat those who are poor with the same assumptions and respect as they do others who are more affluent. Particularly in a case that involves life-and-death decisions, Dr. Barret must carefully evaluate whether his treatment is unfairly biased by inaccurate assumptions about clients who are poor and African American.

Balancing the Code and Foundational Ethical Principles

Dr. Barret may be making one of the most difficult decisions with which he will ever be faced because he may be allowing a human being to end his own life. He will feel the loss, as will Phil's mother and brother, but these feelings and values must be balanced with respect for Phil's right to exercise some control over how his life ends and the potential conse-quences to Phil if he intervenes. In considering his role, Dr. Barret must first ask to what extent he is competent to work with clients like Phil and whether he has been trained to evaluate Phil's competence in decision making. In this case, he has reinforced his own observations regarding Phil's competence by engaging another psychologist to help evaluate Phil. Furthermore, he must decide whether to break confidentiality and intervene against Phil's will. Part of this decision should be based on an evaluation of whether Phil's decision is rational and accurately informed. In this case, using the criteria for rational suicide described above, it appears that it is. He also needs to balance his own values regarding the sanctity of life with Phil's values and consider how stereotypes and biases might be influencing his decision. Last, he must consider the harm and benefits that might occur if he intervenes or if he does not. As in the other cases, meeting Phil with care and compassion may help guide his decisions and be his ultimate gift to Phil. If Dr. Barret decides not to intervene, he should, however, do so with the knowledge that others may strongly disagree with his decision.

IDENTIFY THE LEGAL ISSUES (BY SCOTT BURRIS)

Despite considerable public debate, helping a terminally ill person die remains a crime, at least on paper, almost everywhere in the United States (see chapter 6, Table 6.4). Oregon is the only state that has a law explicitly authorizing and regulating physician-assisted suicide (*Lee v. Oregon*, 1997; The Oregon Death With Dignity Act, 1997). Forty-six states, the District of Columbia, and the territories of Puerto Rico and the Virgin Islands have statutes or court decisions making it a crime to assist in a suicide (*Compassion in Dying v. Washington*, 1996; *Washington v. Glucksberg*, 1997). California has one of the broader provisions: "Every person who deliberately aids, or advises, or encourages another person to commit suicide is guilty of a felony" (Cal. Penal Code, 1998). In two 1997 decisions, the U. S. Supreme Court upheld the authority of states to prohibit assisting a suicide (*Vacco v. Quill*, 1997; *Washington v. Glucksberg*, 1997).

Dr. Jack Kevorkian notwithstanding, these laws are rarely applied and virtually are never used against health care providers practicing discreet euthanasia at the end of a terminal course of disease. In fact, perhaps as many as 6% of U.S. physicians have complied at least once with a patient's request for help in dying (Meier et al., 1998). The few reported cases of prosecution have involved lay defendants who supplied the means of death or who reneged on their side of a suicide pact. In theory, however, a phrase like California's "aids, or advises, or encourages another to commit suicide" could encompass anything from injecting a fatal drug to advising a patient on the best drug to use to supportively counseling a terminally ill patient struggling with the suicide decision. The breadth of these statutes is actually not unusual. Many criminal laws are broadly phrased. Their application is limited in practice by prosecutorial discretion in selecting what cases to pursue.

How might the facts in Phil's case look to a prosecutor? The patient has accumulated a store of pills sufficient to cause death by overdose, but the pills were prescribed by Phil's physician, not Dr. Barret. In the course of his ongoing therapy, Phil has discussed suicide and told Dr. Barret that he plans to use the pills in the very near future, and Dr. Barret has facilitated Phil and his mother in discussing Phil's decision and how to implement it. However, Dr. Barret appears to be certain that Phil will not act immediately, and he has made an appointment for the next visit. Although he believes that Phil is quite ill, Dr. Barret believes that Phil is not in pain and not depressed or otherwise cognitively impaired.

If Phil commits suicide, Dr. Barret's conduct could support a criminal charge only under an extremely broad reading of an assisted suicide law, under which even discussing a patient's thoughts of suicide in a nonjudgmental way is deemed to be "advising" or "aiding." That is a stretch even for the most zealous prosecutor. In some jurisdictions, the case would have to be presented to a grand jury—the body of citizens that supposedly screens criminal charges—and it would have to indict Dr. Barret. Prosecutors usually secure the indictments they want, but a case like this could easily be the exception if the grand jurors sympathized with Dr. Barret or were ambivalent about prosecuting people for helping patients die with dignity. If Dr. Barret were indicted or charged, his lawyer would be able to make very strong arguments to the judge that the prosecutor's interpretation of the statute was far too loose and that some acts beyond words of advice are required before there can be a crime (*In re* Joseph, 1983).

The simplest reason that a prosecutor would never bring such a charge, and a jury would never convict on it, is that Dr. Barret obviously was not trying to help Phil die, but merely, as a therapist, helping Phil and his mother deal with their own feelings and choices. He could not be certain that the talk would lead to action and certainly did not intend his therapeutic assistance to "help" nudge Phil into action. Most prosecutors would be cautious for another reason, too: The morality of assisted suicide is a matter of great social dispute. For a prosecutor, staking out a high-profile position on an issue like this can be a good way to make a name, and a good way to make your name "Mudd." Because this is an important moral and social issue, Dr. Barret may wish to consider whether the chances of being prosecuted, whatever they are, even matter to him.

I have elaborated on the assisted suicide issue because it has been very significant in law and public policy debates in the past few years, and it regularly arises in HIV care. I hope I can make clear to Dr. Barret how low his legal risk is. I do think he may have some legal risk in this case, but that risk comes from letting the drama of the assisted suicide question obscure a much more pressing legal consideration. It is generally the duty of therapists to detect and treat suicidal intentions (*Bellah v. Greenson*, 1978). By helping Phil to "work through" his decision, Dr. Barret exposes himself to any change of heart or mind his mother might have after the event. If she regrets her decision—perhaps out of guilt that her inability to care for Phil hastened his end—she might turn on Dr. Barret, arguing that he breached his professional duty to Phil when he failed to intervene to prevent him from committing suicide. Dr. Barret needs to be sure that his own feelings are not obscuring his assessment of Phil's mental state. This requires him to face the basic question he seems to be struggling with: whether a patient may "rationally" commit suicide under some circumstances, or whether considering suicide is always a symptom of mental illness. If his professional judgment leans toward the latter view, then by his own standards he would be committing malpractice if he did not intervene. If, however, he believes that Phil is not mentally ill, despite his consideration of suicide, then Dr. Barret needs to be sure he can justify his professional judgment and conduct in the probably unlikely event that Phil's mother were to sue.

IDENTIFY AND ASSESS THE OPTIONS (BY BOB BARRET)

This consultation has been helpful, but at this moment I do not like being on the cutting edge of the profession. I know that I have taken a big risk and feel anxious moving forward. Although the risk of being sued may not exist, I am not sure that a licensing board would support my decisions. Some states have had extensive discussions about the legal right to death, but attitudes where I live are very traditional. I may understand these issues, but others probably have made a decision based on traditional values without having been confronted with complex ambiguous situations and flesh-and-blood examples such as Phil's in their own personal and professional lives. No court cases back me up, and the standard of care in such situations is not clear. I do not relish the idea of waking up to a newspaper story that announces I have lost my license to practice. Mr. Burris encourages me by pointing out that my risk of legal charges is low but also warns me that I must consider my ability to justify my professional judgment and conduct before a court of law. In the unlikely event that I might be charged I am aware from both consultants' comments that there is a growing body of literature that supports my decision and that I have taken sound steps to validate my competence by having others evaluate Phil.

When I first started working with clients with HIV disease I knew that situations like this one would eventually come up. There had been a couple of times in the past when clients talked about suicide. But in each instance their death came before they were able to act. These encounters had led me to an intense reflection on what I would do when finally faced with this dilemma. The conclusion of that thinking was that I do believe a person facing death has the right to find the potential for choice as death approaches. Of course, what is difficult is that people with AIDS, like those with cancer, can be extremely ill one day and bounce back to better health fairly quickly. Over the years I have seen many die painful and terrible deaths that seemed deprived of all dignity. I learned that I did not want to ever be in that situation, and I decided that I would not step into another's death with a kind of self-righteousness, at least not without much thought. So, I guess I was somewhat prepared as Phil talked about dying. I know that some physicians have assisted some of their patients when this decision was being made. My value of individual autonomy underlies each step in my interactions with Phil.

Dr. Kitchener's comments are helpful. She raises the issue of my competence and then points out that the consultations support me throughout this process. She also reminds me that I am not really helping Phil die because I chose a role of nonintervention. I am also encouraged by her comments that I am not required by the Ethics Code to break confidentiality. Phil, his mother, and I have talked about hospice care as well as the issues related to pain management. For them, the issue is not pain or even the presence of a care-giving professional. Phil is tired of fighting this illness, and his medical team does not offer hope that he will ever return to reasonable health. He is ready to die, and his mother understands and supports him.

I reflect on the issue Dr. Kitchener raises about the influence of my own cultural and religious values. I know where I stand on this issue in my personal life, and I do not believe I am projecting my personal beliefs onto Phil. His race and economic status are different from mine, but I cannot see that I am either making a negative judgment about the value of his life as a result of those differences. One of the most important aspects of my relationship with Phil has been my respect for the way he has lived his life, his courage and willingness to use himself as an example for others. Over and over I have learned from him, and his death will be a loss on a personal level. At the same time, I respect his autonomy and want him to make the decisions that are best for him.

My options seem clear. I can honor my relationship with Phil by letting him have this final autonomous act. I could accept his decision at our next meeting and hope that there are no negative repercussions. Or, I can call an ambulance and have him admitted to the hospital because he is suicidal. In the end, it comes down to an either–or situation, and I have to make a decision alone and be willing to accept the consequences. I know that I am afraid to just let him die. I worry that I will feel responsible for his death and that I might become unwilling to continue working with persons with HIV. What will happen if he does take the pills and ends up alive but more seriously impaired? What would be my responsibility then?

When I sit down and quietly review the entire situation I can see that the five foundational principles do form a basis for my action. Letting Phil make his own decision clearly respects his autonomy. He is not unduly depressed, nor is he suffering from pain or any mental impairment. The challenge is trying to sort out my beliefs about his right to determine when and how he will die. From my experience with HIV I know that some patients approach death yet often recover and have months or even years of rich life experience. How can I be sure that Phil is right when he believes he is near death this time? On the other hand, cannot I trust him to make that decision? I want him to be in charge as long as possible. And I can see that both Phil and his family have reached the point that they are ready for his death. The principles of beneficence and fidelity also support Phil's making this decision on his own. After a life of so much service to others, Phil deserves the opportunity to die with the kind of dignity he chooses. His physician has indicated that death is near, and both Phil and his family seem ready for the next step. Stopping Phil clearly does not seem benevolent and may add distress to his last days. For Phil to reexperience helplessness and anger during the short time he has left seems cruel. He has the right to the principal role in this decision. So far, so good.

But when I get to the principles of justice and do no harm, I am troubled. I suppose these principles would become important in a legal proceeding, but what about in a hearing before the Board of Psychology? I can state my belief that letting Phil decide to take his life does him no harm. As a matter of fact, stopping him from ending his life could be seen as doing harm to him. And I can also justify my decision on the basis of the principle of justice. I review once again the steps I have taken and remind myself that there is a community of physicians and psychologists who would support my decision and my decision-making process. I am pretty clear that letting Phil be in charge of this decision is appropriate, both legally and ethically. I know that no matter what I do I will have to live with the discomfort.

I also look in the literature to see what the so-called experts in assisted suicide think. Relying on discussions by lawmakers, ethicists, and other mental health professionals, I can see that some would reason differently than I but that there is a significant amount of support for the notion of rational suicide. As I think about acting in my client's best interest I can see that letting him make these decisions with his family seems justifiable ethically and legally.

CHOOSE A COURSE OF ACTION AND
SHARE IT WITH YOUR CLIENT

Soon thereafter, I receive another call from Phil and quickly agree to see him sooner than planned. I am not sure why he called, and I go to see him without hesitation. Although I am aware that we had decided to wait a week for our next appointment, I am just not able to "be too busy" to see him. When I arrive he is home alone. He has deteriorated more but is still able to interact with me and speak with great clarity. He tells me that he is going to take his pills the next day and that he does not intend to share this information with his mother. A social worker is due to make a home visit before his mother comes home. She will find him and do whatever is necessary so his mother would not have to find him dead. He tells me how much he appreciates my support and how much strength he has found in our relationship. Both of us cry as we say goodbye, and I leave knowing I will not see him alive again.

IMPLEMENT THE COURSE OF ACTION:
MONITOR AND ASSESS OUTCOMES

I review my basic assumptions about Phil and his right to determine the way his life ends and decide to leave him to die in peace. I do not call his mother, nor do I alert his physician. Instead I go home and attend to the daily routines of my life, all the while holding Phil near my heart. The next evening Phil's mother calls to tell me that he has died and expresses her gratitude for my assistance during this difficult time. In the following days I visit with his family and feel a kind of bonding and love that is mutually supportive to us in our grief. Phil's family knew that his life had much more meaning than his death and were grateful to Phil for sparing them a prolonged struggle as he died. I carefully document the steps I took in these final sessions with Phil.

I still review this situation from time to time. Was I right in not stopping Phil? I have seen many people with HIV die in agony. That Phil was able to die when he wanted to and in peace is a relief to me. I know that my actions had integrity about them, that my wishes for Phil and his family were noble, and that Phil was grateful that he was able to talk with me about his wishes in the safety of our mutual respect. Would others do what I did? I'll never know the answers to that, nor do I feel the need to expose myself to unnecessary criticism. My decision to write about this case is risky. I decided that it is worth it because I know that others are struggling as I am and I hope that my decision-making process is helpful to them even if they come to decisions that are different from my own.

Having said that, as this book goes to press I am aware that new medications that bring people back from the brink of death may change future decisions. It is one thing to have acted as I did when there was no hope; another decision might be dictated in light of the availability of a wonder drug appearing during a client's struggle with this kind of decision. Over the course of my career as a psychologist I have learned that tolerance of ambiguity is necessary to survive professionally. With clients with terminal illnesses, this ambiguity is amplified. My hope is that by reading about my experience, others will be better able to face such challenges in their work and remain alive and vital professionally and personally, as I have, despite the inherent stress and grief involved in this kind of work.

REFERENCES

American Psychological Association. (1992). Ethical principles of psychologists and code of conduct. *American Psychologist, 47,* 1597–1611.

Beauchamp, T., & Childress, J. (1989). *The principles of biomedical ethics.* Oxford, England: Oxford University Press

Beck, A. T. (1975). *Depression: Causes and treatment.* Philadelphia: University of Pennsylvania Press.

Bellah v. Greenson, 146 Cal. Rptr. 535 (Cal. Ct. App. 1978).

CAL. PENAL CODE § 401 (1998).

Canter, M. B., Bennett, B. E., Jones, S. E., & Nagy, T. F. (1994). *Ethics for psychologists: A commentary on the APA Ethics Code.* Washington, DC: American Psychological Association.

Compassion in Dying v. Washington, 79 F.3d 790, 847 & nn. 10-13 (9th Cir. 1996) (Beezer, J. dissenting).

Faberman, R. K. (1997). Terminal illness and hastened death requests: The important role of the mental health professional. *Professional Psychology, Research and Practice, 28,* 544–547.

Glass, R. M. (1988). AIDS and suicide. *Journal of the American Medical Association, 259,* 1369–1370.

Heyd, D., & Block, S. (1981). The ethics of suicide. In S. Bloch & P. Chodoff (Eds.), *Psychiatric ethics* (pp. 185–202). Oxford, England: Oxford University Press.

In re *Joseph G.,* 34 Cal.3d 429 (1983).

Kalichman, S. C., & Sikkeman, K. J. (1994). Psychological sequella of HIV infection and AIDS: Review of empirical findings. *Clinical Psychology Review, 14,* 611–632.

Lee v. Oregon, 107 F.3d 1382 (9th Cir. 1997).

Mayo, D. (1993, August). *The case for rational suicide*. Paper presented at the 101st Annual Convention of the American Psychological Association, Toronto, Canada.

McIntosh, J. L. (1993, August). *Arguments against rational and assisted suicide*. Paper presented at the 101st Annual Convention of the American Psychological Association, Toronto, Canada.

Meier, D. E., Emmons, C. A., Wallenstein, S., Quill, T., Morrison, R. S., & Cassel, C. K. (1998). A national survey of physician-assisted suicide and euthanasia in the United States. *New England Journal of Medicine, 338*, 1193–1201.

The Oregon Death With Dignity Act, OR. REV. STAT. § 127.800 et seq. (1997).

Pope, K. S., & Vasquez, M. J. T. (1991). *Ethics in psychotherapy and counseling*. San Francisco: Jossey-Bass.

Rogers, J. R., & Britton, P. J. (1994). AIDS and rational suicide: A counseling psychology perspective or a slide on a slippery slope. *The Counseling Psychologist, 22*, 171–178.

Siegel, K. (1986). Psychosocial aspects of rational suicide. *American Journal of Psychotherapy, 40*, 405–418.

Smith, K. (1989). AIDS suicide: Alternate choice or desperate acts? *AIDS Patient Care, 3*(4), 20–22.

Snipe, R. M. (1988). Ethical issues in the assessment and treatment of a rational suicide client. *The Counseling Psychologist, 16*, 128–138.

Vacco v. Quill, 117 S.Ct. 2293 (1997).

Washington v. Glucksberg, 117 S.Ct. 2258 (1997).

Werth, J. L., Jr. (1992). Rational suicide and AIDS: Considerations for the psychotherapist. *The Counseling Psychologist, 20*, 645–659.

Werth, J. L., Jr. (1995). Rational suicide reconsidered: AIDS as an impetus for change. *Death Studies, 19*, 65–80.

Werth, J. L., Jr., & Little, B. J. (1994). Psychotherapists' attitudes towards suicide. *Psychotherapy: Theory, Research, & Practice, 31*, 440–448.

EPILOGUE

It is our hope that the process of reading this book has been as interesting for you as creating it has been for us. Ethics is often one of those topics that receives a lot of attention during graduate studies and then fades to the background until therapists find themselves in a jam or are confronted with a situation with which they have no prior experience. Back in the early 1980s when HIV was just beginning to appear on the landscape, there were very few resources for the many HIV/AIDS practitioners who found themselves in situations with which they had no prior experience. Although there are now a number of good publications available for the HIV/AIDS mental health practitioner, this book provides a unique and substantial contribution to therapists working with people with HIV/AIDS and to therapists with more general concerns about the ethical and legal dimensions of psychotherapy.

Over the years, as the base of knowledge and experience in HIV-related psychotherapy has expanded, veteran HIV/AIDS therapists may experience some of the situations described in this book as rather routine. Disclosing a client's HIV status to his or her sex partners may not invoke the same level of anxiety that it once did, especially when health departments are now initiating programs to assess the feasibility of providing postexposure prophylaxis to exposed individuals (Katz & Gerberding, 1997). Now that the disease is more treatable and fewer people are dying, therapists may not be encountering the drama of end-of-life issues with quite the same force or frequency as they once did. Although the psychological and psychosocial issues of people living with HIV/AIDS are clearly changing, the fact that

315

HIV/AIDS mental health providers must face unprecedented dilemmas with their clients is not changing.

For example, in the months and years to come, HIV/AIDS mental health providers are likely to encounter a new substatus among people living with HIV—those who claim to be HIV infected but noninfectious or "HIV neutral." In the past, this type of proclamation would be readily dismissed as nonsensical and dangerous. However, research showing that combination therapies are associated with reductions in viral load in semen (Vernazza et al., 1997) are beginning to lend some credence to such assertions. Although at present the associations between viral load and infectivity are unclear and providers should continue to emphasize prevention through safer sex and drug use practices (Ostrow & Kalichman, 1999), it is conceivable that this situation may change in the not-too-distant future. If future studies confirm a stable relationship between viral load and infectivity, mental health providers will undoubtedly face many more clients who believe that there is no reason to worry about transmission as long as they take their combination therapies as directed and maintain an undetectable viral load. If this happens, HIV/AIDS providers will again find themselves in uncharted waters seeking strategies for ethical ways in which to respond to their clients and the people who interact with them.

The question of infectivity is not the only "thorny dilemma" on the horizon for HIV/AIDS mental health providers. The time to initiate anti-HIV combination therapies is also a point of considerable controversy (Kalichman & Ramachandran, 1999). Starting early may suppress the propagation of mutant strains of HIV that will ultimately undermine treatment. Slowing the early progress of HIV may therefore alter the course of infection. On the other hand, the effects of combination therapies may diminish over time, with risks for nonadherence, treatment resistance, and cross-resistance increasing and potentially restricting later treatment options. Concerns about the long-term use of combination therapies lead some people to delay starting combination therapies until later in infection. Others think that it is silly to wait. Decisions about when to begin treatment are made in a constantly changing environment that produces high levels of stress and uncertainty for HIV/AIDS clients. As has been the case for nearly two decades, these clients will look to HIV/AIDS mental health providers for guidance and support.

As HIV/AIDS mental health providers struggle to deliver that guidance and support during the next phase of the epidemic, we hope that the experience and wisdom contained in this book will serve as both a practical professional resource and a personal comfort. For most of us, it helps to remember the struggles of those who came before us. As Heitman and Ross (1999) pointed out:

AIDS and its treatment have continually reminded us of the importance of human presence and support in illness, even when no effective therapy is possible. This valuable lesson has come at a high price and should remain the centerpiece of the ethics of HIV care, even as we work to interpret and apply the therapeutic breakthroughs of combination therapy. (p. 132)

REFERENCES

Heitman, E., & Ross, M. W. (1999). Ethical issues in the use of new treatments of HIV. In D. Ostrow & S. Kalichman (Eds.), *Psychosocial and public health impacts of new HIV therapies* (pp. 113–132). New York: Kluwer Academic/Plenum Press.

Kalichman, S. C., & Ramachandran, B. (1999). Mental health implications of new HIV treatments. In D. Ostrow & S. Kalichman (Eds.), *Psychosocial and public health impacts of new HIV therapies* (pp. 137–149). New York: Kluwer Academic/Plenum Press.

Katz, M. H., & Gerberding, J. L. (1997). Post-exposure treatment of people exposed to the human immunodeficiency virus through sexual contact or injection-drug use. *New England Journal of Medicine, 336,* 1097–1100.

Ostrow, D. G., & Kalichman, S. C. (Eds.). (1999). *Psychosocial and public health impacts of new HIV therapies.* New York: Kluwer Academic/Plenum Press.

Vernazza, P. L., Gillian, B., Dyer, M., Fiscus, S., Eron, J., Frank, A., & Cohen, M. (1997). Quantification of HIV in semen: Correlation with antiretroviral treatment and immune status. *AIDS, 11,* 987–993.

APPENDIX:
AMERICAN PSYCHOLOGICAL ASSOCIATION ETHICAL PRINCIPLES OF PSYCHOLOGISTS AND CODE OF CONDUCT

Effective date December 1, 1992.

CONTENTS

1.06 Basis for Scientific and Professional Judgments
1.07 Describing the Nature and Results
of Psychological Services
1.08 Human Differences
1.09 Respecting Others
1.10 Nondiscrimination
1.11 Sexual Harassment
1.12 Other Harassment
1.13 Personal Problems and Conflicts
1.14 Avoiding Harm
1.15 Misuse of Psychologists' Influence
1.16 Misuse of Psychologists' Work
1.17 Multiple Relationships
1.18 Barter (With Patients or Clients)
1.19 Exploitative Relationships
1.20 Consultations and Referrals
1.21 Third-Party Requests for Services
1.22 Delegation to and Supervision of Subordinates
1.23 Documentation of Professional and Scientific Work
1.24 Records and Data
1.25 Fees and Financial Arrangements
1.26 Accuracy in Reports to Payors and Funding Sources
1.27 Referrals and Fees

2. Evaluation, Assessment, or Intervention

2.01 Evaluation, Diagnosis, and Interventions
in Professional Context
2.02 Competence and Appropriate Use of
Assessments and Interventions
2.03 Test Construction
2.04 Use of Assessment in General and With
Special Populations
2.05 Interpreting Assessment Results
2.06 Unqualified Persons
2.07 Obsolete Tests and Outdated Test Results
2.08 Test Scoring and Interpretation Services
2.09 Explaining Assessment Results
2.10 Maintaining Test Security

3. Advertising and Other Public Statements

3.01 Definition of Public Statements
3.02 Statements by Others

INTRODUCTION

The American Psychological Association's (APA's) Ethical Principles of Psychologists and Code of Conduct (hereinafter referred to as the Ethics Code) consists of an Introduction, a Preamble, six General Principles (A–F), and specific Ethical Standards. The Introduction discusses the intent, organization, procedural considerations, and scope of application of the Ethics Code. The Preamble and General Principles are *aspirational* goals to guide psychologists toward the highest ideals of psychology. Although the Preamble and General Principles are not themselves enforceable rules, they should be considered by psychologists in arriving at an ethical course of action and may be considered by ethics bodies in interpreting the Ethical Standards. The Ethical Standards set forth *enforceable* rules for conduct as psychologists. Most of the Ethical Standards are written broadly, in order to apply to psychologists in varied roles, although the application of an Ethical Standard may vary depending on the context. The Ethical Standards are not exhaustive. The fact that a given conduct is not specifically addressed by the Ethics Code does not mean that it is necessarily either ethical or unethical.

Membership in the APA commits members to adhere to the APA Ethics Code and to the rules and procedures used to implement it. Psychologists and students, whether or not they are APA members, should be aware that the Ethics Code may be applied to them by state psychology boards, courts, or other public bodies.

This Ethics Code applies only to psychologists' work-related activities, that is, activities that are part of the psychologists' scientific and professional functions or that are psychological in nature. It includes the clinical or counseling practice of psychology, research, teaching, supervision of trainees, development of assessment instruments, conducting assessments, educational counseling, organizational consulting, social intervention, administration, and other activities as well. These work-related activities can be distinguished from the purely private conduct of a psychologist, which ordinarily is not within the purview of the Ethics Code.

The Ethics Code is intended to provide standards of professional conduct that can be applied by the APA and by other bodies that choose to adopt them. Whether or not a psychologist has violated the Ethics Code does not by itself determine whether he or she is legally liable in a court action, whether a contract is enforceable, or whether other legal consequences occur. These results are based on legal rather than ethical rules. However, compliance with or violation of the Ethics Code may be admissible as evidence in some legal proceedings, depending on the circumstances.

In the process of making decisions regarding their professional behavior, psychologists must consider this Ethics Code, in addition to applicable laws and psychology board regulations. If the Ethics Code establishes a higher standard of conduct than is required by law, psychologists must meet the higher ethical standard. If the Ethics Code standard appears to conflict with the requirements of law, then psychologists make known their commitment to the Ethics Code and take steps to resolve the conflict in a responsible manner. If neither law nor the Ethics Code resolves an issue, psychologists should consider other professional materials[1] and the dictates of their own conscience, as well as seek consultation with others within the field when this is practical.

The procedures for filing, investigating, and resolving complaints of unethical conduct are described in the current Rules and Procedures of the APA Ethics Committee. The actions that APA may take for violations of the Ethics Code include actions such as reprimand, censure, termination of APA membership, and referral of the matter to other bodies. Complainants who seek remedies such as monetary damages in alleging ethical violations by a psychologist must resort to private negotiation, administrative bodies, or the courts. Actions that violate the Ethics Code may lead to the imposition of sanctions on a psychologist by bodies other than APA, including state psychological associations, other professional groups, psychology boards, other state or federal agencies, and payors for health services. In addition to actions for violation of the Ethics Code, the APA Bylaws provide that APA may take action against a member after his or her conviction of a felony, expulsion or suspension from an affiliated state psychological association, or suspension or loss of licensure.

PREAMBLE

Psychologists work to develop a valid and reliable body of scientific knowledge based on research. They may apply that knowledge to human behavior in a variety of contexts. In doing so, they perform many roles, such as researcher, educator, diagnostician, therapist, supervisor, consultant, administrator, social interventionist, and expert witness. Their goal is to broaden knowledge of behavior and, where appropriate, to apply it pragmatically to improve the condition of both the individual and society. Psychologists respect the central importance of freedom of inquiry and expression in research, teaching, and publication. They also strive to help the public

---

[1] Professional materials that are most helpful in this regard are guidelines and standards that have been adopted or endorsed by professional psychological organizations. Such guidelines and standards, whether adopted by the American Psychological Association (APA) or its Divisions, are not enforceable as such by this Ethics Code, but are of educative value to psychologists, courts, and professional bodies. Such materials include, but are not limited to, the APA's *General Guidelines for Providers of Psychological Services* (1987), *Specialty Guidelines for the Delivery of Services by Clinical Psychologists, Counseling Psychologists, Industrial/Organizational Psychologists, and School Psychologists* (1981), *Guidelines for Computer Based Tests and Interpretations* (1987), *Standards for Educational and Psychological Testing* (1985), *Ethical Principles in the Conduct of Research With Human Participants* (1982), *Guidelines for Ethical Conduct in the Care and Use of Animals* (1986), *Guidelines for Providers of Psychological Services to Ethnic, Linguistic, and Culturally Diverse Populations* (1990), and *Publication Manual of the American Psychological Association* (3rd ed., 1983). Materials not adopted by APA as a whole include the APA Division 41 (Forensic Psychology)/American Psychology–Law Society's *Specialty Guidelines for Forensic Psychologists* (1991).

in developing informed judgments and choices concerning human behavior. This Ethics Code provides a common set of values upon which psychologists build their professional and scientific work.

This Code is intended to provide both the general principles and the decision rules to cover most situations encountered by psychologists. It has as its primary goal the welfare and protection of the individuals and groups with whom psychologists work. It is the individual responsibility of each psychologist to aspire to the highest possible standards of conduct. Psychologists respect and protect human and civil rights, and do not knowingly participate in or condone unfair discriminatory practices.

The development of a dynamic set of ethical standards for a psychologist's work-related conduct requires a personal commitment to a lifelong effort to act ethically; to encourage ethical behavior by students, supervisees, employees, and colleagues, as appropriate; and to consult with others, as needed, concerning ethical problems. Each psychologist supplements, but does not violate, the Ethics Code's values and rules on the basis of guidance drawn from personal values, culture, and experience.

GENERAL PRINCIPLES

Principle A: Competence

Psychologists strive to maintain high standards of competence in their work. They recognize the boundaries of their particular competencies and the limitations of their expertise. They provide only those services and use only those techniques for which they are qualified by education, training, or experience. Psychologists are cognizant of the fact that the competencies required in serving, teaching, and/or studying groups of people vary with the distinctive characteristics of those groups. In those areas in which recognized professional standards do not yet exist, psychologists exercise careful judgment and take appropriate precautions to protect the welfare of those with whom they work. They maintain knowledge of relevant scientific and professional information related to the services they render, and they recognize the need for ongoing education. Psychologists make appropriate use of scientific, professional, technical, and administrative resources.

Principle B: Integrity

Psychologists seek to promote integrity in the science, teaching, and practice of psychology. In these activities psychologists are honest, fair, and respectful of others. In describing or reporting their qualifications, services, products, fees, research, or teaching, they do not make statements that are false, misleading, or deceptive. Psychologists strive to be aware of their own belief systems, values, needs, and limitations and the effect of these on their work. To the extent feasible, they attempt to clarify for relevant parties the roles they are performing and to function appropriately in accordance with those roles. Psychologists avoid improper and potentially harmful dual relationships.

Principle C: Professional and Scientific Responsibility

Psychologists uphold professional standards of conduct, clarify their professional roles and obligations, accept appropriate responsibility for their behavior, and adapt their methods to the needs of different populations. Psychologists consult with, refer to, or cooperate with other professionals and institutions to the extent needed to serve the best interests of their patients, clients, or other recipients of their services. Psychologists' moral standards and conduct are personal matters to the same degree as is true for any other person, except as psychologists' conduct may compromise their professional responsibilities or reduce the public's trust in psychology and psychologists. Psychologists are concerned about the ethical compliance of their colleagues' scientific and professional conduct. When appropriate, they consult with colleagues in order to prevent or avoid unethical conduct.

Principle D: Respect for People's Rights and Dignity

Psychologists accord appropriate respect to the fundamental rights, dignity, and worth of all people. They respect the rights of individuals to privacy, confidentiality, self-determination, and autonomy, mindful that legal and other obligations may lead to inconsistency and conflict with the exercise of these rights. Psychologists are aware of cultural, individual, and role differences, including those due to age, gender, race, ethnicity, national origin, religion, sexual orientation, disability, language, and socioeconomic status. Psychologists try to eliminate the effect on their work of biases based on those factors, and they do not knowingly participate in or condone unfair discriminatory practices.

Principle E: Concern for Others' Welfare

Psychologists seek to contribute to the welfare of those with whom they interact professionally. In their professional actions, psychologists weigh the welfare and rights of their patients or clients, students, supervisees, human research participants, and other affected persons, and the welfare of animal subjects of research. When conflicts occur among psychologists' obligations or concerns, they attempt to resolve these conflicts and to perform their roles in a responsible fashion that avoids or minimizes harm. Psychologists are sensitive to real and ascribed differences in power between themselves and others, and they do not exploit or mislead other people during or after professional relationships.

Principle F: Social Responsibility

Psychologists are aware of their professional and scientific responsibilities to the community and the society in which they work and live. They apply and make public their knowledge of psychology in order to contribute to human welfare. Psychologists are concerned about and work to mitigate the causes of human suffering. When undertaking research, they strive to advance human welfare and the science of psychology. Psychologists try to avoid misuse of their work. Psychologists comply with the law and encourage the development of law and social policy that serve the interests of their patients and clients and the public. They are encouraged to contribute a portion of their professional time for little or no personal advantage.

ETHICAL STANDARDS

1. General Standards

These General Standards are potentially applicable to the professional and scientific activities of all psychologists.

1.01 Applicability of the Ethics Code

The activity of a psychologist subject to the Ethics Code may be reviewed under these Ethical Standards only if the activity is part of his or her work-related functions or the activity is psychological in nature. Personal activities having no connection to or effect on psychological roles are not subject to the Ethics Code.

1.02 Relationship of Ethics and Law

If psychologists' ethical responsibilities conflict with law, psychologists make known their commitment to the Ethics Code and take steps to resolve the conflict in a responsible manner.

1.03 Professional and Scientific Relationship

Psychologists provide diagnostic, therapeutic, teaching, research, supervisory, consultative, or other psychological services only in the context of a defined professional or scientific relationship or role. (See also Standards

2.01, Evaluation, Diagnosis, and Interventions in Professional Context, and 7.02, Forensic Assessments.)

1.04 Boundaries of Competence

(a) Psychologists provide services, teach, and conduct research only within the boundaries of their competence, based on their education, training, supervised experience, or appropriate professional experience.

(b) Psychologists provide services, teach, or conduct research in new areas or involving new techniques only after first undertaking appropriate study, training, supervision, and/or consultation from persons who are competent in those areas or techniques.

(c) In those emerging areas in which generally recognized standards for preparatory training do not yet exist, psychologists nevertheless take reasonable steps to ensure the competence of their work and to protect patients, clients, students, research participants, and others from harm.

1.05 Maintaining Expertise

Psychologists who engage in assessment, therapy, teaching, research, organizational consulting, or other professional activities maintain a reasonable level of awareness of current scientific and professional information in their fields of activity, and undertake ongoing efforts to maintain competence in the skills they use.

1.06 Basis for Scientific and Professional Judgments

Psychologists rely on scientifically and professionally derived knowledge when making scientific or professional judgments or when engaging in scholarly or professional endeavors.

1.07 Describing the Nature and Results of Psychological Services

(a) When psychologists provide assessment, evaluation, treatment, counseling, supervision, teaching, consultation, research, or other psychological services to an individual, a group, or an organization, they provide, using language that is reasonably understandable to the recipient of those services, appropriate information beforehand about the nature of such services and appropriate information later about results and conclusions. (See also Standard 2.09, Explaining Assessment Results.)

(b) If psychologists will be precluded by law or by organizational roles from providing such information to particular individuals or groups, they so inform those individuals or groups at the outset of the service.

1.08 Human Differences

Where differences of age, gender, race, ethnicity, national origin, religion, sexual orientation, disability, language, or socioeconomic status significantly affect psychologists' work concerning particular individuals or groups, psychologists obtain the training, experience, consultation, or supervision necessary to ensure the competence of their services, or they make appropriate referrals.

1.09 Respecting Others

In their work-related activities, psychologists respect the rights of others to hold values, attitudes, and opinions that differ from their own.

1.10 Nondiscrimination

In their work-related activities, psychologists do not engage in unfair discrimination based on age, gender, race, ethnicity, national origin, religion, sexual orientation, disability, socioeconomic status, or any basis proscribed by law.

1.11 Sexual Harassment

(a) Psychologists do not engage in sexual harassment. Sexual harassment is sexual solicitation, physical advances, or verbal or nonverbal conduct that is sexual in nature, that occurs in connection with the psychologist's activities or roles as a psychologist, and that either: (1) is unwelcome, is offensive, or creates a hostile workplace environment, and the psychologist knows or is told this; or (2) is sufficiently severe or intense to be abusive to a reasonable person in the context. Sexual harassment can consist of a single intense or severe act or of multiple persistent or pervasive acts.

(b) Psychologists accord sexual-harassment complainants and respondents dignity and respect. Psychologists do not participate in denying a person academic admittance or advancement, employment, tenure, or promotion, based solely upon their having made, or their being the subject of, sexual harassment charges. This does not preclude taking action based upon the outcome of such proceedings or consideration of other appropriate information.

1.12 Other Harassment

Psychologists do not knowingly engage in behavior that is harassing or demeaning to persons with whom they interact in their work based on factors such as those persons' age, gender, race, ethnicity, national origin, religion, sexual orientation, disability, language, or socioeconomic status.

1.13 Personal Problems and Conflicts

(a) Psychologists recognize that their personal problems and conflicts may interfere with their effectiveness. Accordingly, they refrain from undertaking an activity when they know or should know that their personal problems are likely to lead to harm to a patient, client, colleague, student, research participant, or other person to whom they may owe a professional or scientific obligation.

(b) In addition, psychologists have an obligation to be alert to signs of, and to obtain assistance for, their personal problems at an early stage, in order to prevent significantly impaired performance.

(c) When psychologists become aware of personal problems that may interfere with their performing work-related duties adequately, they take appropriate measures, such as obtaining professional consultation or assistance, and determine whether they should limit, suspend, or terminate their work-related duties.

1.14 Avoiding Harm

Psychologists take reasonable steps to avoid harming their patients or clients, research participants, students, and others with whom they work, and to minimize harm where it is foreseeable and unavoidable.

1.15 Misuse of Psychologists' Influence

Because psychologists' scientific and professional judgments and actions may affect the lives of others, they are alert to and guard against personal, financial, social, organizational, or political factors that might lead to misuse of their influence.

1.16 Misuse of Psychologists' Work

(a) Psychologists do not participate in activities in which it appears likely that their skills or data will be misused by others, unless corrective mechanisms are available. (See also Standard 7.04, Truthfulness and Candor.)

(b) If psychologists learn of misuse or misrepresentation of their work, they take reasonable steps to correct or minimize the misuse or misrepresentation.

1.17 Multiple Relationships

(a) In many communities and situations, it may not be feasible or reasonable for psychologists to avoid social or other nonprofessional contacts with persons such as patients, clients, students, supervisees, or research participants. Psychologists must always be sensitive to the potential harmful effects of other contacts on their work and on those persons with whom they deal. A psychologist refrains from entering into or promising another personal, scientific, professional, financial, or other relationship with such persons if it appears likely that such a relationship reasonably might impair the psychologist's objectivity or otherwise interfere with the psychologist's effectively performing his or her functions as a psychologist, or might harm or exploit the other party.

(b) Likewise, whenever feasible, a psychologist refrains from taking on professional or scientific obligations when preexisting relationships would create a risk of such harm.

(c) If a psychologist finds that, due to unforeseen factors, a potentially harmful multiple relationship has arisen, the psychologist attempts to resolve it with due regard for the best interests of the affected person and maximal compliance with the Ethics Code.

1.18 Barter (With Patients or Clients)

Psychologists ordinarily refrain from accepting goods, services, or other nonmonetary remuneration from patients or clients in return for psychological services because such arrangements create inherent potential for conflicts, exploitation, and distortion of the professional relationship. A psychologist may participate in bartering *only* if (1) it is not clinically contraindicated, *and* (2) the relationship is not exploitative. (See also Standards 1.17, Multiple Relationships, and 1.25, Fees and Financial Arrangements.)

1.19 Exploitative Relationships

(a) Psychologists do not exploit persons over whom they have supervisory, evaluative, or other authority such as students, supervisees, employees, research participants, and clients or patients. (See also Standards 4.05–4.07 regarding sexual involvement with clients or patients.)

(b) Psychologists do not engage in sexual relationships with students or supervisees in training over whom the psychologist has evaluative or direct authority, because such relationships are so likely to impair judgment or be exploitative.

1.20 Consultations and Referrals

(a) Psychologists arrange for appropriate consultations and referrals based principally on the best interests of their patients or clients, with appropriate consent, and subject to other relevant considerations, including applicable law and contractual obligations. (See also Standards 5.01, Discussing the Limits of Confidentiality, and 5.06, Consultations.)

(b) When indicated and professionally appropriate, psychologists cooperate with other professionals in order to serve their patients or clients effectively and appropriately.

(c) Psychologists' referral practices are consistent with law.

1.21 Third-Party Requests for Services

(a) When a psychologist agrees to provide services to a person or entity at the request of a third party, the psychologist clarifies to the extent feasible, at the outset of the service, the nature of the relationship with each party. This clarification includes the role of the psychologist (such as therapist, organizational consultant, diagnostician, or expert witness), the probable uses of the services provided or the information obtained, and the fact that there may be limits to confidentiality.

(b) If there is a foreseeable risk of the psychologist's being called upon to perform conflicting roles because of the involvement of a third party, the psychologist clarifies the nature and direction of his or her responsibilities, keeps all parties appropriately informed as matters develop, and resolves the situation in accordance with this Ethics Code.

1.22 Delegation to and Supervision of Subordinates

(a) Psychologists delegate to their employees, supervisees, and research assistants only those responsibilities that such persons can reasonably be expected to perform competently, on the basis of their education, training, or experience, either independently or with the level of supervision being provided.

(b) Psychologists provide proper training and supervision to their employees or supervisees and take reasonable steps to see that such persons perform services responsibly, competently, and ethically.

(c) If institutional policies, procedures, or practices prevent fulfillment of this obligation, psychologists attempt to modify their role or to correct the situation to the extent feasible.

1.23 Documentation of Professional and Scientific Work

(a) Psychologists appropriately document their professional and scientific work in order to facilitate provision of services later by them or by other professionals, to ensure accountability, and to meet other requirements of institutions or the law.

(b) When psychologists have reason to believe that records of their professional services will be used in legal proceedings involving recipients of or participants in their work, they have a responsibility to create and maintain documentation in the kind of detail and quality that would be consistent with reasonable scrutiny in an adjudicative forum. (See also Standard 7.01, Professionalism, under Forensic Activities.)

1.24 Records and Data

Psychologists create, maintain, disseminate, store, retain, and dispose of records and data relating to their research, practice, and other work in accordance with law and in a manner that permits compliance with the requirements of this Ethics Code. (See also Standard 5.04, Maintenance of Records.)

1.25 Fees and Financial Arrangements

(a) As early as is feasible in a professional or scientific relationship, the psychologist and the patient, client, or other appropriate recipient of psychological services reach an agreement specifying the compensation and the billing arrangements.

(b) Psychologists do not exploit recipients of services or payors with respect to fees.

(c) Psychologists' fee practices are consistent with law.

(d) Psychologists do not misrepresent their fees.

(e) If limitations to services can be anticipated because of limitations in financing, this is discussed with the patient, client, or other appropriate recipient of services as early as is feasible. (See also Standard 4.08, Interruption of Services.)

(f) If the patient, client, or other recipient of services does not pay for services as agreed, and if the psychologist wishes to use collection agencies or legal measures to collect the fees, the psychologist first informs the person that such measures will be taken and provides that person an opportunity to make prompt payment. (See also Standard 5.11, Withholding Records for Nonpayment.)

1.26 Accuracy in Reports to Payors and Funding Sources

In their reports to payors for services or sources of research funding, psychologists accurately state the nature of the research or service provided, the fees or charges, and where applicable, the identity of the provider, the findings, and the diagnosis. (See also Standard 5.05, Disclosures.)

1.27 Referrals and Fees

When a psychologist pays, receives payment from, or divides fees with another professional other than in an employer–employee relationship, the payment to each is based on the services (clinical, consultative, administrative, or other) provided and is not based on the referral itself.

2. Evaluation, Assessment, or Intervention

2.01 Evaluation, Diagnosis, and Interventions in Professional Context

(a) Psychologists perform evaluations, diagnostic services, or interventions only within the context of a defined professional relationship. (See also Standards 1.03, Professional and Scientific Relationship.)

(b) Psychologists' assessments, recommendations, reports, and psychological diagnostic or evaluative statements are based on information and techniques (including personal interviews of the individual when appropriate) sufficient to provide appropriate substantiation for their findings. (See also Standard 7.02, Forensic Assessments.)

2.02 Competence and Appropriate Use of Assessments and Interventions

(a) Psychologists who develop, administer, score, interpret, or use psychological assessment techniques, interviews, tests, or instruments do so in a manner and for purposes that are appropriate in light of the research on or evidence of the usefulness and proper application of the techniques.

(b) Psychologists refrain from misuse of assessment techniques, interventions, results, and interpretations and take reasonable steps to prevent others from misusing the information these techniques provide. This includes refraining from releasing raw test results or raw data to persons, other than to patients or clients as appropriate, who are not qualified to use such information. (See also Standards 1.02, Relationship of Ethics and Law, and 1.04, Boundaries of Competence.)

2.03 Test Construction

Psychologists who develop and conduct research with tests and other assessment techniques use scientific procedures and current professional knowledge for test design, standardization, validation, reduction or elimination of bias, and recommendations for use.

2.04 Use of Assessment in General and With Special Populations

(a) Psychologists who perform interventions or administer, score, interpret, or use assessment techniques are familiar with the reliability, validation, and related standardization or outcome studies of, and proper applications and uses of, the techniques they use.

(b) Psychologists recognize limits to the certainty with which diagnoses, judgments, or predictions can be made about individuals.

(c) Psychologists attempt to identify situations in which particular interventions or assessment techniques or norms may not be applicable or may require adjustment in administration or interpretation because of factors such as individuals' gender, age, race, ethnicity, national origin, religion, sexual orientation, disability, language, or socioeconomic status.

2.05 Interpreting Assessment Results

When interpreting assessment results, including automated interpretations, psychologists take into account the various test factors and characteristics of the person being assessed that might affect psychologists' judgments or reduce the accuracy of their interpretations. They indicate any significant reservations they have about the accuracy or limitations of their interpretations.

2.06 Unqualified Persons

Psychologists do not promote the use of psychological assessment techniques by unqualified persons. (See also Standard 1.22, Delegation to and Supervision of Subordinates.)

2.07 Obsolete Tests and Outdated Test Results

(a) Psychologists do not base their assessment or intervention decisions or recommendations on data or test results that are outdated for the current purpose.

(b) Similarly, psychologists do not base such decisions or recommendations on tests and measures that are obsolete and not useful for the current purpose.

2.08 Test Scoring and Interpretation Services

(a) Psychologists who offer assessment or scoring procedures to other professionals accurately describe the purpose, norms, validity, reliability, and applications of the procedures and any special qualifications applicable to their use.

(b) Psychologists select scoring and interpretation services (including automated services) on the basis of evidence of the validity of the program and procedures as well as on other appropriate considerations.

(c) Psychologists retain appropriate responsibility for the appropriate application, interpretation, and use of assessment instruments, whether they score and interpret such tests themselves or use automated or other services.

2.09 Explaining Assessment Results

Unless the nature of the relationship is clearly explained to the person being assessed in advance and precludes provision of an explanation of results (such as in some organizational consulting, preemployment or security screenings, and forensic evaluations), psychologists ensure that an explanation of the results is provided using language that is reasonably understandable to the person assessed or to another legally authorized person on behalf of the client. Regardless of whether the scoring and interpretation are done by the psychologist, by assistants, or by automated or other outside services, psychologists take reasonable steps to ensure that appropriate explanations of results are given.

2.10 *Maintaining Test Security*

Psychologists make reasonable efforts to maintain the integrity and security of tests and other assessment techniques consistent with law, contractual obligations, and in a manner that permits compliance with the requirements of this Ethics Code. (See also Standard 1.02, Relationship of Ethics and Law.)

3. Advertising and Other Public Statements

3.01 *Definition of Public Statements*

Psychologists comply with this Ethics Code in public statements relating to their professional services, products, or publications or to the field of psychology. Public statements include but are not limited to paid or unpaid advertising, brochures, printed matter, directory listings, personal resumes or curricula vitae, interviews or comments for use in media, statements in legal proceedings, lectures and public oral presentations, and published materials.

3.02 *Statements by Others*

(a) Psychologists who engage others to create or place public statements that promote their professional practice, products, or activities retain professional responsibility for such statements.

(b) In addition, psychologists make reasonable efforts to prevent others whom they do not control (such as employers, publishers, sponsors, organizational clients, and representatives of the print or broadcast media) from making deceptive statements concerning psychologists' practice or professional or scientific activities.

(c) If psychologists learn of deceptive statements about their work made by others, psychologists make reasonable efforts to correct such statements.

(d) Psychologists do not compensate employees of press, radio, television, or other communication media in return for publicity in a news item.

(e) A paid advertisement relating to the psychologist's activities must be identified as such, unless it is already apparent from the context.

3.03 Avoidance of False or Deceptive Statements

(a) Psychologists do not make public statements that are false, deceptive, misleading, or fraudulent, either because of what they state, convey, or suggest or because of what they omit, concerning their research, practice, or other work activities or those of persons or organizations with which they are affiliated. As examples (and not in limitation) of this standard, psychologists do not make false or deceptive statements concerning (1) their training, experience, or competence; (2) their academic degrees; (3) their credentials; (4) their institutional or association affiliations; (5) their services; (6) the scientific or clinical basis for, or results or degree of success of, their services; (7) their fees; or (8) their publications or research findings. (See also Standards 6.15, Deception in Research, and 6.18, Providing Participants With Information About the Study.)

(b) Psychologists claim as credentials for their psychological work, only degrees that (1) were earned from a regionally accredited educational institution or (2) were the basis for psychology licensure by the state in which they practice.

3.04 Media Presentations

When psychologists provide advice or comment by means of public lectures, demonstrations, radio or television programs, prerecorded tapes, printed articles, mailed material, or other media, they take reasonable precautions to ensure that (1) the statements are based on appropriate psychological literature and practice, (2) the statements are otherwise consistent with this Ethics Code, and (3) the recipients of the information are not encouraged to infer that a relationship has been established with them personally.

3.05 Testimonials

Psychologists do not solicit testimonials from current psychotherapy clients or patients or other persons who because of their particular circumstances are vulnerable to undue influence.

3.06 In-Person Solicitation

Psychologists do not engage, directly or through agents, in uninvited in-person solicitation of business from actual or potential psychotherapy patients or clients or other persons who because of their particular circumstances are vulnerable to undue influence. However, this does not preclude attempting to implement appropriate collateral contacts with significant others for the purpose of benefiting an already engaged therapy patient.

4. Therapy

4.01 Structuring the Relationship

(a) Psychologists discuss with clients or patients as early as is feasible in the therapeutic relationship appropriate issues, such as the nature and anticipated course of therapy, fees, and confidentiality. (See also Standards 1.25, Fees and Financial Arrangements, and 5.01, Discussing the Limits of Confidentiality.)

(b) When the psychologist's work with clients or patients will be supervised, the above discussion includes that fact, and the name of the supervisor, when the supervisor has legal responsibility for the case.

(c) When the therapist is a student intern, the client or patient is informed of that fact.

(d) Psychologists make reasonable efforts to answer patients' questions and to avoid apparent misunderstandings about therapy. Whenever possible, psychologists provide oral and/or written information, using language that is reasonably understandable to the patient or client.

4.02 Informed Consent to Therapy

(a) Psychologists obtain appropriate informed consent to therapy or related procedures, using language that is reasonably understandable to participants. The content of informed consent will vary depending on many circumstances; however, informed consent generally implies that the person (1) has the capacity to consent, (2) has been informed of significant information concerning the procedure, (3) has freely and without undue influence expressed consent, and (4) consent has been appropriately documented.

(b) When persons are legally incapable of giving informed consent, psychologists obtain informed permission from a legally authorized person, if such substitute consent is permitted by law.

(c) In addition, psychologists (1) inform those persons who are legally incapable of giving informed consent about the proposed interventions in a manner commensurate with the persons' psychological capacities, (2) seek their assent to those interventions, and (3) consider such persons' preferences and best interests.

4.03 Couple and Family Relationships

(a) When a psychologist agrees to provide services to several persons who have a relationship (such as husband and wife or parents and children), the psychologist attempts to clarify at the outset (1) which of the individuals are patients or clients and (2) the relationship the psychologist will have with each person. This clarification includes the role of the psychologist and the probable uses of the services provided or the information obtained. (See also Standard 5.01, Discussing the Limits of Confidentiality.)

(b) As soon as it becomes apparent that the psychologist may be called on to perform potentially conflicting roles (such as marital counselor to husband and wife, and then witness for one party in a divorce proceeding), the psychologist attempts to clarify and adjust, or withdraw from, roles appropriately. (See also Standard 7.03, Clarification of Role, under Forensic Activities.)

4.04 *Providing Mental Health Services to Those Served by Others*

In deciding whether to offer or provide services to those already receiving mental health services elsewhere, psychologists carefully consider the treatment issues and the potential patient's or client's welfare. The psychologist discusses these issues with the patient or client, or another legally authorized person on behalf of the client, in order to minimize the risk of confusion and conflict, consults with the other service providers when appropriate, and proceeds with caution and sensitivity to the therapeutic issues.

4.05 *Sexual Intimacies With Current Patients or Clients*

Psychologists do not engage in sexual intimacies with current patients or clients.

4.06 *Therapy With Former Sexual Partners*

Psychologists do not accept as therapy patients or clients persons with whom they have engaged in sexual intimacies.

4.07 *Sexual Intimacies With Former Therapy Patients*

(a) Psychologists do not engage in sexual intimacies with a former therapy patient or client for at least two years after cessation or termination of professional services.

(b) Because sexual intimacies with a former therapy patient or client are so frequently harmful to the patient or client, and because such intimacies undermine public confidence in the psychology profession and thereby deter the public's use of needed services, psychologists do not engage in sexual intimacies with former therapy patients and clients even after a two-year interval except in the most unusual circumstances. The psychologist who engages in such activity after the two years following cessation or termination of treatment bears the burden of demonstrating that there has been no exploitation, in light of all relevant factors, including (1) the amount of time that has passed since therapy terminated, (2) the nature and duration of the therapy, (3) the circumstances of termination, (4) the patient's or client's personal history, (5) the patient's or client's current mental status, (6) the likelihood of adverse impact on the patient or client and others, and (7) any statements or actions made by the therapist during the course of therapy suggesting or inviting the possibility of a posttermination sexual or romantic relationship with the patient or client. (See also Standard 1.17, Multiple Relationships.)

4.08 Interruption of Services

(a) Psychologists make reasonable efforts to plan for facilitating care in the event that psychological services are interrupted by factors such as the psychologist's illness, death, unavailability, or relocation or by the client's relocation or financial limitations. (See also Standard 5.09, Preserving Records and Data.)

(b) When entering into employment or contractual relationships, psychologists provide for orderly and appropriate resolution of responsibility for patient or client care in the event that the employment or contractual relationship ends, with paramount consideration given to the welfare of the patient or client.

4.09 Terminating the Professional Relationship

(a) Psychologists do not abandon patients or clients. (See also Standard 1.25e, under Fees and Financial Arrangements.)

(b) Psychologists terminate a professional relationship when it becomes reasonably clear that the patient or client no longer needs the service, is not benefiting, or is being harmed by continued service.

(c) Prior to termination for whatever reason, except where precluded by the patient's or client's conduct, the psychologist discusses the patient's or client's views and needs, provides appropriate pretermination counseling, suggests alternative service providers as appropriate, and takes other reasonable steps to facilitate transfer of responsibility to another provider if the patient or client needs one immediately.

5. Privacy and Confidentiality

These Standards are potentially applicable to the professional and scientific activities of all psychologists.

5.01 Discussing the Limits of Confidentiality

(a) Psychologists discuss with persons and organizations with whom they establish a scientific or professional relationship (including, to the extent feasible, minors and their legal representatives) (1) the relevant limitations on confidentiality, including limitations where applicable in group, marital, and family therapy or in organizational consulting, and (2) the foreseeable uses of the information generated through their services.

(b) Unless it is not feasible or is contraindicated, the discussion of confidentiality occurs at the outset of the relationship and thereafter as new circumstances may warrant.

(c) Permission for electronic recording of interviews is secured from clients and patients.

5.02 Maintaining Confidentiality

Psychologists have a primary obligation and take reasonable precautions to respect the confidentiality rights of those with whom they work or consult, recognizing that confidentiality may be established by law, institutional rules, or professional or scientific relationships. (See also Standard 6.26, Professional Reviewers.)

5.03 Minimizing Intrusions on Privacy

(a) In order to minimize intrusions on privacy, psychologists include in written and oral reports, consultations, and the like, only information germane to the purpose for which the communication is made.

(b) Psychologists discuss confidential information obtained in clinical or consulting relationships, or evaluative data concerning patients, individual or organizational clients, students, research participants, supervisees, and employees, only for appropriate scientific or professional purposes and only with persons clearly concerned with such matters.

5.04 Maintenance of Records

Psychologists maintain appropriate confidentiality in creating, storing, accessing, transferring, and disposing of records under their control, whether these are written, automated, or in any other medium. Psychologists maintain and dispose of records in accordance with law and in a manner that permits compliance with the requirements of this Ethics Code.

5.05 Disclosures

(a) Psychologists disclose confidential information without the consent of the individual only as mandated by law, or where permitted by law for a valid purpose, such as (1) to provide needed professional services to the patient or the individual or organizational client, (2) to obtain appropriate professional consultations, (3) to protect the patient or client or others from harm, or (4) to obtain payment for services, in which instance disclosure is limited to the minimum that is necessary to achieve the purpose.

(b) Psychologists also may disclose confidential information with the appropriate consent of the patient or the individual or organizational client (or of another legally authorized person on behalf of the patient or client), unless prohibited by law.

5.06 Consultations

When consulting with colleagues, (1) psychologists do not share confidential information that reasonably could lead to the identification of a patient, client, research participant, or other person or organization with whom they have a confidential relationship unless they have obtained the prior consent of the person or organization or the disclosure cannot be avoided, and (2) they share information only to the extent necessary to achieve the purposes of the consultation. (See also Standard 5.02, Maintaining Confidentiality.)

5.07 Confidential Information in Databases

(a) If confidential information concerning recipients of psychological services is to be entered into databases or systems of records available to persons whose access has not been consented to by the recipient, then psychologists use coding or other techniques to avoid the inclusion of personal identifiers.

(b) If a research protocol approved by an institutional review board or similar body requires the inclusion of personal identifiers, such identifiers are deleted before the information is made accessible to persons other than those of whom the subject was advised.

(c) If such deletion is not feasible, then before psychologists transfer such data to others or review such data collected by others, they take reasonable steps to determine that appropriate consent of personally identifiable individuals has been obtained.

5.08 Use of Confidential Information for Didactic or Other Purposes

(a) Psychologists do not disclose in their writings, lectures, or other public media, confidential, personally identifiable information concerning their patients, individual or organizational clients, students, research participants, or other recipients of their services that they obtained during the course of their work, unless the person or organization has consented in writing or unless there is other ethical or legal authorization for doing so.

(b) Ordinarily, in such scientific and professional presentations, psychologists disguise confidential information concerning such persons or organizations so that they are not individually identifiable to others and so that discussions do not cause harm to subjects who might identify themselves.

5.09 Preserving Records and Data

A psychologist makes plans in advance so that confidentiality of records and data is protected in the event of the psychologist's death, incapacity, or withdrawal from the position or practice.

5.10 Ownership of Records and Data

Recognizing that ownership of records and data is governed by legal principles, psychologists take reasonable and lawful steps so that records and data remain available to the extent needed to serve the best interests of patients, individual or organizational clients, research participants, or appropriate others.

5.11 Withholding Records for Nonpayment

Psychologists may not withhold records under their control that are requested and imminently needed for a patient's or client's treatment solely because payment has not been received, except as otherwise provided by law.

6. Teaching, Training Supervision, Research, and Publishing

6.01 Design of Education and Training Programs

Psychologists who are responsible for education and training programs seek to ensure that the programs are competently designed, provide the proper experiences, and meet the requirements for licensure, certification, or other goals for which claims are made by the program.

6.02 Descriptions of Education and Training Programs

(a) Psychologists responsible for education and training programs seek to ensure that there is a current and accurate description of the program content, training goals and objectives, and requirements that must be met for satisfactory completion of the program. This information must be made readily available to all interested parties.

(b) Psychologists seek to ensure that statements concerning their course outlines are accurate and not misleading, particularly regarding the subject matter to be covered, bases for evaluating progress, and the nature of course experiences. (See also Standard 3.03, Avoidance of False or Deceptive Statements.)

(c) To the degree to which they exercise control, psychologists responsible for announcements, catalogs, brochures, or advertisements describing workshops, seminars, or other non-degree-granting educational programs ensure that they accurately describe the audience for which the program is intended, the educational objectives, the presenters, and the fees involved.

6.03 Accuracy and Objectivity in Teaching

(a) When engaged in teaching or training, psychologists present psychological information accurately and with a reasonable degree of objectivity.

(b) When engaged in teaching or training, psychologists recognize the power they hold over students or supervisees and therefore make reasonable efforts to avoid engaging in conduct that is personally demeaning to students or supervisees. (See also Standards 1.09, Respecting Others, and 1.12, Other Harassment.)

6.04 Limitation on Teaching

Psychologists do not teach the use of techniques or procedures that require specialized training, licensure, or expertise, including but not limited to hypnosis, biofeedback, and projective techniques, to individuals who lack the prerequisite training, legal scope of practice, or expertise.

6.05 Assessing Student and Supervisee Performance

(a) In academic and supervisory relationships, psychologists establish an appropriate process for providing feedback to students and supervisees.

(b) Psychologists evaluate students and supervisees on the basis of their actual performance on relevant and established program requirements.

6.06 Planning Research

(a) Psychologists design, conduct, and report research in accordance with recognized standards of scientific competence and ethical research.

(b) Psychologists plan their research so as to minimize the possibility that results will be misleading.

(c) In planning research, psychologists consider its ethical acceptability under the Ethics Code. If an ethical issue is unclear, psychologists seek to resolve the issue through consultation with institutional review boards, animal care and use committees, peer consultations, or other proper mechanisms.

(d) Psychologists take reasonable steps to implement appropriate protections for the rights and welfare of human participants, other persons affected by the research, and the welfare of animal subjects.

6.07 Responsibility

(a) Psychologists conduct research competently and with due concern for the dignity and welfare of the participants.

(b) Psychologists are responsible for the ethical conduct of research conducted by them or by others under their supervision or control.

(c) Researchers and assistants are permitted to perform only those tasks for which they are appropriately trained and prepared.

(d) As part of the process of development and implementation of research projects, psychologists consult those with expertise concerning any special population under investigation or most likely to be affected.

6.08 Compliance With Law and Standards

Psychologists plan and conduct research in a manner consistent with federal and state law and regulations, as well as professional standards governing the conduct of research, and particularly those standards governing research with human participants and animal subjects.

6.09 Institutional Approval

Psychologists obtain from host institutions or organizations appropriate approval prior to conducting research, and they provide accurate information about their research proposals. They conduct the research in accordance with the approved research protocol.

6.10 Research Responsibilities

Prior to conducting research (except research involving only anonymous surveys, naturalistic observations, or similar research), psychologists enter into an agreement with participants that clarifies the nature of the research and the responsibilities of each party.

6.11 Informed Consent to Research

(a) Psychologists use language that is reasonably understandable to research participants in obtaining their appropriate informed consent (except as provided in Standard 6.12, Dispensing with Informed Consent). Such informed consent is appropriately documented.

(b) Using language that is reasonably understandable to participants, psychologists inform participants of the nature of the research; they inform participants that they are free to participate or to decline to participate or to withdraw from the research; they explain the foreseeable consequences of declining or withdrawing; they inform participants of significant factors that may be expected to influence their willingness to participate (such as risks, discomfort, adverse effects, or limitations on confidentiality, except as provided in Standard 6.15, Deception in Research); and they explain other aspects about which the prospective participants inquire.

(c) When psychologists conduct research with individuals such as students or subordinates, psychologists take special care to protect the prospective participants from adverse consequences of declining or withdrawing from participation.

(d) When research participation is a course requirement or opportunity for extra credit, the prospective participant is given the choice of equitable alternative activities.

(e) For persons who are legally incapable of giving informed consent, psychologists nevertheless (1) provide an appropriate explanation, (2) obtain the participant's assent, and (3) obtain appropriate permission from a legally authorized person, if such substitute consent is permitted by law.

6.12 Dispensing With Informed Consent

Before determining that planned research (such as research involving only anonymous questionnaires, naturalistic observations, or certain kinds of archival research) does not require the informed consent of research participants, psychologists consider applicable regulations and institutional review board requirements, and they consult with colleagues as appropriate.

6.13 Informed Consent in Research Filming or Recording

Psychologists obtain informed consent from research participants prior to filming or recording them in any form, unless the research involves simply naturalistic observations in public places and it is not anticipated that the recording will be used in a manner that could cause personal identification or harm.

6.14 Offering Inducements for Research Participants

(a) In offering professional services as an inducement to obtain research participants, psychologists make clear the nature of the services, as well as the risks, obligations, and limitations. (See also Standard 1.18, Barter [With Patients or Clients].)

(b) Psychologists do not offer excessive or inappropriate financial or other inducements to obtain research participants, particularly when it might tend to coerce participation.

6.15 Deception in Research

(a) Psychologists do not conduct a study involving deception unless they have determined that the use of deceptive techniques is justified by the study's prospective scientific, educational, or applied value and that equally effective alternative procedures that do not use deception are not feasible.

(b) Psychologists never deceive research participants about significant aspects that would affect their willingness to participate, such as physical risks, discomfort, or unpleasant emotional experiences.

(c) Any other deception that is an integral feature of the design and conduct of an experiment must be explained to participants as early as is feasible, preferably at the conclusion of their participation, but no later than at the conclusion of the research. (See also Standard 6.18, Providing Participants With Information About the Study.)

6.16 Sharing and Utilizing Data

Psychologists inform research participants of their anticipated sharing or further use of personally identifiable research data and of the possibility of unanticipated future uses.

6.17 Minimizing Invasiveness

In conducting research, psychologists interfere with the participants or milieu from which data are collected only in a manner that is warranted by an appropriate research design and that is consistent with psychologists' roles as scientific investigators.

6.18 Providing Participants With Information About the Study

(a) Psychologists provide a prompt opportunity for participants to obtain appropriate information about the nature, results, and conclusions of the research, and psychologists attempt to correct any misconceptions that participants may have.

(b) If scientific or humane values justify delaying or withholding this information, psychologists take reasonable measures to reduce the risk of harm.

6.19 Honoring Commitments

Psychologists take reasonable measures to honor all commitments they have made to research participants.

6.20 Care and Use of Animals in Research

(a) Psychologists who conduct research involving animals treat them humanely.

(b) Psychologists acquire, care for, use, and dispose of animals in compliance with current federal, state, and local laws and regulations, and with professional standards.

(c) Psychologists trained in research methods and experienced in the care of laboratory animals supervise all procedures involving animals and are responsible for ensuring appropriate consideration of their comfort, health, and humane treatment.

(d) Psychologists ensure that all individuals using animals under their supervision have received instruction in research methods and in the care, maintenance, and handling of the species being used, to the extent appropriate to their role.

(e) Responsibilities and activities of individuals assisting in a research project are consistent with their respective competencies.

(f) Psychologists make reasonable efforts to minimize the discomfort, infection, illness, and pain of animal subjects.

(g) A procedure subjecting animals to pain, stress, or privation is used only when an alternative procedure is unavailable and the goal is justified by its prospective scientific, educational, or applied value.

(h) Surgical procedures are performed under appropriate anesthesia; techniques to avoid infection and minimize pain are followed during and after surgery.

(i) When it is appropriate that the animal's life be terminated, it is done rapidly, with an effort to minimize pain, and in accordance with accepted procedures.

6.21 Reporting of Results

(a) Psychologists do not fabricate data or falsify results in their publications.

(b) If psychologists discover significant errors in their published data, they take reasonable steps to correct such errors in a correction, retraction, erratum, or other appropriate publication means.

6.22 Plagiarism

Psychologists do not present substantial portions or elements of another's work or data as their own, even if the other work or data source is cited occasionally.

6.23 Publication Credit

(a) Psychologists take responsibility and credit, including authorship credit, only for work they have actually performed or to which they have contributed.

(b) Principal authorship and other publication credits accurately reflect the relative scientific or professional contributions of the individuals involved, regardless of their relative status. Mere possession of an institutional position, such as Department Chair, does not justify authorship credit. Minor contributions to the research or to the writing for publications are appropriately acknowledged, such as in footnotes or in an introductory statement.

(c) A student is usually listed as principal author on any multiple-authored article that is substantially based on the student's dissertation or thesis.

6.24 Duplicate Publication of Data

Psychologists do not publish, as original data, data that have been previously published. This does not preclude republishing data when they are accompanied by proper acknowledgment.

6.25 Sharing Data

After research results are published, psychologists do not withhold the data on which their conclusions are based from other competent professionals who seek to verify the substantive claims through reanalysis and who intend to use such data only for that purpose, provided that the confidentiality of the participants can be protected and unless legal rights concerning proprietary data preclude their release.

6.26 Professional Reviewers

Psychologists who review material submitted for publication, grant, or other research proposal review respect the confidentiality of and the proprietary rights in such information of those who submitted it.

7. Forensic Activities

7.01 Professionalism

Psychologists who perform forensic functions, such as assessments, interviews, consultations, reports, or expert testimony, must comply with all other provisions of this Ethics Code to the extent that they apply to such activities. In addition, psychologists base their forensic work on appropriate knowledge of and competence in the areas underlying such work, including specialized knowledge concerning special populations. (See also Standards 1.06, Basis for Scientific and Professional Judgments; 1.08, Human Differences; 1.15, Misuse of Psychologists' Influence; and 1.23, Documentation of Professional and Scientific Work.)

7.02 Forensic Assessments

(a) Psychologists' forensic assessments, recommendations, and reports are based on information and techniques (including personal interviews of the individual, when appropriate) sufficient to provide appropriate substantiation for their findings. (See also Standards 1.03, Professional and Scientific Relationship; 1.23, Documentation of Professional and Scientific Work; 2.01, Evaluation, Diagnosis, and Interventions in Professional Context; and 2.05, Interpreting Assessment Results.)

(b) Except as noted in (c), below, psychologists provide written or oral forensic reports or testimony of the psychological characteristics of an individual only after they have conducted an examination of the individual adequate to support their statements or conclusions.

(c) When, despite reasonable efforts, such an examination is not feasible, psychologists clarify the impact of their limited information on the reliability and validity of their reports and testimony, and they appropriately limit the nature and extent of their conclusions or recommendations.

7.03 Clarification of Role

In most circumstances, psychologists avoid performing multiple and potentially conflicting roles in forensic matters. When psychologists may be called on to serve in more than one role in a legal proceeding—for example, as consultant or expert for one party or for the court and as a fact witness—they clarify role expectations and the extent of confidentiality in advance to the extent feasible, and thereafter as changes occur, in order to avoid compromising their professional judgment and objectivity and in order to avoid misleading others regarding their role.

7.04 Truthfulness and Candor

(a) In forensic testimony and reports, psychologists testify truthfully, honestly, and candidly and, consistent with applicable legal procedures, describe fairly the bases for their testimony and conclusions.

(b) Whenever necessary to avoid misleading, psychologists acknowledge the limits of their data or conclusions.

7.05 Prior Relationships

A prior professional relationship with a party does not preclude psychologists from testifying as fact witnesses or from testifying to their services to the extent permitted by applicable law. Psychologists appropriately take into account ways in which the prior relationship might affect their professional objectivity or opinions and disclose the potential conflict to the relevant parties.

7.06 Compliance With Law and Rules

In performing forensic roles, psychologists are reasonably familiar with the rules governing their roles. Psychologists are aware of the occasionally competing demands placed upon them by these principles and the requirements of the court system, and attempt to resolve these conflicts by making known their commitment to this Ethics Code and taking steps to resolve the conflict in a responsible manner. (See also Standard 1.02, Relationship of Ethics and Law.)

8. Resolving Ethical Issues

8.01 Familiarity With Ethics Code

Psychologists have an obligation to be familiar with this Ethics Code, other applicable ethics codes, and their application to psychologists' work. Lack of awareness or misunderstanding of an ethical standard is not itself a defense to a charge of unethical conduct.

8.02 Confronting Ethical Issues

When a psychologist is uncertain whether a particular situation or course of action would violate this Ethics Code, the psychologist ordinarily consults with other psychologists knowledgeable about ethical issues, with state or national psychology ethics committees, or with other appropriate authorities in order to choose a proper response.

8.03 Conflicts Between Ethics and Organizational Demands

If the demands of an organization with which psychologists are affiliated conflict with this Ethics Code, psychologists clarify the nature of the conflict, make known their commitment to the Ethics Code, and to the extent feasible, seek to resolve the conflict in a way that permits the fullest adherence to the Ethics Code.

8.04 Informal Resolution of Ethical Violations

When psychologists believe that there may have been an ethical violation by another psychologist, they attempt to resolve the issue by bringing it to the attention of that individual if an informal resolution appears appropriate and the intervention does not violate any confidentiality rights that may be involved.

8.05 Reporting Ethical Violations

If an apparent ethical violation is not appropriate for informal resolution under Standard 8.04 or is not resolved properly in that fashion, psychologists take further action appropriate to the situation, unless such action conflicts with confidentiality rights in ways that cannot be resolved. Such action might include referral to state or national committees on professional ethics or to state licensing boards.

8.06 Cooperating With Ethics Committees

Psychologists cooperate in ethics investigations, proceedings, and resulting requirements of the APA or any affiliated state psychological association to which they belong. In doing so, they make reasonable efforts to resolve any issues as to confidentiality. Failure to cooperate is itself an ethics violation.

8.07 Improper Complaints

Psychologists do not file or encourage the filing of ethics complaints that are frivolous and are intended to harm the respondent rather than to protect the public.

HISTORY AND EFFECTIVE DATE

This version of the APA Ethics Code was adopted by the American Psychological Association's Council of Representatives during its meeting, August 13 and 16, 1992, and is effective beginning December 1, 1992. Inquiries concerning the substance or interpretation of the APA Ethics Code should be addressed to the Director, Office of Ethics, American Psychological Association, 750 First Street, NE, Washington, DC 20002-4242.

This Code will be used to adjudicate complaints brought concerning alleged conduct occurring after the effective date. Complaints regarding conduct occurring prior to the effective date will be adjudicated on the basis of the version of the Code that was in effect at the time the conduct occurred, except that no provisions repealed in June 1989, will be enforced even if an earlier version contains the provision. The Ethics Code will undergo continuing review and study for future revisions; comments on the Code may be sent to the above address.

The APA has previously published its Ethical Standards as follows:

American Psychological Association. (1953). *Ethical standards of psychologists*. Washington, DC: Author.

American Psychological Association. (1958). Standards of ethical behavior for psychologists. *American Psychologist, 13*, 268–271.

American Psychological Association. (1963). Ethical standards of psychologists. *American Psychologist, 18*, 56–60.

American Psychological Association. (1968). Ethical standards of psychologists. *American Psychologist, 23*, 357–361.

American Psychological Association. (1977, March). Ethical standards of psychologists. *APA Monitor*, pp. 22–23.

American Psychological Association. (1979). Ethical standards of psychologists. Washington, DC: Author.

American Psychological Association. (1981). Ethical principles of psychologists. *American Psychologist, 36*, 633–638.

American Psychological Association. (1990). Ethical principles of psychologists (Amended June 2, 1989). *American Psychologist, 45*, 390–395.

Request copies of the APA's Ethical Principles of Psychologists and Code of Conduct from the APA Order Department, 750 First Street, NE, Washington, DC 20002-4242, or phone (202) 336–5510.

AUTHOR INDEX

Numbers in italics refer to listings in reference sections.

SUBJECT INDEX

ABOUT THE EDITORS

John R. Anderson received his PhD in clinical psychology in 1988 from the University of Kansas. He was the director of the American Psychological Association (APA) AIDS Community Training Project, and he is currently director of the APA HIV Office for Psychology Education and director of the APA Office on AIDS, which provides training and technical assistance on a wide range of HIV/AIDS-related topics associated with coping, mental health services, prevention, technology transfer, community collaboration, public policy, and ethics. His primary area of research and writing has focused on the relationships among hope, coping, adjustment, and health. In addition, he has authored numerous articles and training curricula on the mental health and psychosocial aspects of HIV/AIDS. Since 1986, he has conducted a private, mental health services practice in Washington, DC, where he specializes in individual, couples, family, and hypnosis therapies for people living with or affected by HIV/AIDS.

Bob Barret is professor of counseling at the University of North Carolina–Charlotte. He received his PhD in counseling psychology from Georgia State University. His professional career extends from business to high school teaching, university appointments, and clinical practice as a psychologist in San Francisco and Charlotte, NC. After working with cancer patients for several years, he began to do volunteer work with persons with HIV/AIDS and eventually became known as a skilled HIV/AIDS trainer and practitioner. He was a senior faculty member of the AIDS Community Training Project and the HOPE Program, both sponsored by the APA, and he has worked with the APA's Office on AIDS in several capacities. He is the coauthor of three books; the latest, *Counseling Gay Men and Lesbians* (with Colleen Logan), is to be published in 2001. His research articles cover topics such as gay fathers, gay and lesbian spirituality, and social advocacy for sexual minorities. He has served as president of the Association for Gay, Lesbian, and Bisexual Issues in Counseling, a division of the American Counseling Association. In addition to his teaching he participates in a clinical practice that focuses on gay and lesbian counseling, grief and loss, and relationship enhancement.